HYPERTENSIVE DISORDERS IN WOMEN

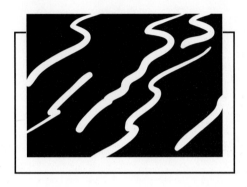

HYPERTENSIVE DISORDERS IN WOMEN

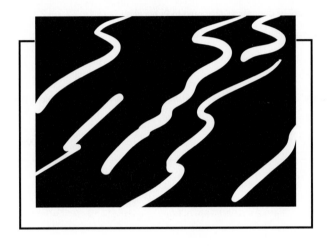

Baha M. Sibai, MD

Professor and Chairman
Department of Obstetrics and Gynecology
University of Cincinnati College of Medicine
Cincinnati, Ohio

W.B. SAUNDERS COMPANY

A Harcourt Health Sciences Company
Philadelphia   London   New York   St. Louis   Sydney   Toronto

W.B. SAUNDERS COMPANY
A Harcourt Health Sciences Company

The Curtis Center
Independence Square West
Philadelphia, Pennsylvania 19106

Library of Congress Cataloging-in-Publication Data

Hypertensive disorders in women/[edited by] Baha M. Sibai.—1st ed.

p.   cm.

ISBN 0–7216–7374–0

1. Hypertension in pregnancy.   2. Heart diseases in women.   3. Hypertension.   I. Sibai, Baha M.

RG580.H9 H95 2001

616.1′32′0082—dc21   00-049272

Acquisitions Editor: Judith Fletcher
Manuscript Editor: Carol Robins
Production Editor: Natalie Ware
Designer: Matt Andrews
Illustration Specialist: John Needles

HYPERTENSIVE DISORDERS IN WOMEN   ISBN 0–7216–7374–0

Printed in the United States of America

Last digit is the print number: 9   8   7   6   5   4   3   2   1

DEDICATION

This book is dedicated to my wife and children, who were always supportive and understanding for all the time I missed spending with them. In addition, I dedicate this book to women all over the world who might benefit from the information summarized in this textbook.

NOTICE

Obstetrics/Gynecology is an ever-changing field. Standard safety precautions must be followed, but as new research and clinical experience broaden our knowledge, changes in treatment and drug therapy may become necessary or appropriate. Readers are advised to check the most current product information provided by the manufacturer of each drug to be administered to verify the recommended dose, the method and duration of administration, and contraindications. It is the responsibility of the treating physician, relying on experience and knowledge of the patient, to determine dosages and the best treatment for each individual patient. Neither the publisher nor the editor assumes any liability for any injury and/or damage to persons or property arising from this publication.

THE PUBLISHER

CONTRIBUTORS

PHYLLIS AUGUST, MD
Professor of Medicine and Chief, Division of Hypertension, The Hypertension Center, New York Presbyterian Hospital–Weill Medical College of Cornell University, New York, New York
ACUTE AND LONG-TERM MANAGEMENT OF HYPERTENSION IN NONPREGNANT WOMEN

JOHN R. BARTON, MD
Volunteer Professor, Department of Obstetrics and Gynecology, University of Cincinnati College of Medicine, Cincinnati, Ohio; Director, Maternal-Fetal Medicine, Central Baptist Hospital, Perinatal Diagnostic Center, Lexington, Kentucky
HELLP SYNDROME

MICHAEL A. BELFORT, MD
Associate Professor, Department of Obstetrics and Gynecology, University of Utah School of Medicine, Provo, Utah
PREECLAMPSIA, ECLAMPSIA, AND THE CEREBRAL CIRCULATION: ABNORMALITIES IN AUTOREGULATION AND PERFUSION

GUSTAAF A. DEKKER, MD, PhD, FRANZCOG
Professor, University of Adelaide; Divisional Head, Obstetrics, Gynaecology, and Paediatrics, North Western Adelaide Health Service, Lyell McEwin Health Service, Australia
PREVENTION OF PREECLAMPSIA; MEDICAL CONDITIONS ASSOCIATED WITH HYPERTENSIVE DISORDERS OF PREGNANCY

ROBERT S. EGERMAN, MD
Associate Professor, Department of Obstetrics and Gynecology, University of Tennessee, Memphis, College of Medicine, Memphis, Tennessee
PRECONCEPTION COUNSELING FOR WOMEN WITH A HISTORY OF HYPERTENSIVE DISORDERS

STEVEN A. FRIEDMAN, MD
Clinical Associate Professor, Department of Obstetrics and Gynecology, Oregon Health Sciences University School of Medicine; Staff Perinatologist, Kaiser Permanente, Northwest Region, Portland, Oregon
MILD GESTATIONAL HYPERTENSION AND PREECLAMPSIA

BASSAM HADDAD, MD
Department of Obstetrics and Gynecology, C.H.I. Creteil, Creteil, France
CHRONIC HYPERTENSION IN PREGNANCY

KEE-HAK LIM, MD
Assistant Professor, Department of Obstetrics, Gynecology, and Reproductive Biology, Harvard Medical School; Staff Perinatologist, Beth Israel Deaconess Medical Center, Boston, Massachusetts
MILD GESTATIONAL HYPERTENSION AND PREECLAMPSIA

SUZANNE L. LUBARSKY, MD
Clinical Assistant Professor, Department of Obstetrics and Gynecology, Oregon Health Sciences University School of Medicine; Staff Perinatologist, Kaiser Permanente, Northwest Region, Portland, Oregon
MILD GESTATIONAL HYPERTENSION AND PREECLAMPSIA

WILLIAM C. MABIE, MD
Professor, Department of Obstetrics and Gynecology, University of Tennessee, Memphis, College of Medicine, Memphis, Tennessee
LIFE-THREATENING COMPLICATIONS OF HYPERTENSION IN PREGNANCY

NICHOLAS H. MORRIS, MB BS, MRCOG
Senior Clinical Research Fellow and Consultant Obstetrician and Gynaecologist, Central Middlesex Hospital and Imperial College School of Medicine at Chelsea and Westminster Hospital, London, United Kingdom
MEDICAL CONDITIONS ASSOCIATED WITH HYPERTENSIVE DISORDERS OF PREGNANCY

HEIN J. ODENDAAL, MBCHB, FCOG(SA), FRCOG, MD
Professor and Head, Department of Obstetrics and Gynaecology University of Stellenbosch, Stellenbosch, South Africa
SEVERE PREECLAMPSIA AND ECLAMPSIA

SUZANNE OPARIL, MD
Director, Vascular Biology and Hypertension Program, University of Alabama at Birmingham, School of Medicine, Birmingham, Alabama
ACUTE AND LONG-TERM MANAGEMENT OF HYPERTENSION IN NONPREGNANT WOMEN

LAUREN A. PLANTE, MD
Assistant Professor, Departments of Obstetrics and Gynecology and Anesthesiology, MCP Hahnemann University School of Medicine, Philadelphia, Pennsylvania
THE HYPERTENSIVE DIABETIC WOMAN

E. ALBERT REECE, MD
Professor and Chair, Department of Obstetrics, Gynecology, and Reproductive Sciences, Temple University School of Medicine, Philadelphia, Pennsylvania
THE HYPERTENSIVE DIABETIC WOMAN

JOHN T. REPKE, MD
Chris J. and Marie A. Olson Professor of Obstetrics and Gynecology, University of Nebraska College of Medicine; Chairman, Department of Obstetrics and Gynecology, University of Nebraska Medical Center, Omaha, Nebraska
CONTRACEPTION FOR THE WOMAN WITH HYPERTENSION

BAHA M. SIBAI, MD
Professor and Chairman, Department of Obstetrics and Gynecology, University of Cincinnati College of Medicine, Cincinnati, Ohio
EPIDEMIOLOGY AND CLASSIFICATION OF HYPERTENSION IN WOMEN; HELLP SYNDROME; CHRONIC HYPERTENSION IN PREGNANCY; RANDOMIZED TRIALS FOR PREVENTION AND TREATMENT OF ECLAMPTIC CONVULSIONS; PRECONCEPTION COUNSELING FOR WOMEN WITH A HISTORY OF HYPERTENSIVE DISORDERS

JAMES J. WALKER, MD, FRCP, FRCOG
Professor and Chairman, University of Leeds; Consultant, St. James University Hospital, Leeds, United Kingdom
ANTIHYPERTENSIVE DRUGS IN PREGNANCY

ANDREA WITLIN, DO
Assistant Professor, University of Texas Medical Branch, University of Texas Medical School at Galveston, Galveston, Texas
EPIDEMIOLOGY AND CLASSIFICATION OF HYPERTENSION IN WOMEN; RANDOMIZED TRIALS FOR PREVENTION AND TREATMENT OF ECLAMPTIC CONVULSIONS

FOREWORD

• • • • •

This book on hypertension in women will bring a breath of fresh air and knowledge to a problem experienced by many childbearing women. The hypertensive diseases affecting pregnant women constitute the most common medical problem seen during pregnancy; 4% to 7% of pregnant women experience preeclampsia, and an equal number of them experience chronic hypertension, for a total incidence of 8% to 10% in the United States. This incidence is governed by a woman's age at childbearing and by geographic location. In many developing countries hypertension accounts for one third of the total pregnancies.

One thing is for certain: We do not know the specific etiologic mechanism of preeclampsia and eclampsia. Much progress has been made during the past 30 years in bringing a better understanding of the pathophysiology of the disease, but the cause still eludes the clinical scientist. Dr. Joseph B. DeLee, founder of the Chicago Lying-in Hospital at the University of Chicago, was so concerned about finding the cause that when the "new hospital" was constructed, he designed an empty plaque for the person who will discover the cause of eclampsia. The plaque rests beside plaques dedicated to other great scientists who made major contributions to women's

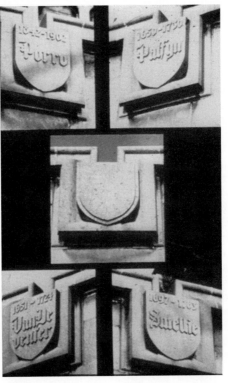

health, such as Palfyn, vandeVenter, and Smellie. The plaque remains empty—will a name ever be inscribed? Scholars in the world know that such a plaque exists.

The Chicago Lying-in Hospital is one of the institutions that has always been dedicated to research in the area of hypertension in pregnancy. One of the early chairmen, Fred Adair, M.D., was concerned about maternal and fetal health; next came William Dieckmann, M.D., one of the early scientific scholars on "toxemias of pregnancy." The first edition of his book with that title was published in 1941, the second edition in 1952. Much can be learned by reading both of these texts.

Our current clinical scientists often overlook the wonderful, dedicated scholars and their work prior to 1964, when information was computerized. A look into the past may show important directions for the future. It may even be that readers of this book will realize that their projects have already been done, but not with today's sophisticated scientific techniques now available.

Next came Edith Potter, M.D., Ph.D., whom I call the "Mother of Perinatal Pathology." She made significant contributions to our understanding of maternal mortality and other areas pertaining to the fetus. Charles McCartney, M.D., along with Ben Spargo, M.D., a renal patholo-gist, discovered the "toxemic lesion of the kidney" by performing renal biopsies in pregnancy and during the immediate post-partum period. Most recently, a nephrolo-gist, Marshall Lindheimer, M.D., has con-tinued the legacy at Chicago Lying-in Hospital.

In 1974, Dr. Lindheimer and I hosted an invitational closed meeting of 25 to 30 individuals from around the world at the University of Chicago. This nucleus of people met the following year in Germany and formed the International Society for the Study of Hypertension in Pregnancy (ISSHP) to bring together those interested in this entity. Marshall and I feel that it has been a privilege to be part of a move-ment, now worldwide, that embraces 65 countries. Ideas are shared every two years at an international meeting. This relation-ship has underscored the differences in various countries in the hypertensive dis-eases of pregnancy. We often think that the problem is easily solved in developed countries, but in fact the incidence has changed very little. Eclampsia is now seen less frequently in developed countries be-cause of prenatal care and early diagnosis of severe preeclampsia, but we often forget that Dr. Dieckmann pointed out more than 50 years ago that 20% of patients with eclampsia do not have hypertension or proteinuria when they experience an eclamptic seizure.

Most of the scholars in this textbook are members of ISSHP and have enjoyed fellowship and exchanged ideas on a worldwide basis. One example of idea ex-change has been treatment of severe pre-eclampsia and eclampsia. For more than 40 years, the standard of care in the United States has been the use of paren-teral magnesium sulfate and the control of the blood pressure, usually by hydrala-zine. Most physicians from other coun-tries never accepted this form of therapy, even though many of us have spoken throughout the world describing our methods. The group at Oxford, England, established a multicentered study and compared magnesium sulfate (methods of Zuspan [IV] or of Pritchard [IM]), pheny-toin, and diazepam in a randomized, pro-spective trial of good magnitude (more than 1650 eclamptic patients). The results clearly demonstrate that magnesium sul-fate is superior for both mother and fetus, thus making magnesium sulfate the ther-apy of choice for the world when avail-able. Neither magnesium sulfate nor hy-dralazine cures severe preeclampsia or eclampsia but does help control the mater-nal problem until delivery—the only cure.

Over the past 30 years, my friend, Leon Chesley, Ph.D., was a true scholar of hy-pertensive diseases of pregnancy. He au-thored a wonderful textbook on this topic, which I understand will now be rewritten. It would be wonderful to have two books dedicated to the hypertensive diseases of pregnancy, and I am assuming that each will be different from the other.

Dr. Sibai has been the most prolific clin-ical scientist in the study of hypertensive diseases of pregnancy in the United States for more than 15 years. It is fitting that he is the editor of this textbook, since his life has been dedicated to hypertension in pregnant women. He has assembled a banner group of clinical scientists as con-tributors. All of them have made contribu-tions to the subject area in which they write. The book should become a "classic" for those interested in the hypertensive diseases of pregnancy and women.

FREDERICK P. ZUSPAN, M.D.
Professor and Chairman Emeritus
Department of Obstetrics and Gynecology
The Ohio State University College of Medicine

PREFACE

• • • •

This textbook, *Hypertensive Disorders in Women,* focuses on recent developments in the prevention and management of hypertension in young women. The chapters are written by national and international experts who have dedicated their careers to the management and study of hypertension in nonpregnant women as well as in women who develop hypertension in pregnancy. These chapters are designed to take the reader beyond what can be found in general textbooks. In addition, they include references published as recently as December 2000.

The topics covered include hypertension in nonpregnant women, hypertensive disorders of pregnancy, and preconception counseling of women with hypertensive disorders. The emphasis in each chapter is on evidence-based data regarding prevention and management of the various disorders covered. It may become apparent, as one reads some of these chapters, that there is a definite need for research in young women with hypertension, particularly as it relates to the use of antihypertensive drugs, including their pharmacokinetics and pharmacodynamics as well as the efficacy and safety of the various antihypertensive drugs used in pregnancy.

In my editing of this book, my goal was to have available a comprehensive source on hypertension in women that would be useful to physicians in training as well as practicing physicians who take care of women with hypertension, including those with hypertension of pregnancy. I have spent the past few years developing this book and hope that the reader will find it informative.

BAHA M. SIBAI

CONTENTS

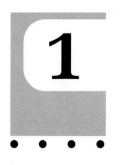

1

EPIDEMIOLOGY and CLASSIFICATION of HYPERTENSION in WOMEN

Andrea Witlin and Baha M. Sibai

Heart disease and stroke are among the leading causes of death in the United States and are responsible for an excess of $259 billion in direct and indirect costs.[1] As health care providers for women, we are challenged to improve upon these statistics. It is important to understand the distribution, determinants, and prevention of hypertension because it is a major etiologic factor for the development of heart disease and stroke. Issues for the 21st century include increasing the awareness and detection of hypertension, improving blood pressure control, increasing the recognition of controlled systolic hypertension, and decreasing the age-related rise of blood pressure.

More generic issues include reduction of cardiovascular risk factors and the recognition of the importance of high-normal blood pressure. Societal issues include reduction of ethnic, socioeconomic, and regional variations in hypertension, improved opportunities for treatment, and enhanced community programs.[1] As obstetrician/gynecologists and primary health care providers for women, we need to be aware of the pertinent differences between the disease processes and their respective therapies in women versus men. Existing differences will be highlighted; otherwise, conclusions may be assumed to pertain equally to women as to men.

EPIDEMIOLOGY AND CLASSIFICATION OF HYPERTENSION IN NONGRAVID WOMEN

Classification of Hypertension

Hypertension for adults aged 18 years and older is classified according to systolic and diastolic blood pressure (Table 1–1) into categories of optimal, normal, high-normal, and hypertension.[1] For nonpregnant individuals, hypertension is further classified into risk groups (see Table 1–1)[1]:

- A, no risk factors
- B, at least one risk factor not including diabetes
- C or blood pressure stages (high-normal [130–139/85–89 mmHg], stage 1 [140–159/90–99 mmHg], and stages 2 and 3 [160/100 mmHg]).

For therapeutic decisions, patients with hypertension are additionally classified into risk groups according to presence or absence of cardiovascular disease or target organ damage.[2]

Insulin Resistance

The role of insulin resistance in the epidemiology of hypertension has been attracting attention. It is likely that the debate regarding the role of insulin resistance and hypertension will continue in the literature as we see more written about syndrome X *(insulin-resistance syndrome)* and its far-reaching effects. Syndrome X includes insulin resistance associated with hyperlipidemia, hypertension, obesity, and cardiovascular disease.[3]

Beginning in the early 1900s, observations were made connecting obesity with hypertension.[4] Likewise, the assumption arose that obesity was associated with impaired glucose metabolism and fasting hyperinsulinemia.[4] For the current discussion, it is important to remember that *insulin resistance* is an imprecise term used to describe

TABLE 1–1. CLASSIFICATION OF HYPERTENSION

BLOOD PRESSURE STAGES (mmHg)	RISK GROUP A (NO RISK FACTORS)	RISK GROUP B (AT LEAST 1 RISK FACTOR NOT INCLUDING DIABETES)	RISK GROUP C
High-normal (130–139/85–89)	Lifestyle modification	Lifestyle modification	Drug therapy
Stage 1 (140–159/90–99)	Lifestyle modification (up to 12 mo)	Lifestyle modification (up to 6 mo)	Drug therapy
Stages 2 and 3 (160/100)	Drug therapy	Drug therapy	Drug therapy

widely disparate types of insulin resistance.[4] Confusion also exists because of the confounding variables of type of obesity (central versus overall), genetic determinants, weight loss, exercise training, and drug treatment.[3] Lifestyle changes with regard to therapy for hypertension will be revisited later in this chapter.

Hepatic insulin resistance (or impaired insulin-mediated suppression of hepatic glucose output) is the primary cause of fasting hyperinsulinemia. Hepatic insulin resistance is also associated with obesity-related hypertension. However, it is unclear whether this is the etiologic factor in hypertension induced by obesity.[4] Peripheral insulin resistance (or impaired insulin-mediated glucose uptake, primarily related to an acute glucose load in skeletal muscle) is also present in essential hypertension in lean individuals.[4] Because of these widely disparate pathophysiologic states, it can be difficult to link insulin resistance to hypertension per se. An easier association may be to link obesity, hypertension, and insulin resistance to long-term cardiovascular morbidity and mortality.

Insulin resistance and compensatory hyperinsulinemia are common in both obese and nonobese patients with hypertension. Furthermore, these changes of insulin resistance and hyperinsulinemia may persist despite reduction in blood pressure. Up to half of patients with hypertension may manifest these changes. These changes are also present in normotensive first-degree relatives of hypertensive patients, but not in patients with secondary hypertension. The resistance to the effects of insulin on glucose uptake does not necessarily imply resistance to the insulin-stimulated renal tubular reabsorption of sodium.[5] It does not appear that insulin resistance is responsible for all cases of hypertension because insulin resistance is not present in all patients with hypertension nor does hypertension occur in all patients with hyperinsulinemia.[5] Nondiabetic hypertensive patients with insulin resistance have an increased risk of coronary artery disease relative to those patients with hypertension alone. Proposed etiologic explanations for the association of insulin resistance and hypertension include insulin-induced vasodilation and decreased peripheral resistance, and alteration of vascular responsiveness to vasoactive agents (perhaps through a calcium-dependent mechanism).[6]

Dyslipidemia

Dyslipidemia (elevated triglycerides and lower high-density lipoprotein [HDL] levels) tends to be present in patients with hypertension. Dyslipidemia appears to be an independent risk factor for the development of coronary artery disease and is linked to hyperinsulinemia. Likewise, treatment of hypertension has decreased the risk of stroke to a greater extent than the risk of coronary artery disease, thus suggesting an additional role for abnormalities in lipoprotein metabolism in morbidity secondary to coronary artery disease.[5] In addition, certain antihypertensive agents may worsen lipoprotein profiles, thus suggesting a need to modify drug therapy in patients with dyslipidemia.

The Treatment of Mild Hypertension study (TOMHS)[7] research group compared plasma lipid changes among six antihypertensive regimens: placebo, the β-blocker acebutolol, the calcium antagonist amlodipine, the diuretic chlorthalidone, the α_1 antagonist doxazosin, and the angiotensin-converting enzyme inhibitor enalapril. In addition to antihypertensive drug regimens, lifestyle counseling regarding weight loss, dietary sodium and alcohol reduction, and exercise were included as therapeutic interventions.[7] The results were as follows.

Decreases in plasma total cholesterol and low-density lipoprotein (LDL) cholesterol were greater with doxazosin and acebutolol and less with chlorthalidone and placebo. Decreases in triglycerides were greater with doxazosin and enalapril and least with acebutolol. Increases in HDL cholesterol were greater with enalapril and doxazosin and least with acebutolol. Also, low-dose chlorthalidone therapy demonstrated no adverse effects on lipid profile.[7]

In general, the TOMHS group[7] found that participants were moderately successful in maintaining weight loss for 4 years with an accompanying improvement in the lipid profile in these patients. These results should encourage clinicians to pursue lifestyle modification with their patients and additionally conclude that antihypertensive therapy should be tailored to the patient's lipoprotein profile and degree of dyslipidemia.

Dietary Calcium

Epidemiologic evidence exists for an inverse relationship between dietary calcium intake and blood pressure.[8] Meta-analysis[9] suggests a statistically significant decrease in systolic blood pressure with calcium supplementation for hypertensive individuals—a reduction of 1.68 mmHg (95% confidence interval [CI] -3.18, -0.18), with a nonsignificant trend for normotensive individuals—a reduction of 0.53 mmHg (95% CI -1.56, 0.49). However, a similar beneficial effect of calcium supplementation was not observed for reduction of diastolic blood pressure. The median calcium supplementation per day in these trials was 1 g/day. Further evaluation of the data revealed a greater antihypertensive effect in women and older individuals. However, the authors of the meta-analysis[9] do not recommend routine calcium supplementation at this time for either hypertensive or normotensive patients. Furthermore, in reviewing these data, al-though statistically significant results are observed, one may question the clinical significance of an approximately 2-mmHg reduction in systolic blood pressure without any decrease in diastolic pressure. The recommendations for calcium supplementation should be based on general health considerations such as for those women who have added risk factors for osteoporosis and would benefit from calcium supplementation, or for those patients with nephrolithiasis, in which case calcium supplementation would be detrimental.

In general, although there may be evidence suggesting an inverse relationship between dietary calcium intake and development of hypertension, there is no compelling evidence at present that routine calcium supplementation would reduce the incidence of hypertension.

Lifestyle Modifications

Lifestyle modifications (Table 1–2) as reviewed by the Joint National Committee on Prevention, Detection, Evaluation, and Treatment of High Blood Pressure[1] and TOMHS group[7] have been shown to be effective in reducing blood pressure and decreasing cardiovascular risk factors. In many cases, especially in those individuals with borderline or high-normal blood pressure, lifestyle modifications including diet and exercise may suffice for control of hypertension. In addition, lifestyle modifications may reduce the need or dosage of antihypertensive agents.

Dietary Protein

Historical data have suggested a hypertensive effect to increased dietary protein in-

---

TABLE 1–2. LIFESTYLE MODIFICATIONS FOR PREVENTION AND MANAGEMENT OF HYPERTENSION

Weight loss
Limiting alcohol intake
Increasing aerobic physical activity
Reducing dietary sodium intake
Adequate intake of dietary calcium
Smoking cessation

Adapted from The Sixth Report of the Joint National Committee on Prevention, Detection, Evaluation, and Treatment of High Blood Pressure. Arch Intern Med 1997;157:2422.

take.[10] However, most studies have been observational, population-based studies that evaluated the level of dietary protein intake and attempted to correlate dietary protein with blood pressure measurements. The researchers themselves have questioned the mechanism whereby the amount and type of dietary protein could affect blood pressure.[10] The metabolic pathways involving degradation of dietary proteins into the various amino acids and the subsequent synthesis of neurotransmitters and biologic peptides (from these amino acids) that in turn modify the mechanisms involved in blood pressure regulation are quite complex and have not yet been delineated. Therefore, insufficient data and limitations of study design limit any conclusions regarding the link between dietary protein and blood pressure.[10]

Dietary Sodium

The literature provides conflicting information regarding the effect of dietary sodium reduction on blood pressure.[11, 12] In a meta-analysis of randomized controlled trials, Midgley and associates[11] suggested that dietary sodium restriction for older hypertensive individuals may have merit; however, routine dietary sodium restriction in the normotensive population is not supported. Furthermore, Midgley's group[11] noted an increase in mortality from cardiovascular disease in those patients with low urinary sodium excretion and, by extension, reduction in dietary sodium.

In contrast, Messerli and colleagues[12] suggested that 24-hour urinary sodium excretion correlated not only with the degree of hypertensive heart disease (as measured by left ventricular hypertrophy) but also with the degree of end-organ renal, cerebral, and vascular disease. The group[12] further suggested that sodium can have a direct toxic effect on the cerebral vasculature independent of its hypertensive effect. In addition, high salt intake may promote left ventricular hypertrophy by insufficiently suppressing the activity of the renin-angiotensin system.[12] This overall detrimental effect of dietary sodium is probably magnified in salt-sensitive patients. To further confound the issue, normotensive salt sensitivity may be a precursor to hypertension in African Americans and may occur less frequently in Caucasians but appears to be related to deficient dietary potassium.[13] Makaritsis and coworkers[14] have studied the β_2-adrenergic receptor as putative in the development of salt-sensitive hypertension.

From these contrasting reports, it appears that further studies are needed before definitive conclusions can be reached regarding sodium restriction or salt sensitivity in the epidemiology of hypertension in adults.

Blood Pressure Measurement

Noninvasive ambulatory blood pressure monitoring has been available for more than 30 years.[15] Target organ damage in patients with essential hypertension has been more closely correlated with ambulatory than clinic blood pressure.[16] Verdecchia and associates[16] compared 1187 patients with essential hypertension and 205 healthy normotensive controls. Cardiovascular risk was quantified by echocardiographic findings of left ventricular hypertrophy. Patients with "white coat" hypertension (elevated clinic hypertension despite normal ambulatory readings) did not have significantly different morbidity as compared with normotensive individuals.

DiPette and Townsend[17] have reviewed the issues of ambulatory blood pressure monitoring and hypertensive target organ damage. They concluded that ambulatory blood pressures were important in discriminating between high-risk and low-risk patients for cardiovascular complications and in those patients with borderline pressure where treatment decisions become controversial. Furthermore, with 24-hour ambulatory blood pressure determinations, nocturnal blood pressure variations may be observed. Those patients who do not show the "normal" nocturnal "dipping" may be at greater risk for the development of left ventricular hypertrophy.[17]

Recommended indications for ambulatory monitoring include persistently elevated clinic blood pressure as well as monitoring and adjustment of therapy. Other situations in which ambulatory blood pressure monitoring is helpful have included suspected white coat hypertension in patients with mild hypertension and no target organ damage, apparent drug resistance, hypotensive symptoms with antihypertensive medication, episodic hypertension, and autonomic dysfunction.[15] The office or clinic pressure may not be representative of usual ambulatory pressure in the prior situations.[15]

A further issue that favors ambulatory blood pressure monitoring for the "correct" diagnosis of hypertension includes insurance concerns and the stigma of being labeled as hypertensive when this diagnosis may not be correct. It is incumbent upon us as health care providers to make the correct diagnosis and then provide appropriate therapy.

HYPERTENSION IN PREGNANCY

Epidemiology

Hypertension during pregnancy, including chronic hypertension, is the most common medical disorder in pregnancy. The exact incidence of chronic hypertension during pregnancy in the United States is unknown, and reported rates have ranged from 1% to 5%.[2] Using data from the National Hospital Discharge Survey, Samadi and coworkers[18] reported an incidence of 1.3% among more than 12 million women who delivered in-hospital during the years 1988 to 1992. The incidence of chronic hypertension during pregnancy was 2.5% among African Americans and 1% among other racial groups.[18]

The prevalence of hypertension in women of reproductive age varies according to age, race/ethnicity, and body mass index.[19] According to data derived from the Third National Health and Nutrition Examination Survey, 1988–1991, the prevalence of chronic hypertension among women 18 to 29 years of age was 2.0% for African Americans, 0.6% for Caucasians, and 1.0% for Mexican Americans. For women 30 to 39 years old, the respective rates were 22.3%, 4.6%, and 6.2%. For women 40 to 49 years of age, the prevalence was 30.5% for African Americans, 12.7% for Caucasians, and 10.6% for Mexican Americans.[19] In addition, according to data derived from United States natality statistics for 1993, the total number of pregnancies among women 35 or older is increasing.[20] Indeed, the birth rate for women aged 40 to 44 years increased by 56% from 1980 to 1993. This shift in childbearing patterns among women 35 or older may be due to marriage or remarriage later in life or because of delaying pregnancy until completion of educational or career goals.[21] Therefore, given the current trend of childbearing at an older age, it is expected that the incidence of chronic hypertension in pregnancy will continue to rise. Given an estimated prevalence of chronic hypertension during pregnancy of 2%, it is expected that at least 80,000 women will be treated with chronic hypertension per year.

Economic Impact

The costs of managing women with chronic hypertension during pregnancy are enormous. Treatment costs include not only the costs of prenatal care and delivery but also the expense of multiple laboratory tests, antenatal fetal surveillance testing, emergency room or labor and delivery visits to control hypertension, prolonged antenatal hospitalization, and time lost from work because of recommendations for bedrest. In addition, pregnancies complicated by chronic hypertension are associated with increased rates of fetal and maternal complications such as fetal growth restriction, preterm delivery, superimposed preeclampsia, and abruptio placentae.[22, 23] The frequency of these complications is particularly increased in women with severe hypertension,[24, 25] longstanding hypertension, and those with preexisting cardiovascular and renal disease.[26, 27]

In general, most of the adverse maternal and fetal outcomes in such pregnancies are related to superimposed preeclampsia or abruptio placentae, or both.[24–30] Indeed, some studies suggest that pregnancy outcome is not adversely affected in the absence of superimposed preeclampsia.[28–30] Other authors found that even without superimposed preeclampsia, women with chronic hypertension have significantly higher rates of small-for-gestational-age (SGA) infants and fetal deaths as compared with women with normotensive pregnancies.[31]

The triad of superimposed preeclampsia, abruptio placentae (placental abruption), and fetal growth restriction when it develops in women with chronic hypertension is an important cause of fetal death, delivery before 34 weeks' gestation, admission to the neonatal intensive care unit, and long-term infant complications. In addition, the combination of superimposed preeclampsia and abruptio placentae is a leading cause of disseminated intravascular coagulopathy (DIC), acute renal failure, pulmonary edema, and intracerebral hemorrhage in pregnant women.[32] The direct and indirect costs attributable to the above complications are extremely high considering the acute and long-term costs for infants born prior to 34 weeks' gestation and the costs attributable to management and long-term care of women with the above complications.

Definition and Classification

Approximately 10% of pregnancies are complicated by hypertension. The incidence varies according to the population studied and the criteria used for diagnosis. Apart from being the most common medical complication of pregnancy, hypertensive disorders are associated with significant maternal, fetal, and neonatal morbidity and mortality.[33, 34] Preeclampsia accounts for 70% of hypertension in pregnancy, and chronic essential hypertension accounts for most of the remaining 30%.

Hypertension is defined as a systolic blood pressure of 140 mmHg or greater, a diastolic blood pressure of 90 mmHg or greater, or the condition of a woman receiving antihypertensive medication.[1] The diagnosis of chronic hypertension in pregnancy is usually based on either a history of hypertension before pregnancy or the presence of hypertension before 20 weeks' gestation.[2] In reviewing the literature on chronic hypertension in pregnancy, one is faced with several problems:

1. The inconsistency in the criteria used to define or classify chronic hypertension. Some European and Australian studies tend to include patients with all forms of hypertension during pregnancy (chronic, gestational, preeclampsia) as well as at various gestational ages up to 32 weeks.

2. Differences regarding the criteria used to classify hypertension (mild or severe) as well as the criteria used to diagnose superimposed preeclampsia (a major primary outcome for most clinical trials).[2]

3. Differences regarding inclusion of patients with essential hypertension only versus patients with all forms of chronic hypertension with or without clinical cardiovascular disease or target organ damage, or both.

4. The classification of chronic hypertension as mild or severe—mild if systolic blood pressure is 140 to 169 mmHg or diastolic pressure is 90 to 109 mmHg and severe if systolic pressure is at least 170 mmHg or diastolic pressure at least 110 mmHg.

Preeclampsia is a disorder peculiar to human pregnancy. Reported incidence ranges from 2% to 7%, depending on the diagnostic criteria and the population studied. It is principally a disease of primigravidas (women giving birth for the first time) and rarely presents before 20 weeks' gestation. Early presentation is more likely to be associated with unrecognized renal disease,[35] whereas onset at term or intrapartum is more often associated with transient or latent hypertension. Although geographic and racial differences in incidence have been reported, it is difficult to be certain that other influences (e.g., socioeconomic status) are not involved. Several risk factors have been identified as predisposing to the development of preeclampsia.

Eclampsia is the occurrence of seizures or coma (not attributable to any other cause) in a woman with preeclampsia (Table 1–3). Antepartum eclampsia occurs in about 75% of cases, with the remaining 25% of cases occurring post partum. Eclampsia rarely oc-

---

TABLE 1–3. DIFFERENTIAL DIAGNOSIS OF ECLAMPSIA

CEREBROVASCULAR ACCIDENTS
Cerebrovenous thrombosis
Cerebroarterial occlusion
Cerebroarterial embolism
Intracerebral hemorrhage

HYPERTENSIVE DISEASE
Hypertensive encephalopathy
Pheochromocytoma

SPACE-OCCUPYING CENTRAL NERVOUS SYSTEM LESIONS
Tumor
Abscess

INFECTIOUS DISEASE
Meningitis
Encephalitis

METABOLIC DISEASE
Hypoglycemia
Hypocalcemia
Water intoxication
Epilepsy

curs prior to 20 weeks' gestation.[36] Late postpartum eclampsia is defined as that beginning more than 48 hours post partum, but less than 4 weeks after delivery.[37] In our series, late postpartum eclampsia comprised 56% of postpartum eclampsia and 16% of all cases of eclampsia.[37]

Why convulsions or coma occurs in some women with symptoms of preeclampsia and not others is unknown. Several mechanisms have been suggested as predisposing factors: cerebral vasospasm, cerebral hemorrhage, cerebral ischemia, cerebral edema, hypertensive encephalopathy, and metabolic encephalopathy.

The reported incidence of eclampsia varies between 0.5% and 0.2% of all deliveries. In Memphis, the incidence is 1 in 300, and this figure has not changed over the past 30 years.[38] Eclampsia is associated with multiple organ dysfunction. Factors determining the degree of dysfunction include a delay in the treatment of preeclampsia and the presence of complicating obstetric and medical factors.

Eclampsia is associated with a wide spectrum of signs and symptoms, ranging from extreme hypertension, hyperreflexia, 4+ proteinuria, and generalized edema to isolated mild hypertension. Laboratory findings also vary. Levels of serum uric acid and creatinine are usually elevated, and creatinine clearance is reduced. Hemoconcentration reflected by an increased hematocrit and reduced plasma volume is common. Elevated liver function tests are found in 11% to 74% of eclamptic patients. *HELLP syndrome* (*h*emolysis, *el*evated *l*iver enzymes, and *l*ow *p*latelets) complicates about 10% of eclampsia and usually occurs in longstanding disease and in women with medical complications. DIC may develop if treatment is delayed or abruptio placentae with fetal demise has occurred.

Hypertensive disorders including preeclampsia and eclampsia are multietiologic, elusive disorders unique to human pregnancy. They affect women of all races without regard to socioeconomic status and are responsible for significant maternal and fetal morbidity and mortality.

References

1. The Sixth Report of the Joint National Committee on Prevention, Detection, Evaluation, and Treatment of High Blood Pressure. Arch Intern Med 1997;157:2413–2446.
2. Sibai BM. Hypertension in pregnancy. Obstet Gynecol Clin North Am 1992;19(4):615–632.
3. Chisholm DJ, Campbell LV, Kraegen EW. Pathogenesis of the insulin resistance syndrome (Syndrome X). Clin Exp Pharmacol Physiol 1997;24:782–784.
4. Brands MW, Hall JE, Keen HL. Is insulin resistance linked to hypertension? Clin Exp Pharmacol Physiol 1998;25:70–76.
5. Reaven GM, Lithell H, Landsberg L. Hypertension and associated metabolic abnormalities—the role of insulin resistance and the sympathoadrenal system. N Engl J Med 1996;334:374–381.
6. Scherrer U, Sartori C. Insulin as a vascular and sympathoexcitatory hormone. Circulation 1997;96:4104–4113.
7. Grimm RH Jr, Flack JM, Grandits GA, et al, for the Treatment of Mild Hypertension Study (TOMHS) Research Group. Long-term effects on plasma lipids of diet and drugs to treat hypertension. JAMA 1996;275(20):1549–1556.
8. Cappuccio FP, Elliott P, Allender PS, et al. Epidemiologic association between dietary calcium intake and blood pressure: A meta-analysis of published data. Am J Epidemiol 1995;142(9):935–945.
9. Allender PS, Cutler JA, Follmann D, et al. Dietary calcium and blood pressure: A meta-analysis of randomized clinical trials. Ann Intern Med 1996;124(9):825–831.
10. Obarzanek E, Velletri PA, Culter JA. Dietary protein and blood pressure. JAMA 1996;275(20):1598–1603.
11. Midgley JP, Matthew AG, Greenwood CMT, Logan AG. Effect of reduced dietary sodium on blood pressure: A meta-analysis of randomized controlled trials. JAMA 1996;275(20):1590–1597.
12. Messerli FH, Schmieder RE, Weir MR. Salt: A perpetrator of hypertensive target organ disease? Arch Intern Med 1997;157:2449–2452.
13. Morris RC, Sebastian A, Forman A, et al. Normotensive salt sensitivity: Effects of race and dietary potassium. Hypertension 1999;33:18–33.
14. Makaritsis KP, Handy DE, Johns C, et al. Role of the α_{2B}-adrenergic receptor in the development of salt-induced hypertension. Hypertension; 1999; 33:14–17.
15. Pickering T, for an American Society of Hypertension Ad Hoc Panel. Recommendations for the use of home (self) and ambulatory blood pressure monitoring. Am J Hypertens 1995;9:1–11.
16. Verdecchia P, Porcellati C, Schillaci G, et al. Ambulatory blood pressure: An independent predictor of prognosis in essential hypertension. Hypertension 1994;24:793–801.
17. DiPette DJ, Townsend RR. Classic papers symposium: Ambulatory blood pressure monitoring and hypertensive target organ damage. Am J Med Sci 1996;312(5):221–224.
18. Samadi AR, Mayberry RM, Zaidi AA, et al. Maternal hypertension and associated pregnancy complications among African-American and other women in the United States. Obstet Gynecol 1996;87:557–563.
19. Burt VL, Whelton P, Rocella EJ, et al. Prevalence of hypertension in the U.S. adult population. Results from the Third National Health and Nutrition Examination Survey, 1988–1991. Hypertension 1995;25:305–313.

20. Ventura SJ, Martin JA, Taftel SM, et al. Advance report of final natality statistics, 1993. Monthly Vital Statistics Report, National Center for Health Statistics 1995;44(Suppl):1–88.

21. Barton JR, Bergauer NK, Jacques DL, et al. Does advanced maternal age affect pregnancy outcome in women with mild hypertension remote from term? Am J Obstet Gynecol 1997;176:1236–1243.

22. Sibai BM. Treatment of hypertension in pregnant women. N Engl J Med 1996;335:257–265.

23. Sibai BM. Diagnosis and management of chronic hypertension in pregnancy. Obstet Gynecol 1991;78:451–461.

24. Sibai BM, Anderson GD. Pregnancy outcome of intensive therapy in severe hypertension in first trimester. Obstet Gynecol 1986;67:517–522.

25. McCowan LME, Buist RE, North RA, Gamble G. Perinatal morbidity in chronic hypertension. Br J Obstet Gynaecol 1996;103:123–129.

26. Ferrazzani S, Caruso A, DeCarolis S, et al. Proteinuria and outcome of 444 pregnancies complicated by hypertension. Am J Obstet Gynecol 1990; 162:366–371.

27. Sibai BM, Lindheimer M, Hauth J, et al. Risk factors for preeclampsia, abruptio placentae, and adverse neonatal outcomes among women with chronic hypertension. N Engl J Med 1998;339:667–671.

28. Sibai BM, Abdella TN, Anderson GD. Pregnancy outcome in 211 patients with chronic hypertension. Obstet Gynecol 1983;61:571–576.

29. Sibai BM, Mabie WC, Shamsa F, et al. A comparison of no medication versus methyldopa or labetalol in chronic hypertension during pregnancy. Am J Obstet Gynecol 1990;162:960–967.

30. Mabie WC, Pernoll ML, Biswas MK. Chronic hypertension in pregancy. Obstet Gynecol 1986;67:197–205.

31. Rey E, Couturier A: The prognosis of pregnancy in women with chronic hypertension. Am J Obstet Gynecol 1994;171:410–416.

32. Sibai BM, Villar MA, Mabie BC. Acute renal failure in hypertensive disorders of pregnancy: Pregnancy outcome and remote prognosis in thirty-one consecutive cases. Am J Obstet Gynecol 1990;162:777–783.

33. Quilligan EJ, Little AB, Oh W. Pregnancy, Birth and the Infant. Washington, DC: U.S. Department of Health and Human Services, Public Health Services, National Institutes of Health, 1981, p 11.

34. Department of Health and Social Security. Report on confidential inquiries into maternal deaths in England and Wales in 1979–81. London: HM Stationary Office, 1986.

35. Ihle J, Long P, Oats J. Early onset preeclampsia—recognition of underlying renal disease. Br Med J 1987;294:78.

36. Sibai BM, Abdella TH, Taylor HA. Eclampsia in the first half of pregnancy: A report of three cases and review of the literature. J Reprod Med 1982;27:706.

37. Lubarsky SL, Barton JR, Friedman SA, et al. Late postpartum eclampsia revisited. Obstet Gynecol 1994;83;502–505.

38. Mattar F, Sibai BM. Eclampsia VIII: Risk factors for maternal morbidity. Am J Obstet Gynecol 2000;82:307–313.

2 MILD GESTATIONAL HYPERTENSION and PREECLAMPSIA

Steven A. Friedman, Suzanne L. Lubarsky, and Kee-Hak Lim

Hypertension is the most common medical disorder encountered in pregnancy, complicating approximately 7% to 10% of all pregnancies. Although there are numerous classifications of hypertension in pregnancy, all acknowledge two basic types of hypertension: (1) that which precedes pregnancy (*chronic* hypertension), and (2) that which is first manifested during pregnancy (*gestational* hypertension). For a detailed discussion of chronic hypertension in pregnancy, see Chapter 8. This chapter focuses on the two most common forms of mild gestational hypertension: *transient* hypertension and *mild* preeclampsia.

DEFINITIONS

The most widely used definition of *hypertension* in pregnancy is a systolic blood pressure of 140 mmHg or above, or a diastolic blood pressure of 90 mmHg or above, on two occasions 6 hours apart. Formerly, threshold increases in blood pressure ($\geq$30 mmHg systolic, $\geq$15 mmHg diastolic, or $\geq$20 mmHg mean arterial pressure) were used to diagnose new-onset hypertension, but these findings are too prevalent and nonspecific in normal women to be useful.[1, 2] In women with chronic hypertension, whose blood pressure may already exceed 140 mmHg systolic or 90 mmHg diastolic, the above threshold increases may be used to aid in the diagnosis of exacerbated hypertension preeclampsia.

Abnormal *proteinuria* in pregnancy is the excretion of 300 mg or more of protein in 24 hours. This diagnosis is most accurate when confirmed with a 24-hour urine collection. Semiquantitative dipstick measurements are often used to identify abnormal proteinuria rapidly, and measurements of 1+ or greater are considered positive. Although dipstick measurements are acceptable when a prompt determination is required, they are not definitive. Several studies have shown a poor correlation between semiquantitative dipstick measurements on spot urine samples and 24-hour urinary protein measurements.[3–5] Similarly, the protein/creatinine ratio is highly variable[6] and should be substituted for a 24-hour urine collection only when a rapid determination is essential.

Approximately 50% of all women have detectable *edema* during pregnancy.[7, 8] Consequently, for edema to be considered pathologic, it should be present in nondependent areas such as the face, hands, or lungs. Another manifestation of abnormal fluid retention is rapid excessive weight gain ($\geq$3 pounds/week using the same scale and equivalent clothing).

Preeclampsia is a complex multisystemic disorder without any clinically apparent pathognomonic signs or symptoms. For the purposes of research studies, in which a high degree of diagnostic specificity is essential, the definition of preeclampsia is necessarily more strict than it is in the clinical arena, where high sensitivity (not missing women who have disease) is more important. For clinical management, therefore, preeclampsia is usually defined as the occurrence of hypertension and proteinuria after 20 weeks' gestation. In some cases, hypertension plus other signs of preeclampsia (such as thrombocytopenia, elevated serum transaminase levels, or seizures) may be sufficient for the diagnosis in the absence of proteinuria.

CLASSIFICATION

In the United States, the most frequently used classification of hypertension during

TABLE 2–1. CLASSIFICATION OF HYPERTENSION IN PREGNANCY

DISORDER	DEFINITION
Gestational hypertension	Hypertension appearing in the second half of pregnancy or in the first 24 hours post partum, without other signs of preeclampsia
Preeclampsia/eclampsia	Hypertension usually appearing after 20 weeks of pregnancy, in combination with proteinuria and/or abnormal edema; eclampsia denotes the development of seizures or coma that have no other identifiable cause
Chronic hypertension	Hypertension that antedates pregnancy or is first manifested before 20 weeks' gestation or after 6 weeks post partum
Preeclampsia superimposed on chronic hypertension	The development of preeclampsia/eclampsia in a woman with preexisting chronic hypertension

Data from Hughes EC (ed). Obstetric-Gynecologic Terminology: With Section on Neonatology and Glossary of Congenital Anomalies. Philadelphia: FA Davis, 1972; and from Consensus Report. National High Blood Pressure Education Program Working Group report on high blood pressure in pregnancy. Am J Obstet Gynecol 2000;183:S1–S18.

pregnancy was proposed by the American College of Obstetricians and Gynecologists Committee on Terminology in 1972[9] and subsequently modified by the National High Blood Pressure Education Program Working Group in 2000.[10] This classification recognizes the four major categories of hypertension in pregnancy depicted in Table 2–1.

Traditionally, preeclampsia has been categorized as mild or severe. The presence of any one of the features listed in Table 2–2 constitutes severe disease.[11]

DIFFERENTIAL DIAGNOSIS

Gestational hypertension is generally a benign condition characterized by late-pregnancy hypertension in the absence of signs or symptoms suggesting preeclampsia or preexisting hypertension. It has little effect on maternal or perinatal morbidity or mortality.[12] Gestational hypertension may be the preproteinuric phase of preeclampsia, the return to baseline chronic hypertension after a mid-pregnancy nadir, or the unmasking by pregnancy of incipient essential hypertension.[10] Redman and Jeffries[13] reported that adopting a stricter definition of hypertension increases the likelihood that a woman with hypertension in pregnancy would have preeclampsia. The criteria that they advocated were an initial diastolic blood pressure below 90 mmHg, a rise of 25 mmHg or more, and a maximum reading of 90 mmHg or higher.

Hypocalciuria may be effective in distinguishing transient hypertension from preeclampsia. Sanchez-Ramos and coworkers[14] measured urinary calcium excretion in healthy women suspected of having preeclampsia. After pregnancy, women were classified as having had preeclampsia (hypertension and proteinuria), gestational hypertension (hypertension alone, or transient hypertension), or normal pregnancy. Hypocalciuria was defined as a urinary calcium concentration below 12 mg/dL in a 24-hour collection. They reported a sensitivity of 85% and a specificity of 91% for detecting preeclampsia. Although 24-hour urinary collections are cumbersome, this test is widely available, inexpensive, and highly practical, particularly when a 24-hour urine specimen is already being collected for the measurement of protein excretion.

Hyperuricemia, on the other hand, is not

TABLE 2–2. CRITERIA FOR THE DIAGNOSIS OF SEVERE PREECLAMPSIA

Presence of one or more of the following in a patient with preeclampsia:

Blood pressure >160–180 mmHg systolic or >110 mmHg diastolic
Proteinuria >5 g/24 hr
Elevated serum creatinine
Grand mal seizures (eclampsia)
Pulmonary edema
Oliguria < 500 mL/24 hr
Microangiopathic hemolysis
Thrombocytopenia
Hepatocellular dysfunction (elevated alanine or aspartate aminotransferase level)
Symptoms suggesting significant end-organ involvement: headache, visual disturbances, or epigastric or right upper quadrant pain

Modified from American College of Obstetricians and Gynecologists. Hypertension in Pregnancy. ACOG Educational Bulletin No. 219. Washington, DC: The College, 1996, pp 1–8.

helpful in distinguishing preeclampsia from transient hypertension (likelihood ratio 1.4).[15] Similarly, Weenink and colleagues[16] found no difference in antithrombin III levels in newly hypertensive pregnant women with and without proteinuria. Although circulating concentrations of both plasma[17] and cellular[18] fibronectin are higher in women with preeclampsia than in women with transient hypertension, predictive statistics were not provided to assess their clinical utility. These tests are not widely available in hospital-based clinical laboratories and are unlikely to prove useful. Activin A, advocated as a highly specific marker of preeclampsia,[19, 20] has been reported in one study[19] to be significantly higher in preeclampsia than in chronic hypertension, transient hypertension, and normal pregnancy. This finding awaits confirmation by other investigators. In the meantime, this test is not widely available for clinical use.

PREDICTION

In the past, efforts to devise screening tests to predict the subsequent development of preeclampsia centered on attempts to detect the known manifestations of disease (hypertension, proteinuria, hyperuricemia, increased vascular resistance, excessive weight gain) at an earlier time in the pregnancy. Later efforts have focused on detection of more proximal events in the pathogenesis of preeclampsia (faulty placentation, reduced placental perfusion, endothelial dysfunction, and activation of coagulation).

Using the Papanicolaou smear as a prototype, Grimes[21] described 10 attributes of an ideal screening test. The test should be safe, acceptable to the population, reproducible, valid (sensitive and specific), appropriate for the population, and economical (relative to expected benefits). The disease should be important, treatable, discernible in a preclinical stage, and prevalent.

Preeclampsia is an appropriate disease for which to develop a screening test. It is certainly an important disease, inasmuch as it increases maternal mortality threefold and perinatal mortality fivefold. Although the only definitive therapy available is delivery, intensified maternal and fetal surveillance could be offered to women at high risk of developing the disease. There is ample evidence that a preclinical phase of disease

exists, during which women destined to develop preeclampsia exhibit biochemical and biophysical signs of impending disease.[22] Finally, preeclampsia is relatively common, complicating 6% to 7% of pregnancies in healthy nulliparas[23, 24] and up to 25% of pregnancies in high-risk populations.[25]

For several decades, investigators have attempted to develop screening tests that would predict the onset of preeclampsia several weeks or months before clinically apparent disease. The major problem with the preponderance of literature on predictive tests lies in the definition of the outcome of interest, preeclampsia. Until the 1990s, the outcome reported in most large studies was merely hypertension that occurred in the second half of pregnancy, what would be termed *gestational hypertension* today. In most cases, no mention was made of proteinuria, so that the major causes of gestational hypertension—transient hypertension, chronic hypertension, and preeclampsia—cannot be distinguished, even retrospectively. Such a distinction is extremely important because proteinuric hypertension is associated with increased maternal and fetal morbidity and mortality, whereas mild isolated hypertension (transient hypertension) is not.[10] Thus, the bulk of the past literature on predictive tests reflects the ability of those tests to predict gestational hypertension, which is of little consequence unless other findings of preeclampsia are present.

Table 2–3 lists the major predictive tests reported in the English-language literature. Because most studies in the past used the occurrence of hypertension in late pregnancy as their primary outcome, they actually predict the development of gestational hypertension rather than preeclampsia, as originally intended. Table 2–4 contains data from those studies that used true preeclampsia (new-onset proteinuric hypertension) as their primary outcome. Results of several studies have been pooled when the reports contained the same tests applied to similar populations.

Careful review of these studies reveals that there is currently no screening test for preeclampsia that is safe, acceptable to the population, reliable, valid, appropriate for the population, and economical. It is hoped that advances in the understanding of the underlying pathophysiology of preeclamp-

TABLE 2–3. SCREENING TESTS FOR GESTATIONAL HYPERTENSION

1. **Routine components of antepartum care performed in the second trimester**
   a. Measurement of blood pressure
   b. Detection of proteinuria (microalbuminuria)
   c. Measurement of weight
   d. Measurement of serum β-hCG

2. **Early detection of vasoconstriction**
   a. Intravenous infusion of angiotensin II
   b. Roll-over test
   c. Hand grip (isometric exercise) test
   d. Platelet angiotensin II receptors
   e. Platelet calcium response to arginine vasopressin

3. **Early detection of altered renal function**
   a. Serum (plasma) uric acid
   b. Urinary excretion of calcium
   c. Urinary kallikrein

4. **Early detection of altered hemodynamics**
   a. Cardiac output

5. **Detection of placental hypoperfusion/ischemia**
   a, Doppler waveforms of uterine arteries
   b. Fetal fibronectin in plasma or amniotic fluid

6. **Detection of endothelial activation, disruption, or injury**
   a. Plasma fibronectin (soluble, cellular)
   b. Urinary excretion of prostacyclin metabolites
   c. Plasma endothelial cell adhesion molecules

7. **Detection of an activated coagulation/fibrinolytic system**
   a. Plasma antithrombin III
   b. Plasma thrombomodulin
   c. Platelet count
   d. Platelet volume
   e. Platelet activation (CD63 expression)
   f. Factor VIII–related antigen/coagulant
   g. Plasminogen activator inhibitor-1

β-hCG, beta-human chorionic gonadotropin.
Modified from Friedman SA, Lindheimer MD. Prediction and differential diagnosis. *In* Lindheimer MD, Roberts JM, Cunningham FG (eds). Chesley's Hypertensive Disorders in Pregnancy, 2nd ed. Stamford, CT: Appleton & Lange, 1999, p 206.

sia will ultimately lead to the development of effective screening tests.

MANAGEMENT

Despite decades of intensive research, delivery remains the only definitive cure for preeclampsia. Consequently, when mild preeclampsia occurs at term, there is widespread agreement that delivery is appropriate. When gestational hypertension or preeclampsia occurs prior to term, however, the most appropriate management may be controversial. Optimal treatment of such patients depends on a variety of factors, including:

- Gestational age
- Severity of maternal and fetal disease
- Patient compliance
- Availability of facilities for prolonged maternal and fetal surveillance
- Prevailing neonatal outcome data

Once the diagnosis of mild hypertension or preeclampsia is made, perhaps the most basic question is whether the patient requires delivery. If the pregnancy is preterm, ordinarily the answer is no. The next question that immediately arises is the most appropriate setting—inpatient or outpatient—for subsequent care. Traditionally, such patients have been managed in-hospital with the hope of reducing the incidence of eclampsia and improving perinatal outcome.[53, 54]

Gilstrap and coworkers[54] reported a descriptive study of 545 women with "pregnancy-induced hypertension" whose pregnancies were managed on the High Risk Pregnancy Unit at Parkland Memorial Hospital, Dallas. Although the precise incidence was not mentioned, most of the women in this series probably did not have proteinuria. Management consisted of hospitalization until delivery, ambulation as desired, and close observation. Antihypertensive medications and diuretics were not used. Nearly 80% of the women were at 33 weeks' gestation or greater at the time of admission. Pregnancies were prolonged by a mean of 24 days. There were five cases of abruptio placentae (placental abruption) (0.9%) and one case of eclampsia (0.2%). The perinatal mortality rate was 9.2/1000 (corrected 7.3/1000). In contrast, 31 women with mild "pregnancy-induced hypertension" refused hospitalization on the High Risk Unit. There were four antepartum fetal deaths in this (nonrandomized) group, for a perinatal mortality rate of 129/1000.

Similarly, Sibai and associates[55] studied 200 healthy nulliparous women with preeclampsia (hypertension, proteinuria, and hyperuricemia) who were hospitalized and randomized to receive either labetalol or no medication. The patients were allowed unrestricted activity. One hundred eighty-six women completed the study. Administration of labetalol reduced the incidence of delivery for severe hypertension but had no effect on overall maternal or perinatal out-

TABLE 2–4. SCREENING TESTS FOR TRUE PREECLAMPSIA (HYPERTENSION PLUS PROTEINURIA)*

TEST	CUTOFF	FIRST AUTHOR	NO. OF PATIENTS	SENS	SPEC	PPV	NPV
MAP 2nd trimester	≥90 mmHg	Friedman[26]	22,582	64	62	6	98
	≥87 mmHg	Massé[27]	504	47	80	23	92
	≥85 mmHg	Ales[28]	730	67	81	3	99.7
	≥85 mmHg	Conde-Agudelo[29]	580	43	78	8	97
		Combined MAP ≥ 85	1310	48	80	5	99
Systolic BP	120–134 mmHg	Sibai[30]	1500	36	82	12	95
	120–136 mmHg	Sibai[31]	4314	13	94	14	93
		Combined	5814	18	91	13	93
Ambulatory BP	mean diastolic ≥ 71 mmHg	Higgins[32]	1048	22	97	15	98
Weight gain	≥10 lb from 20–30 wk	Nelson[33]	1492	73	43	10	94
	≥8 lb from 20–30 wk	Thomson[34]	4214	85	25	7	96
	≥12 lb from 20–30 wk		4214	53	66	10	95
Serum β-hCG	≥2 MoM	Sorensen[35]	426	69	70	7	99
	≥3 MoM		426	15	94	7	97
	≥2 MoM	Vaillant[36]	434	69	85	15	99
	≥2 MoM	Ashour[37]	2737	12	89	5	96
	≥3 MoM		2737	5	97	8	96
		Combined ≥ 2 MoM	3597	23	86	7	96
		Combined ≥ 3 MoM	3163	6	97	8	96
Angiotensin II infusion	≥8 ng/kg/min	Morris[38]	26	33	39	7	82
	≥10 ng/kg/min		26	67	30	11	88
	≥10 ng/kg/min	Öney[39]	231	85	82	38	98
	≥8 ng/kg/min	Dekker[40]	90	78	96	70	9
	≥10 ng/kg/min		90	89	83	36	99
	≥10 ng/kg/min	Kyle[41]	495	25	84	6	96
	≥8 ng/kg/min	Combined	116	67	84	32	96
	≥10 ng/kg/min	Combined	842	64	82	21	97
Roll-over	↑ diastolic ≥ 20 mmHg	Dekker[40]	90	33	93	33	93
Hand-grip	↑ diastolic ≥ 20 mmHg	Baker[42]	200	80	92	20	99
Uric acid (plasma) (serum)	≥350 μmol/L (≥5.9 mg/dL)	Jacobson[43]	135	54	89	33	95
	Not specified	Conde-Agudelo[44]	387	53	65	6	97
Urinary calcium	≤195 mg/day	Sanchez-Ramos[45]	103	88	84	32	99
	Not specified	Conde-Agudelo[44]	387	33	77	5	96
Urinary kallikrein	IUK:creatinine ratio ≤ 170	Millar[46]	307	83	99.7	91	99
	IUK:creatinine ratio ≤ 170	Kyle[47]	458	80	71	11	99
Uterine artery Doppler	RI ≥ 0.58	Jacobson[43]	136	64	64	17	94
	RI ≥ 0.58	Steel[48]	1014	63	89	10	99
	Early diastolic notch	Bower[49]	2026	78	96	28	99.5
	Placental-side RI > 0.57	North[50]	446	27	89	8	97
	Placental-side AC > 90th percentile		446	53	88	14	98
Fibronectin (plasma)	≥230 mg/L	Paarlberg[51]	376	69	59	12	96
Platelet count	?	Conde-Agudelo[44]	387	47	59	5	96
Platelet activation	Platelet CD63 2%	Konijnenberg[52]	244	47	76	13	95

*Including sensitivity (SENS), specificity (SPEC), and positive and negative predictive values.

PPV, positive predictive value; NPV, negative predictive value; MAP, mean arterial pressure; BP, blood pressure; β-hCG, beta-human chorionic gonadotropin; IUK, inactive urinary kallikrein; RI, resistance index; AC, systolic to early diastolic ratio.

Modified from Friedman SA, Lindheimer MD. Prediction and differential diagnosis. *In* Lindheimer MD, Roberts JM, Cunningham FG (eds). Chesley's Hypertensive Disorders in Pregnancy, 2nd ed. Stamford, CT: Appleton & Lange, 1999, pp 208–209.

come. Outcomes were similar to those described by Gilstrap and colleagues[54]: Mean pregnancy prolongation for the entire study population was 21 days, the incidence of abruptio placentae was 1.1%, and the perinatal mortality rate was 5.4/1000.

Mathews and associates[56, 57] conducted a randomized clinical trial comparing bed rest to unrestricted activity in 40 women hospitalized with preeclampsia ("proteinuric hypertension"). As measured by plasma urea and urate concentrations, there was no difference in renal function between the two groups.[56] Similarly, there was no significant difference between maternal or perinatal outcome in the two groups.[56] In a subset of 10 women with particularly severe disease (as measured by hyperuricemia and fetal growth restriction), bed rest "seemed to encourage the development of the premonitory symptoms of eclampsia, but was associated with a better prognosis for the fetus."[57] The significance of this observation in this small group of women is uncertain.

Hospitalization Versus Routine Outpatient Management

For many years, inpatient management of women with signs of mild gestational hypertension or preeclampsia was based largely on empirical observations rather than on the results of controlled randomized trials. As noted earlier, hospitalization was believed to result in improved maternal and perinatal outcome.

In 1971, Mathews and associates[58] reported on a change in practice at one hospital from inpatient to outpatient management of gestational hypertension (without proteinuria). Two years after institution of the new policy, they noted similar rates of perinatal mortality (4.8% inpatient versus 3.1% outpatient), maternal eclampsia (2.8% inpatient versus 0% outpatient), and maternal mortality (0% inpatient versus 0.8% outpatient). The hospital bed days utilized by women with "toxaemia" were reduced by 72%.

Crowther and coworkers[59] conducted a randomized study in which 218 women with nonproteinuric hypertension between 28 and 38 weeks' gestation were treated by hospital bed rest or routine outpatient care. The hospitalized women were encouraged to rest in bed but were allowed ambulation

as desired. Women at home were encouraged to continue normal activity and to check urine daily for the appearance of protein. Weekly outpatient visits were arranged. Women in the outpatient group were admitted to the hospital for any of the following indications: (1) blood pressure of 160/110 mmHg; (2) proteinuria ($\geq 1+$ on dipstick testing); (3) decreased fetal movement; or (4) symptoms suggestive of preeclampsia, such as headache, visual changes, and abdominal pain. The authors found a lower incidence of development of severe hypertension in the hospitalized women; otherwise, there were no significant differences in maternal outcome. Although the mean gestational age at delivery was similar in the two groups (38.3 weeks hospital, 38.2 weeks home), the preterm delivery rate was lower in the hospitalized group (11.8% versus 22.2%, odds ratio [OR] 0.48, 95% confidence interval [CI] 0.24–0.97). Otherwise, there was no difference in neonatal morbidity. The authors concluded that outpatient management of gestational (nonproteinuric) hypertension is a safe alternative to hospitalization.

Day Care Programs

In an attempt to decrease hospital bed occupancy yet maintain close maternal and fetal surveillance, several authors[60–63] have described hospital-based day care (fetal surveillance) units run by a midwife and staffed by an attending physician. Women were referred to these units for several indications, as determined by their referring clinician. Typically, maternal blood pressure, weight, and requested laboratory studies, as well as fetal monitoring, were performed as indicated during periodic visits. The referring clinicians would continue to manage the patients based on the results obtained at the day care unit.

Tuffnell and colleagues[62] randomized 54 women with nonproteinuric hypertension after 26 weeks' gestation to either day care or routine care (inpatient or outpatient management, according to the established practice of the referring clinician without access to the day care unit). Women in the routine care group spent an average of 4.6 times longer as inpatients (difference in mean stay between routine care and day care patients 4.0 days [95% CI 2.1–5.9 days]) and were 8.8 (95% CI 3.0–25.8) times more likely to be admitted to the hospital. The authors concluded that day care safely reduces the need for hospital admissions in women with mild gestational hypertension.

Twaddle and Harper[63] compared the costs and pregnancy outcomes of women with mild gestational hypertension at two teaching hospitals, one in Glasgow (with a day care unit) and one in Aberdeen (with no day care unit). The average cost of managing pregnancy in women with mild gestational hypertension was lower in Glasgow because of the availability of day care management. Other pregnancy outcome measures were similar in the two groups.

Monitored Home Management

A monitored home management scheme was intended to reproduce many of the aspects of day care management in a patient's own home. Outpatient evaluation included measurement of blood pressure and pulse four times per day; monitoring of maternal weight, fetal kick counts, duration of rest/sleep periods; and assessment of proteinuria daily. In addition, patients received non-stress testing and amniotic fluid index measurement twice weekly. Indications for hospitalization included worsening blood pressure, abnormal hematologic parameters, and deteriorating fetal condition. Indications for delivery included worsening maternal or fetal condition, spontaneous labor, and a favorable cervix at term. Utilizing the database of Healthdyne Perinatal Services, Barton and coworkers[64-66] reported the results of this monitored home management protocol in three observational studies.

The first study[64] comprised 592 women between 24 and 36 weeks' gestation with mild gestational hypertension. At the time of enrollment, 68% had no proteinuria (dipstick negative or trace), 26% had 1+ or more, and 6% had inadequate documentation of proteinuria. The mean number of inpatient days was 1.7. The average gestational age at delivery was 36.7 ± 3.6 weeks. The corrected perinatal mortality rate was 3.4/1000. Pregnancy was prolonged by 27.4 ± 3.3 days. The authors indicated that the pregnancy prolongation in this study compared favorably to that in earlier studies performed in inpatients.[55,67] This comparison is not entirely appropriate, however, because the latter studies contained only patients

with preeclampsia (hypertension plus proteinuria or hyperuricemia, or both), whereas the former study contained a majority of patients with isolated hypertension only.

The second study[65] applied this management scheme to a population of 60 adolescents. The authors compared outcomes in the adolescents with those in a group of 120 adults aged 20 to 42 years. The groups were matched for race, gestational age, and proteinuria status at the time of enrollment. The mean number of inpatient days was 1.4. The average gestational age at delivery was 37.0 ± 2.0 weeks. There were no perinatal deaths. Pregnancy was prolonged by 23.5 ± 19.0 days. This study demonstrated the feasibility of outpatient management of gestational hypertension remote from term in the adolescent population.

The third study[66] compared outpatient evaluation of mild gestational hypertension remote from term in mature gravidas (age 35 years or over) and younger adult controls (age 20 to 30 years). The groups were matched for race, gestational age, and proteinuria status at enrollment. The mean number of inpatient days after enrollment was 1.0 (0.9 in controls). The average gestational age at delivery was 37.2 ± 2.3 weeks. There were five perinatal deaths (zero in the control group), for a corrected perinatal mortality rate of 13.2/1000. Although this rate was not significantly different from that in the control group (P = .063), the clinical importance of this finding cannot be overlooked. Furthermore, a type II error is certainly possible. The authors reported that noncompliance with antepartum testing and other medical recommendations was a problem in four of the five pregnancies complicated by perinatal death. This study demonstrates the importance of patient selection, rather than maternal age per se, in judging the suitability of outpatient evaluation of mild gestational hypertension remote from term.

Antihypertensive Therapy

Many studies, both retrospective and prospective, have described the use of a variety of antihypertensive drugs in women with mild gestational hypertension and preeclampsia. These drugs include methyldopa, hydralazine, dihydralazine, labetalol, pure β-blockers (atenolol, metoprolol, oxprenolol, pindolol, acebutolol, timolol), calcium channel blockers (nifedipine, nicardipine), prazosin, and diuretics. The purpose of using antihypertensive drugs in these studies was not to treat severe maternal hypertension but to improve perinatal outcome.

In individual studies, certain benefits of drug therapy have been reported. For example, Rubin and associates[68] reported that atenolol prevented the development of maternal proteinuria and reduced the incidence of neonatal respiratory distress syndrome by allowing prolongation of pregnancy. Pickles and colleagues[69] found a reduction in neonatal respiratory distress syndrome and jaundice in a group of women with mild to moderate gestational hypertension treated with labetalol.

Phippard and associates[70] found a higher incidence of delivery after 38 weeks' gestation and a lower requirement for neonatal intensive care in patients receiving clonidine with or without hydralazine compared to controls. However, these studies were relatively small and these benefits have not been consistently substantiated in subsequent large studies.

Table 2–5 contains the results of randomized clinical trials of antihypertensive therapy to improve perinatal outcome in women with mild gestational hypertension (proteinuria absent) or preeclampsia (proteinuria present) prior to term. Within individual studies, none of the important measures of perinatal outcome contained in the table is significantly improved by prophylactic treatment of mild hypertension.

Antepartum Management

The patient with findings consistent with preeclampsia but without a definite diagnosis should be warned about the signs and symptoms of disease progression and should be evaluated with serial measurements of clinical and laboratory markers of disease. So-called "preeclampsia warnings" should be given verbally and, when possible, in writing.

Figure 2–1 contains a sample patient instruction sheet. The patient should be instructed to maintain relative rest at home. Urine protein measurements by dipstick, fetal movement counts, and blood pressure measurements should be made daily, if possible. Initial outpatient laboratory evaluation includes a 24-hour urine collection for protein, creatinine clearance, and calcium; hematocrit and platelet count; and serum creatinine, aspartate aminotransferase (AST), and uric acid. On the basis of the results, as well as those from maternal blood pressure and fetal monitoring, these tests may be repeated serially (weekly or twice weekly) or they may necessitate hospitalization. New-onset proteinuria in excess of 500 to 1000 mg/day, thrombocytopenia ($<150,000/\mu L$), elevated serum creatinine (≥ 1.2 mg/dL), or elevated AST is considered an indication for hospitalization.

Women who are considered to have probable or certain preeclampsia or who have other coexisting medical problems may be admitted directly to the hospital for initial evaluation as an inpatient. While in the hospital, they are given a regular diet with no salt restriction or activity limits. Antihypertensive drugs, diuretics, and sedatives are not used. Inpatient evaluation for preeclampsia includes measurement of blood pressure daily; weight daily; fetal monitoring; 24-hour urine collection for protein; hematocrit and platelet count twice per week.

Once a patient is determined by inpatient or outpatient evaluation to have stable disease, further outpatient management can be undertaken if reliable follow-up is ensured. Any evidence of significant disease progression (exacerbation of hypertension or proteinuria, laboratory abnormalities, nonreassuring fetal testing, fetal growth restriction) demands (re)hospitalization with consideration of delivery. At any time after 34 weeks' gestation, the diagnosis of severe preeclampsia (see Table 2–2) warrants delivery.

With continued mild disease and reassuring fetal monitoring twice per week (nonstress testing with amniotic fluid index), we usually manage pregnancy as outlined in Figure 2–2. Before 37 weeks' gestation, we usually manage mild disease expectantly with careful outpatient or inpatient monitoring. In individual cases, however, we might recommend delivery with or without documentation of fetal lung maturity. After 37 weeks' gestation, the condition of the cervix may determine whether a patient with otherwise stable hypertension or preeclampsia will be managed by delivery or continued monitoring.

TABLE 2–5. RANDOMIZED TRIALS OF ANTIHYPERTENSIVE THERAPY FOR WOMEN WITH GESTATIONAL HYPERTENSION OR MILD PREECLAMPSIA

AUTHOR	YEAR	GROUP	MOTHERS (NO.)	INFANTS (NO.)	GESTA-TIONAL AGE AT ENTRY (WK)	GESTA-TIONAL AGE AT DELIVERY (WK)	ABRUPTIO PLACENTAE (%)	IUGR (%)	PERI-NATAL DEATHS (%)
Rubin et al[68]	1983	Atenolol	46	46	33.8±4.9	39.1±1.5	—	15.2	2.2
		Placebo	39	39	33.8±4.3	38.7±1.8	—	17.9	5.1
Wichman et al[71]	1984	Metoprolol	26	26	33±4	38±3	—	—	0
		Placebo	26	26	33±3	38±2	—	—	3.8†
Sibai et al[55]	1987	Labetalol	92	94	32.6±2.4	35.4±3.0	2.1	19.1	0
		Bed rest	94	97	32.4±2.4	35.5±3.0	0	9.3	1.1
Plouin et al[72]	1988	Labetalol	91	91	25.8±7.5	37.8±2.6	—	12.1	1.1
		Methyldopa	85	85	26.2±6.8	37.8±2.5	—	16.5	4.7
Pickles et al[69]	1989	Labetalol	70	70	34.0±2.7	37.8±2.2	—	14.3	0
		Placebo	74	74	34.2±2.6	37.5±1.9	—	6.8	0
Plouin et al[73]	1990	Oxprenolol ± dihydral-azine	78	78	28.0±5	38.4±2	—	9.0	2.6
		Placebo	76	76	28.2±5	38.1±3	—	11.8	3.9†
Phippard et al[70]	1991	Clonidine ± hydralazine	25	25	30.7±1.7	—	0	4.0	0
		Placebo	27	27	31.6±1.6	—	0	7.4	0
Cruickshank et al[74]	1992	Labetalol	51	51	33.4	—	—	—	—
		No therapy	63	63	34.6	—	—	—	—
Sibai et al[67]	1992	Nifedipine	98	99	32.8±2.8	36.1±2.8	3.0	15.2	0
		No therapy	99	101	33.4±2.7	36.7±2.5	2.0	12.9	0
Jannet et al[75]	1994	Nicardipine	50	50	29.6±6.7	—	0	—	2.0†
		Metoprolol	50	50	28.8±7.2	—	0	—	2.0
Italian Study Group[76]	1998	Nifedipine	132	132	24.4±6.9	—	—	20.2	2.3
		No therapy	129	129	24.6±6.9	—	—	25.2	1.6

*For all comparisons within studies, $P > .05$.
†Includes one perinatal death in a fetus/infant with congenital anomalies.
IUGR, intrauterine growth restriction (<10th percentile).

Women with a Bishop's score of 6 or greater usually undergo induction of labor. Women with a less favorable cervix may undergo either cervical ripening, followed by induction of labor, or continued close monitoring, usually according to the patient's preference. If gestational age is questionable and delivery or expectant management is equally advisable, we might perform an amniocentesis to document fetal lung maturity. After 40 weeks' gestation, we manage women who have gestational hypertension or preeclampsia with delivery.

Because preeclampsia is a disease cured only by delivery, delivery is always appropriate therapy for the mother. When it occurs before term, however, delivery may not

be optimal for the fetus. The primary purpose of prolonging pregnancy in the presence of preeclampsia is to benefit the fetus. It is therefore essential to ensure fetal well-being during expectant management of preeclampsia before term.

We usually begin with an ultrasound study for growth and fluid at the time of diagnosis, repeating the study every 3 to 4 weeks thereafter. At the time of diagnosis, we also initiate fetal monitoring. No studies indicate which women or their fetuses benefit most from monitoring, although the presence of proteinuria worsens the maternal and fetal prognosis.[10] Similarly, no data have proved that certain methods of fetal monitoring are superior to others in these pa-

---

Preeclampsia Instructions

You (may) have preeclampsia, which is also known as pregnancy-induced hypertension or toxemia. This condition is characterized by high blood pressure, swelling, and protein in the urine. In unusually severe cases seizures, kidney failure, liver damage, uncontrolled bleeding, or fetal distress may result.

The cause of this disease is unknown. Although bed rest may temporarily improve your symptoms, only delivery can provide a cure. Because you have not yet reached your due date, we are allowing your pregnancy to continue so long as it is safe for you and your fetus.

As part of your continued care as an outpatient, you should do and record the following:
1. Take your blood pressure 2–4 times per day.
2. Weigh yourself every morning.
3. Dip your first urine of the morning for protein.
4. Remain at home on bed rest, except to go to the bathroom and eat your meals.

You should contact us immediately for ANY ONE or more of the following:
1. Your blood pressure is persistently greater than ___*___ systolic.
2. Your blood pressure is persistently greater than ___*___ diastolic.
3. Your urine protein is ___*___ or greater on dipstick.
4. You have weight gain of more than 2 lb in one day or 5 lb in one week.
5. You have a severe, lasting headache that is not relieved by acetaminophen.
6. You have lasting pain in your abdomen, particularly in the upper middle or right side, that is not relieved by antacid.
7. You have visual disturbances, such as blurry vision or seeing spots ("flashing lights").
8. You have vaginal bleeding.
9. You notice watery fluid leaking from the vagina.
10. You experience regular uterine contractions.
11. Your baby doesn't move as much as usual.
12. You have any other symptoms that cause you concern, such as nausea and vomiting.

Contact our office at any time of the day or night by calling ___*___ . If you are unable to contact us promptly, call the hospital Labor and Delivery Unit at ___*___ and discuss your condition with a nurse or doctor. You may also request that the hospital personnel contact your doctor. When calling our office or the hospital, remember to state first that you may have preeclampsia and are being monitored for it at home.

If you cannot reach anyone and you feel your condition is an emergency, call 911 and go to the hospital by ambulance.

*To be filled in based on individual circumstances.

FIGURE 2–1. Sample instructions for outpatients suspected of having preeclampsia. (Modified from Barton JR, Witlin AG, Sibai BM. Management of mild preeclampsia. Clin Obstet Gynecol 1999;42:465.)

---

tients. We prefer to perform twice-weekly non-stress tests. A biophysical profile (or, in unusual cases, a contraction stress test) is used for further evaluation when the non-stress test is nonreactive.

Intrapartum Management

Vaginal delivery is the preferred route unless other indications for cesarean section are present. In women with an unfavorable cervix, ripening agents (prostaglandins, Foley catheter, oxytocin) may be used as in the normal patient. Continuous electronic fetal heart rate monitoring is recommended. While in labor, women receive an intravenous (IV) physiologic saline solution (e.g., lactated Ringer's with 5% dextrose) at 100 to 150 mL/hr. Fluid intake and urinary output are monitored hourly. Maternal analgesia, as in the normotensive woman, may include IV doses of narcotic (e.g., fentanyl 50–100 µg) or regional anesthesia (epidural or intrathecal).

To prevent complications of hypertension such as stroke, we recommend antihypertensive therapy when the systolic blood pressure persistently exceeds 160 mmHg or the diastolic 110 mmHg. The goal of therapy is a blood pressure of 130 to 155 mmHg systolic and 90 to 105 mmHg diastolic. The drug we use most commonly for this purpose is IV labetalol or hydralazine or oral labetalol or nifedipine. An excessive decline in blood pressure (>20% reduction in mean arterial pressure) may worsen maternal cerebral ischemia, maternal renal function, and placental blood flow.

Magnesium sulfate ($MgSO_4$) is used to prevent seizures. For decades, the use of $MgSO_4$ in the United States was based on empirical

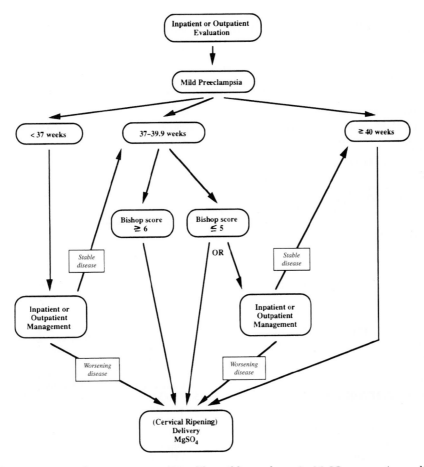

FIGURE 2–2. Management of pregnancy complicated by mild preeclampsia. MgSO$_4$, magnesium sulfate.

reports of its success.[77, 78] During the 1990s, data from randomized clinical trials demonstrated its superiority over classic anticonvulsants (phenytoin, diazepam) in both eclamptic[79–81] and preeclamptic[82] women.

Lucas and colleagues[82] randomly assigned more than 2000 hypertensive parturients to receive intrapartum seizure prophylaxis with either MgSO$_4$ or phenytoin. The incidence of seizure in the group receiving phenytoin (10/1089) was significantly higher than that in the group receiving MgSO$_4$ (0/1049, $P = .004$). Despite the reduced incidence of seizure, no data demonstrate an improvement in overall maternal and perinatal outcome for women with mild preeclampsia or gestational hypertension who receive MgSO$_4$ versus phenytoin or versus placebo. Nevertheless, the use of MgSO$_4$ for seizure prophylaxis in women with preeclampsia has become standard practice in the United States.[11] In women with transient hypertension, without other signs of pre-

eclampsia (proteinuria, hyperuricemia, thrombocytopenia, headache), it is reasonable to forgo MgSO$_4$.

Several MgSO$_4$ regimens have been published. The most commonly used today are the IV regimens popularized by Zuspan and Sibai and the intramuscular/IV regimen promoted by Pritchard (Table 2–6).

There is considerable debate about when MgSO$_4$ therapy should commence during the intrapartum period. For women with mild gestational hypertension or preeclampsia, some clinicians prefer to begin the infusion at admission (or at initiation of labor induction); others prefer to wait until regular contractions have been established; and still others prefer to begin when active labor ($\geq$4 cm cervical dilation) has been achieved. Because no firm data have supported or refuted any of these preferences, we believe that an individualized approach is appropriate. Conflicting reports about the effects of MgSO$_4$ on term labor have been pub-

---

TABLE 2–6. ACCEPTABLE REGIMENS FOR THE ADMINISTRATION OF MAGNESIUM SULFATE

INTRAVENOUS REGIMEN

Loading dose: 4–6 g $MgSO_4$ in 100 mL fluid over 15–20 min
Maintenance dose: 2 g $MgSO_4$/h which may be adjusted according to serum magnesium levels (target 4–8 mEq/L [4.8–9.6 mg/dL]) or patient symptoms (depressed but not absent deep tendon reflexes)

INTRAMUSCULAR/INTRAVENOUS REGIMEN[77, 82]

Loading dose: 4 g $MgSo_4$ in a 20% solution infused at a rate not to exceed 1 g/min (severe preeclampsia and eclampsia only) plus 10 g $MgSO_4$ as a 50% solution, half of which is injected deeply into upper outer quadrant of each buttock
Maintenance dose: 5 g $MgSO_4$ in a 50% solution injected deeply into upper outer quadrant of alternate buttocks every 4 hours, provided:
1. Patellar reflex present
2. Respirations not depressed
3. Urine output during the previous 4 hours exceeding 100 mL

$MgSO_4$, magnesium sulfate.

lished.[83–86] The best interpretation of the literature is that $MgSO_4$ may (or may not) have a dilatory effect on labor, which would be surmountable with oxytocin administration (see Chapter 13).

Postpartum Management

After delivery, the patient with mild gestational hypertension or preeclampsia should be observed closely for 12 to 24 hours. Hypertension should be treated as in the intrapartum period. Because 29% of eclamptic patients have their first seizure in the postpartum period,[78] $MgSO_4$ should be continued for 12 to 24 hours after delivery in most cases. One exception is the patient with mild hypertension or preeclampsia with postpartum hemorrhage caused by uterine atony. In such patients, the risk of seizure ($<1\%$) may be outweighed by the greater risk of hemorrhage. If $MgSO_4$ is withheld, it should be readily available for rapid administration should the need arise.

At the time of hospital discharge, a minority of women may require continued antihypertensive therapy. Prophylactic anticonvulsant medications are not needed. The patient may then be seen weekly until blood pressure returns to normal without medications. When the patient becomes normotensive, whether in the hospital or several weeks after discharge, she may receive a prescription for oral contraceptives. If hypertension persists for more than 6 weeks post partum, the possibility of chronic hypertension should be evaluated.

References

1. Villar MA, Sibai BM. Clinical significance of elevated mean arterial blood pressure in second trimester and threshold increase in systolic or diastolic blood pressure during third trimester. Am J Obstet Gynecol 1989;160:419–423.
2. MacGillivray I, Rose GA, Rowe B. Blood pressure survey in pregnancy. Clin Sci 1969;37:395–407.
3. Kuo VS, Koumantakis G, Gallery EDM. Proteinuria and its assessment in normal and hypertensive pregnancy. Am J Obstet Gynecol 1992;167:723–728.
4. Meyer NL, Mercer BM, Friedman SA, Sibai BM. Urinary dipstick protein: A poor predictor of absent or severe proteinuria. Am J Obstet Gynecol 1994;170:137–141.
5. Brown MA, Buddle ML. Inadequacy of dipstick proteinuria in hypertensive pregnancy. Aust N Z J Obstet Gynaecol 1995;35:366–369.
6. Lindow SW, Davey DA. The variability of urinary protein and creatinine excretion in patients with gestational proteinuric hypertension. Br J Obstet Gynaecol 1992;99:869–872.
7. Thomson AM, Hytten FE, Billewicz WZ. The epidemiology of oedema during pregnancy. J Obstet Gynaecol Br Commonw 1967;74:1–10.
8. Robertson EG. The natural history of oedema during pregnancy. J Obstet Gynaecol Br Commonw 1971;78:520–529.
9. Hughes EC (ed). Obstetric-Gynecologic Terminology: With Section on Neonatology and Glossary of Congenital Anomalies. Philadelphia: FA Davis, 1972.
10. National High Blood Pressure Education Program Working Group report on high blood pressure in pregnancy. Am J Obstet Gynecol 2000;183:S1–S22.
11. American College of Obstetricians and Gynecologists (ACOG). Hypertension in Pregnancy. ACOG Educational Bulletin No. 219. Washington: ACOG, 1996, pp 1–8.
12. Redman CWG, Jeffries M. Revised definition of preeclampsia. Lancet 1988;1:809–812.
13. Hauth JC, Ewell MG, Levine RJ, Sibai B, et al. Pregnancy outcome in healthy nulliparas who subsequently developed hypertension. Obstet Gynecol 2000;95:24–28.

14. Sanchez-Ramos L, Sandroni S, Andres FJ, Kaunitz AM. Calcium excretion in preeclampsia. Obstet Gynecol 1991;77:510–513.

15. Lim K-H, Friedman SA, Ecker JL, et al. The clinical utility of serum uric acid measurements in hypertensive diseases of pregnancy. Am J Obstet Gynecol 1998;178:1067–1071.

16. Weenink GH, Borm JJJ, Ten Cate JW, Treffers PE. Antithrombin III levels in normotensive and hypertensive pregnancy. Gynecol Obstet Invest 1983; 16:230–242.

17. Paarlberg KM, De Jong CLD, Van Geijn HP, et al. Total plasma fibronectin as a marker of pregnancy-induced hypertensive disorders: A longitudinal study. Obstet Gynecol 1998;91:383–388.

18. Taylor RN, Crombleholme WR, Friedman SA, et al. High plasma cellular fibronectin levels correlate with biochemical and clinical features of preeclampsia but cannot be attributed to hypertension alone. Am J Obstet Gynecol 1991;165:895–901.

19. Petraglia F, Aguzzoli L, Gallinelli A, et al. Hypertension in pregnancy: Changes in activin A maternal serum concentration. Placenta 1995;16:447–454.

20. Muttukrishna S, Knight PG, Redman CWG, Ledger WL. Activin A and inhibin A as possible endocrine markers for pre-eclampsia. Lancet 1997;349:1285–1288.

21. Grimes DA. Understanding screening tests: The key to avoiding pitfalls in interpretation. Contemp Obstet Gynecol 2000;45:46–68.

22. Friedman SA, Taylor RN, Roberts JM. Pathophysiology of preeclampsia. Clin Perinatol 1991;18:661–682.

23. Sibai BM, Caritis SN, Thom E, et al. Prevention of preeclampsia with low-dose aspirin in healthy, nulliparous pregnant women. N Engl J Med 1993;329:1213–1218.

24. Levine RJ, Hauth JC, Curet LB, et al. Trial of calcium to prevent preeclampsia. N Engl J Med 1997;337:69–76.

25. Caritis SN, Sibai BM, Hauth J, et al. Low-dose aspirin to prevent preeclampsia in women at high risk. N Engl J Med 1998;338:701–705.

26. Friedman EA, Neff RK. Pregnancy hypertension: A systematic evaluation of clinical diagnostic criteria. Littleton, MA: PSG, 1977, pp 212–219.

27. Massé J, Forest J-C, Moutquin J-M, et al. A prospective study of several potential biologic markers for early prediction of the development of preeclampsia. Am J Obstet Gynecol 1993;169:501–508.

28. Ales KL, Norton ME, Druzin ML. Early prediction of antepartum hypertension. Obstet Gynecol 1989;73:928–933.

29. Conde-Agudelo A, Belizán JM, Lede R, Bergel EF. What does an elevated mean arterial pressure in the second half of pregnancy predict—gestational hypertension or preeclampsia? Am J Obstet Gynecol 1993;169:509–514.

30. Sibai BM, Gordon T, Thom E, et al. Risk factors for preeclampsia in healthy nulliparous women: A prospective multicenter study. Am J Obstet Gynecol 1995;172:642–648.

31. Sibai BM, Ewell M, Levine RJ, et al. Risk factors associated with preeclampsia in healthy nulliparous women. Am J Obstet Gynecol 1997;177:1003–1010.

32. Higgins JR, Walshe JJ, Halligan A, et al. Can 24-hour ambulatory blood pressure measurement predict the development of hypertension in primigravidae? Br J Obstet Gynaecol 1997;104:356–362.

33. Nelson TR. A clinical study of pre-eclampsia. J Obstet Gynaecol Br Commonw 1955;62:48–57.

34. Thomson AM, Billewicz WZ. Clinical significance of weight trends during pregnancy. Br Med J 1957;1:243–247.

35. Sorensen TK, Williams MA, Zingheim RW, Clement SJ, Hickok DE. Elevated second-trimester human chorionic gonadotropin and subsequent pregnancy-induced hypertension. Am J Obstet Gynecol 1993;169:834–838.

36. Vaillant P, David E, Constant I, et al. Validity in nulliparas of increased β-human chorionic gonadotrophin at mid-term for predicting pregnancy-induced hypertension complicated with proteinuria and intrauterine growth retardation. Nephron 1996;72:557–563.

37. Ashour AMN, Lieberman ES, Wilkins Haug LE, Repke JT. The value of elevated second-trimester β-human chorionic gonadotropin in predicting development of preeclampsia. Am J Obstet Gynecol 1997;176:438–442.

38. Morris JA, O'Grady JP, Hamilton CJ, Davidson EC. Vascular reactivity to angiotensin II infusion during gestation. Am J Obstet Gynecol 1978;130:379–384.

39. Öney T, Kaulhausen H. The value of the angiotensin sensitivity test in the early diagnosis of hypertensive disorders in pregnancy. Am J Obstet Gynecol 1982;142:17–20.

40. Dekker GA, Makovitz JW, Wallenburg HCS. Prediction of pregnancy-induced hypertensive disorders by angiotensin II sensitivity and supine pressor test. Br J Obstet Gynaecol 1990;97:817–821.

41. Kyle PM, Buckley D, Kissane J, et al. The angiotensin sensitivity test and low-dose aspirin are ineffective methods to predict and prevent hypertensive disorders in nulliparous pregnancy. Am J Obstet Gynecol 1995;173:865–872.

42. Baker PN, Johnson IR. The use of the hand-grip test for predicting pregnancy-induced hypertension. Eur J Obstet Gynecol Reprod Biol 1994; 56:169–172.

43. Jacobson S-L, Imhof R, Manning N, et al. The value of Doppler assessment of the uteroplacental circulation in predicting preeclampsia or intrauterine growth retardation. Am J Obstet Gynecol 1990; 162:110–114.

44. Conde-Agudelo A, Belizán JM, Lede R, Bergel E. Prediction of hypertensive disorders of pregnancy by calcium/creatinine ratio and other laboratory tests [letter]. Int J Gynecol Obstet 1994;47:285–286.

45. Sanchez-Ramos L, Jones DC, Cullen MT. Urinary calcium as an early marker for preeclampsia. Obstet Gynecol 1991;77:685–688.

46. Millar JGB, Campbell SK, Albano JDM, et al. Early prediction of pre-eclampsia by measurement of kallikrein and creatinine on a random urine sample. Br J Obstet Gynaecol 1996;103:421–426.

47. Kyle P, Redman C, de Swiet M, Millar G. A comparison of the inactive urinary kallikrein:creatinine ratio and the angiotensin sensitivity test for the prediction of pre-eclampsia [letter reply]. Br J Obstet Gynaecol 1997;104:969–974.

48. Steel SA, Pearce JM, McParland P, Chamberlain GVP. Early doppler ultrasound screening in prediction of hypertensive disorders of pregnancy. Lancet 1990;335:1548–1551.

49. Bower S, Bewley S, Campbell S. Improved predic-

tion of preeclampsia by two-stage screening of uterine arteries using the early diastolic notch and color Doppler imaging. Obstet Gynecol 1994;82:78–83.

50. North RA, Ferrier C, Long D, et al. Uterine artery Doppler flow velocity waveforms in the second trimester for the prediction of preeclampsia and fetal growth retardation. Obstet Gynecol 1994; 83:378–386.

51. Paarlberg KM, De Jong CLD, Van Geijn HP, et al. Total plasma fibronectin as a marker of pregnancy-induced hypertensive disorders: A longitudinal study. Obstet Gynecol 1998;91:383–388.

52. Konijnenberg A, van der Post JAM, Mol BW, et al. Can flow cytometric detection of platelet activation early in pregnancy predict the occurrence of preeclampsia? A prospective study. Am J Obstet Gynecol 1997;177:434–442.

53. Hamlin RHJ. The prevention of eclampsia and preeclampsia. Lancet 1952;i:64–68.

54. Gilstrap LC III, Cunningham FG, Whalley PJ. Management of pregnancy-induced hypertension in the nulliparous patient remote from term. Semin Perinatol 1978;2:73–81.

55. Sibai BM, Gonzalez AR, Mabie WC, Moretti M. A comparison of labetalol plus hospitalization versus hospitalization alone in the management of preeclampsia remote from term. Obstet Gynecol 1987;70:323–327.

56. Mathews DD, Agarwal V, Shuttleworth TP. The effect of rest and ambulation on plasma urea and urate levels in pregnant women with proteinuric hypertension. Br J Obstet Gynaecol 1980;87:1095–1098.

57. Mathews DD, Agarwal V, Shuttleworth TP. A randomized controlled trial of complete bed rest versus ambulation in the management of proteinuric hypertension during pregnancy. Br J Obstet Gynaecol 1982;89:128–131.

58. Mathews DD, Patel IR, Sengupta SM. Out-patient management of toxaemia. J Obstet Gynaecol Br Commonw 1971;78:610–619.

59. Crowther CA, Bouwmeester AM, Ashurst HM. Does admission to hospital for bed rest prevent disease progression or improve fetal outcome in pregnancy complicated by non-proteinuric hypertension? Br J Obstet Gynaecol 1992;99:13–17.

60. Dawson AJ, Middlemiss C, Coles EC, et al. A randomized study of a domiciliary antenatal care scheme: The effect on hospital admissions. Br J Obstet Gynaecol 1989;96:1319–1322.

61. Soothill PW, Ajayi R, Campbell S, et al. Effect of a fetal surveillance unit on admission of antenatal patients to hospital. BMJ 1991;303:269–271.

62. Tuffnell DJ, Lilford RJ, Buchan PC, et al. Randomised controlled trial of day care for hypertension in pregnancy. Lancet 1992;339:224–227.

63. Twaddle S, Harper V. An economic evaluation of daycare in the management of hypertension in pregnancy. Br J Obstet Gynaecol 1992;99:459–463.

64. Barton JR, Stanziano GJ, Sibai BM. Monitored outpatient management of mild gestational hypertension remote from term. Am J Obstet Gynecol 1994;170:765–769.

65. Barton JR, Stanziano GJ, Jacques DL, et al. Monitored outpatient management of mild gestational hypertension remote from term in teenage pregnancies. Am J Obstet Gynecol 1995;173:1865–1868.

66. Barton JR, Bergauer NK, Jacques DL, et al. Does advanced maternal age affect pregnancy outcome in women with mild hypertension remote from term? Am J Obstet Gynecol 1997;176:1236–1240.

67. Sibai BM, Barton JR, Akl S, et al. A randomized prospective comparison of nifedipine and bed rest versus bed rest alone in the management of preeclampsia remote from term. Am J Obstet Gynecol 1992;167:879–884.

68. Rubin PC, Butters L, Clark DM, et al. Placebo-controlled trial of atenolol in treatment of pregnancy-associated hypertension. Lancet 1983;i:431–434.

69. Pickles CJ, Symonds EM, Broughton Pipkin F. The fetal outcome in a randomized double-blind controlled trial of labetalol versus placebo in pregnancy-induced hypertension. Br J Obstet Gynaecol 1989;96:38–43.

70. Phippard AF, Fischer WE, Horvath JS, et al. Early blood pressure control improves pregnancy outcome in primigravid women with mild hypertension. Med J Aust 1991;154:378–382.

71. Wichman K, Rydén G, Karlberg BE. A placebo controlled trial of metoprolol in the treatment of hypertension in pregnancy. Scand J Clin Lab Invest Suppl 1984;169:90–95.

72. Plouin P-F, Breart G, Maillard F, et al. Comparison of antihypertensive efficacy and perinatal safety of labetalol and methyldopa in the treatment of hypertension in pregnancy: A randomized controlled trial. Br J Obstet Gynaecol 1988;95:868–876.

73. Plouin P-F, Breart G, Llado J, et al. A randomized comparison of early with conservative use of antihypertensive drugs in the management of pregnancy-induced hypertension. Br J Obstet Gynaecol 1990;97:134–141.

74. Cruickshank DJ, Robertson AA, Campbell DM, MacGillivray I. Does labetalol influence the development of proteinuria in pregnancy hypertension? A randomised controlled study. Eur J Obstet Gynaecol Reprod Biol 1992;45:47–51.

75. Jannet D, Carbonne B, Sebban E, Milliez J. Nicardipine versus metoprolol in the treatment of hypertension during pregnancy: A randomized comparative trial. Obstet Gynecol 1994;84:354–359.

76. Gruppo di Studio Ipertensione in Gravidanza. Nifedipine versus expectant management in mild to moderate hypertension in pregnancy. Br J Obstet Gynaecol 1998;105:718–722.

77. Pritchard JA, Cunningham FG, Pritchard SA. The Parkland Memorial Hospital protocol for treatment of eclampsia: Evaluation of 245 cases. Am J Obstet Gynecol 1984;148:951–963.

78. Sibai BM. Eclampsia. VI. Maternal-perinatal outcome in 254 consecutive cases. Am J Obstet Gynecol 1990;163:1049–1054.

79. Dommisse J. Phenytoin sodium and magnesium sulphate in the management of eclampsia. Br J Obstet Gynaecol 1990;97:104–109.

80. Crowther C. Magnesium sulphate versus diazepam in the management of eclampsia: A randomized controlled trial. Br J Obstet Gynaecol 1990;97:110–117.

81. Eclampsia Trial Collaborative Group. Which anticonvulsant for women with eclampsia? Evidence from the Collaborative Eclampsia Trial. Lancet 1995;345:1455–1463.

82. Lucas MJ, Leveno KJ, Cunningham FG. A comparison of magnesium sulfate with phenytoin for the prevention of eclampsia. N Engl J Med 1995; 333:201–205.

83. Friedman SA, Lim K-H, Baker CA, Repke JT. Phenytoin versus magnesium sulfate in preeclampsia: A pilot study. Am J Perinatol 1993;10:233–238.

84. Atkinson MW, Guinn D, Owen J, Hauth JC. Does magnesium sulfate affect the length of labor induction in women with pregnancy-associated hypertension? Am J Obstet Gynecol 1995;173:1219–1222.

85. Witlin AG, Friedman SA, Sibai BM. The effect of magnesium sulfate therapy on the duration of labor in women with mild preeclampsia at term: A randomized, double-blind, placebo-controlled trial. Am J Obstet Gynecol 1997;176:623–627.

86. Leveno KJ, Alexander JM, McIntyre DD, Lucas MJ. Does magnesium sulfate given for prevention of eclampsia affect the outcome of labor? Am J Obstet Gynecol 1998;178:707–712.

3

HELLP SYNDROME

John R. Barton and Baha M. Sibai

• • • •

For many years, hemolysis, abnormal liver function tests, and thrombocytopenia have been recognized as complications of preeclampsia-eclampsia.[1-4] According to Chesley,[1] some of these components had been reported in the obstetric literature for almost a century (in 1893, coagulation defects and microthrombi were first described by Schmorl). In 1982, Weinstein described 29 cases of severe preeclampsia-eclampsia complicated by thrombocytopenia, abnormal peripheral smear, and abnormal liver function tests.[5] He suggested that this collection of signs and symptoms constituted an entity separate from severe preeclampsia and coined the term *HELLP syndrome: H* for hemolysis, *EL* for elevated liver enzymes, and *LP* for low platelets.

Since 1982, numerous articles and case reports describing HELLP syndrome have appeared in the medical literature. In addition, the presence of this syndrome has become a major cause of litigation against obstetricians, involving cases of alleged misdiagnosed preeclampsia, particularly in cases complicated by severe liver involvement. This chapter reviews the diagnosis, pathologic findings, hepatic manifestations, and current management recommendations for pregnancies complicated by HELLP syndrome.

TERMINOLOGY AND DIAGNOSIS

A review of the literature by Sibai and associates[6] revealed considerable difference concerning the terminology, incidence, cause, diagnosis, and management of HELLP syndrome. Goodlin[2] considered it an early form of severe preeclampsia and labeled it as a great imitator and impending EPH (edema, proteinuria, hypertension) gestosis type B. Weinstein[5] considered it a "unique variant" of preeclampsia, whereas MacKenna and

colleagues[7] considered it to be misdiagnosed preeclampsia. Conversely, several authors have considered HELLP syndrome to be mild disseminated intravascular coagulation (DIC) that was missed because of inadequate laboratory investigation.

The reported incidence of HELLP syndrome ranges from 2% to 12%, reflecting the different diagnostic criteria and methods used in studies describing this syndrome. In addition, there are considerable differences regarding its time of onset and the type and degree of laboratory abnormalities used to make the diagnosis. Evidence of hemolysis was documented in few of the early studies, and the definition of thrombocytopenia ranged from less than $75,000/mm^3$ to less than $150,000/mm^3$. Moreover, there is no consensus in the literature regarding which liver function test abnormalities should be used in the diagnosis of the HELLP syndrome. Weinstein[5, 8] did not indicate whether it was necessary to attain specific concentrations of bilirubin, serum aspartate transaminase (AST), or serum alanine transaminase (ALT) before reaching a diagnosis of HELLP syndrome. Furthermore, he made no mention of lactate dehydrogenase (LDH) as a diagnostic feature.

Martin and coworkers,[9] in a retrospective review of 302 cases of HELLP syndrome at the University of Mississippi, Jackson, have devised the following classification of subpopulations based on platelet count nadir:

Class 1: a platelet nadir below $50,000/mm^3$
Class 2: a platelet nadir between 51,000 and $100,000/mm^3$
Class 3: a platelet nadir between 101,000 and $150,000/mm^3$

These classes have been used to predict the rapidity of postpartum disease recovery,[9] risk of recurrence of HELLP syndrome,[10] perinatal outcome, and the need for plasmapheresis.[11]

Miles and associates,[12] also from the University of Mississippi, Jackson, reported a strong association between the presence of HELLP syndrome and eclampsia. HELLP syndrome was present in 30% of patients with postpartum eclampsia and in 28% of patients having eclampsia before delivery. As a result, the authors suggested that the presence of HELLP syndrome might be a predisposing factor in the development of eclampsia.

Hemolysis, defined as the presence of microangiopathic hemolytic anemia, is the hallmark of HELLP syndrome. The role of DIC in preeclampsia is controversial. Most authors do not regard HELLP syndrome to be a variant of DIC because coagulation parameters (prothrombin time, partial thromboplastin time, serum fibrinogen level) are normal.

Many authors now advocate that LDH and bilirubin values be included in the diagnosis of hemolysis and that the degree of liver enzyme abnormality be defined as a certain number of standard deviations (SDs) from normal values for each hospital. At the University of Tennessee, Memphis, a cut-off value of more than twice the upper limits of normal for the population is used to indicate abnormality.[6] These criteria for the diagnosis of the HELLP syndrome include the laboratory findings summarized in Table 3–1 and are compared with the criteria of other investigators in Table 3–2.

CLINICAL PRESENTATION

In the series reported by Sibai and associates,[6] patients with HELLP syndrome were significantly older (mean age, 25 years) than patients with severe preeclampsia-eclamp-

TABLE 3–2. CLASSIFICATIONS OF HELLP SYNDROME

STUDY	PLATELET COUNT	AST	LDH
Sibai et al[6]	<100,000/mm³	≥70 U/L	≥600 U/L
Martin et al[9]	<150,000/mm³	≥40 U/L	≥600 U/L
van Pampus et al[35]	<100,000/mm³	>50 U/L	>600 U/L
Visser and Wallenburg[36]	<100,000/mm³	>30 U/L	*

*Not included in their criteria.
AST, aspartate transaminase; LDH, lactate dehydrogenase.

sia without features of HELLP syndrome (mean age, 19 years). The incidence of the syndrome was significantly higher in the Caucasian population and among multiparous patients. The incidence of HELLP syndrome is also higher in preeclamptic patients with conservative management of their disease. Coincidentally, medical complications (notably diabetes mellitus and lupus nephritis) were no more common among the patients with HELLP syndrome. Other authors have made similar observations.[7, 8, 13]

Patients with HELLP syndrome may present with various signs and symptoms, none of which are diagnostic, and all of which may be found in patients with severe preeclampsia-eclampsia without HELLP syndrome. Sibai[14] noted that the patient usually presents remote from term, complaining of epigastric or right upper quadrant pain; some have nausea or vomiting, and others have nonspecific viral syndrome–like symptoms. Most patients (90%) give a history of malaise for the past few days prior to presentation. In Weinstein's reports,[5, 8] nausea or vomiting and epigastric pain were the most common symptoms. Right upper quadrant or epigastric pain is thought to result from obstruction to blood flow in the hepatic sinusoids, which are blocked by intravascular fibrin deposition.

Patients with HELLP syndrome usually demonstrate significant weight gain with generalized edema. It is important to appreciate that *severe* hypertension (systolic blood pressure > 160 mmHg; diastolic blood pressure > 110 mmHg) is not a constant or even a frequent finding in HELLP syndrome. Although 68.8% of the 112 patients studied by Sibai and associates[6] had a diastolic blood pressure above 110 mmHg at hospital

TABLE 3–1. UNIVERSITY OF TENNESSEE, MEMPHIS, CRITERIA FOR HELLP SYNDROME

HEMOLYSIS
Abnormal peripheral smear
Total bilirubin ≥ 1.2 mg/dL
Lactate dehydrogenase > 600 U/L

ELEVATED LIVER ENZYMES
Serum aspartate aminotransferase ≥ 70 U/L
Lactate dehydrogenase > 600 U/L

LOW PLATELETS
Platelet count < 100,000/mm³

HELLP, *h*emolysis, *e*levated *l*iver enzymes, *l*ow *p*latelets.

admission, 14.5% had a diastolic blood pressure below 90 mmHg.

In Weinstein's initial report of 29 patients,[5] fewer than half (13) had blood pressure greater than 160/110 mmHg on admission. Only 66% of the 18 primigravidas and 44% of the 9 multigravidas studied by MacKenna and coworkers[7] had severe hypertension on admission. Aarnoudse and colleagues[15] described six women presenting with severe epigastric pain in the third trimester who had significantly elevated liver enzymes, a low platelet count, and evidence of hemolysis. None of these patients had a blood pressure greater than 140/90 mmHg or proteinuria.

DIFFERENTIAL DIAGNOSIS

Patients with HELLP syndrome may present with a variety of signs and symptoms, none of which are diagnostic of severe preeclampsia. As a result, they are often misdiagnosed as having various medical and surgical disorders (Table 3–3). For these reasons, Sibai[14] recommended that pregnant women thought to have preeclampsia with any of these symptoms should undergo a complete blood count, platelet count, and liver enzyme determinations irrespective of maternal blood pressure.

A rare but interesting complication of HELLP syndrome is transient nephrogenic diabetes insipidus. Unlike central diabetes insipidus, which occurs as a result of diminished or absent secretions of arginine vasopressin by the hypothalamus, transient nephrogenic diabetes insipidus is characterized by a resistance to arginine vasopressin mediated by excessive vasopressinase.[16] It is postulated that elevated circulating vaso-

TABLE 3–4. CLINICAL AND LABORATORY CHARACTERISTICS OF HELLP SYNDROME, TTP/HUS, AND AFLP

	HELLP	TTP/HUS	AFLP
Hypertension	+ +	±	±
Proteinuria	+ +	±	±
Thrombocytopenia	+ + +	+ + +	±
Lactate dehydrogenase	>>	>>>	>>
Anemia	+	+ +	±
Bilirubin	>	>>	>>
Aspartate transaminase	>>	±	>>
Fibrinogen	=	=	<
Antithrombin III	<	=	<
Ammonia	=	=	+
Glucose	=	=	<
Creatinine	>	>>	>>

Key: ±, equivocal; +, possible; + +, likely; + + +, definitely; =, normal; <, decreased; >, increased; >>, more increased; >>>, very increased.

TTP, thrombotic thrombocytopenic purpura; HUS, hemolytic uremic syndrome; AFLP, acute fatty liver of pregnancy.

pressinase may result from impaired hepatic metabolism of the enzyme.

Acute fatty liver of pregnancy (AFLP) is a rare but potentially fatal complication of the third trimester. It occurs in about 1 of 13,000 pregnancies. In a study of 14 patients with AFLP, Usta and colleagues[17] reported a mean gestational age of onset at 34.5 weeks (range, 28–39 weeks). In its early presentation, AFLP may be difficult to differentiate from HELLP syndrome. Patients with AFLP typically present with nausea, vomiting, abdominal pain, and jaundice. HELLP syndrome and AFLP are both characterized by elevated liver function values; however, the abnormalities tend to be greater in HELLP syndrome. Furthermore, prothrombin and partial thromboplastin times are usually prolonged in AFLP, although normal in HELLP syndrome. Microscopic examination of the liver is the definitive diagnostic test for determining AFLP. Microvesicular change (steatosis most prominent in the centrizonal region) is pathognomonic for AFLP. Table 3–4 details clinical and laboratory differences between AFLP and HELLP syndrome.

An association exists between AFLP and autosomal recessive long-chain 3-hydroxyacyl–coenzyme A dehydrogenase (LCHAD) deficiency.[18–20] In a study from Finland of women heterozygous for LCHAD deficiency,[19] pregnancies in which the infants were affected with LCHAD deficiency showed a significantly greater frequency of preeclampsia, HELLP syndrome, smallness for gestational age, and hypoxia compared

TABLE 3–3. MEDICAL AND SURGICAL DISORDERS CONFUSED WITH THE HELLP SYNDROME

Acute fatty liver of pregnancy	Hyperemesis gravidarum
Appendicitis	Idiopathic thrombocytopenia
Diabetes insipidus	Kidney stones
Gallbladder disease	Peptic ulcer
Gastroenteritis	Pyelonephritis
Glomerulonephritis	Systemic lupus erythematosus
Hemolytic uremic syndrome	Thrombotic thrombocytopenic purpura
Hepatic encephalopathy	Viral hepatitis

with pregnancies in which the infants were unaffected.

Ibdah and coworkers[20] studied 24 children with LCHAD deficiency. They used deoxyribonucleic acid (DNA) amplification and nucleotide-sequence analyses to identify mutations in the α subunit of the trifunctional protein. The investigators then correlated the results with the presence of liver disease during pregnancy in the mothers. Nineteen children had a deficiency of LCHAD only and presented with hypoketotic hypoglycemia and fatty liver. In eight children, a homozygous mutation was identified in which the glutamic acid (Glu) at residue 474 was changed to glutamine (Gln). While carrying fetuses with the Glu474Gln mutation, 79% of the heterozygous mothers had AFLP or the HELLP syndrome.[20]

Management of AFLP includes supportive care and delivery after maternal stabilization, including correction of hypoglycemia or coagulopathy. Vaginal delivery is preferred, and a cesarean section should be used as necessary for standard obstetric indications. Major risks to the mother include hepatic encephalopathy, renal failure, metabolic acidosis, coagulopathy, and infection.

Much rarer than HELLP syndrome, thrombotic thrombocytopenic purpura (TTP) and hemolytic uremic syndrome (HUS) are remarkably similar to one another and have even thought to be one and the same. HUS characteristically has been a disease of children, impairing renal function and causing platelet and erythrocyte destruction. When it occurs in association with pregnancy, the presentation typically has occurred post partum.

TTP is more commonly recognized among adults, with similar manifestations to HUS. The classic pentad of TTP includes thrombocytopenia, microangiopathic hemolysis, neurologic symptoms, renal impairment, and fever. Table 3–4 details the clinical and laboratory differences between HELLP syndrome, TTP, HUS, and AFLP.

Plasma transfusions and exchanges have revolutionized the management of TTP/HUS, increasing survival to 80% to 90%. Plasma infusions have been suggested as first-line therapy during pregnancy, with response rates of 64%, but many have proposed that plasma exchange be used as initial therapy.[21, 22] Initial plasma replacement dose is 30 to 40 mL/kg, which can be reduced to 15 to 20 mL/kg for maintenance.[23]

PATHOLOGIC FINDINGS

Microangiopathic hemolytic anemia is the hallmark of HELLP syndrome. It is thought to result from the passage of red blood cells through small blood vessels with damaged intima and fibrin deposition,[5, 24] leading to the appearance on peripheral smear of triangular cells, burr cells, echinocytes, and spherocytes. Microangiopathic hemolytic anemia is not specific to HELLP syndrome and is also found in association with TTP, renal disease, HUS, eclampsia, and carcinomatosis.

In a study published by our group,[25] the microscopic findings from liver biopsies obtained under direct visualization after cesarean delivery from pregnancies complicated by HELLP syndrome were categorized and correlated with the severity of the concurrent clinical and laboratory abnormalities. In comparing the histologic findings with the laboratory findings, we found that periportal hemorrhage correlated with the presence of fibrin deposition but with none of the laboratory parameters measured. Similarly, fibrin deposition was not statistically correlated with any measured laboratory parameter. Although steatosis occurred in only one third of the patients, it correlated significantly with abnormalities in platelet count, AST, and total bilirubin but not with periportal hemorrhage or fibrin deposition.

To further test for a relationship between the severity of histologic, clinical, and biochemical parameters in patients with HELLP syndrome, the study group was divided into two subgroups on the basis of histologic criteria; six patients were classified as having mild HELLP syndrome and five were considered to have severe HELLP syndrome. Statistical analysis demonstrated a significant difference for periportal hemorrhage and fibrin deposition between these two histologic criteria groups but failed to show any statistically significant difference in gestational age, mean arterial blood pressure, or any laboratory parameter.

In the case report by Hannah and colleagues,[26] frozen sections of liver from a patient with elevated liver enzymes and thrombocytopenia that were stained with hematoxylin and eosin and oil red O showed many small orangeophilic globules considered to be fat in hepatocytes, comparable with that seen in AFLP. Similarly, we noted steatosis in several of the liver biopsy specimens from our study population.[25] Although there is overlap both clinically and pathologically between AFLP and HELLP syndrome, we believe that these syndromes can be distinguished histopathologically. On light microscopy in AFLP, the vacuolization and necrosis is more prominent in the central zone, whereas in HELLP syndrome the necrosis is predominantly periportal. Although fat droplets may be present on electron microscopy in hepatocytes from patients with the HELLP syndrome, fat droplets are much more numerous in AFLP.

From our study[25] and from previous case reports[3, 15, 26–28] describing the histopathologic findings of hepatic lesions associated with HELLP syndrome, the classic hepatic lesion associated with the HELLP syndrome is periportal or focal parenchymal necrosis in which hyaline deposits of fibrin-like material can be seen in the sinusoids. In addition, immunofluorescence studies show fibrin microthrombi and fibrinogen deposits in the sinusoids in areas of hepatocellular necrosis and in sinusoids of histologically normal parenchyma.[15, 27] These histopathologic findings may be related to the elevated liver enzymes and the right upper quadrant pain and tenderness seen in patients with this syndrome. In certain cases, the cellular necrosis and infarction may be severe enough to be seen by computed tomography (CT) of the liver (Fig. 3–1).

MANAGEMENT

Patients with HELLP syndrome who are remote from term should be referred to a ter-

TABLE 3–5. MANAGEMENT OF ANTEPARTUM HELLP SYNDROME

1. Assess and stabilize the maternal condition:
   a. If disseminated intravascular coagulation is present, correct coagulopathy
   b. Antiseizure prophylaxis with magnesium sulfate
   c. Treatment of severe hypertension
   d. Transfer to tertiary care center if appropriate
   e. Computed tomography or ultrasound of the abdomen if subcapsular hematoma of the liver is suspected
2. Evaluate fetal well-being:
   a. Non-stress testing
   b. Biophysical profile
3. Evaluate fetal lung maturity if <35 weeks' gestation:
   a. If mature, delivery
   b. If immature, give steroids, then induce delivery in 48 hours

tiary care center, and initial management should be as for any patient with severe preeclampsia. The first priority is to assess and stabilize maternal condition, particularly coagulation abnormalities (Table 3–5). The next step is to evaluate fetal well-being using the non-stress test or biophysical profile and to obtain ultrasonographic biometry for assessment of possible intrauterine growth retardation. Finally, a decision must be made as to whether immediate delivery is indicated. Amniocentesis may be performed in these patients without risk of bleeding complications.

A review of the literature highlights the confusion surrounding the management of HELLP syndrome.[6] Some authors consider its presence to be an indication for immediate delivery by cesarean section, whereas

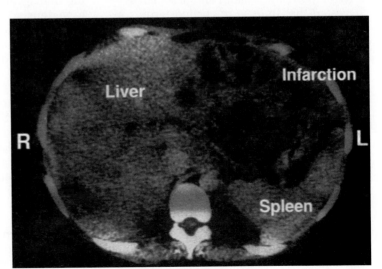

FIGURE 3–1. Computed tomography axial image through liver and spleen. *R,* Maternal right. *L,* Maternal left. (From Barton JR, Sibai B. Hepatic imaging in HELLP syndrome [hemolysis, elevated liver enzymes, and low platelet count]. Am J Obstet Gynecol 1996; 174:1823.)

others recommend a more conservative approach to prolong pregnancy in cases of fetal immaturity. Consequently, several therapeutic modalities have been described for treatment of or reversal of the HELLP syndrome. Most of these therapeutic modalities are similar to those used in the management of severe preeclampsia remote from term.

Goodlin and Holdt[29] described five patients with features of HELLP syndrome who were treated conservatively with bed rest in an attempt to increase plasma volume. Three women also received intravenous (IV) infusions of 5% or 25% albumin. The authors felt that their efforts at plasma volume expansion were in part beneficial as measured by a fall in hemoglobin concentration, rise in platelet count, and resolution of some of the symptoms of severe toxemia. Thiagarajah and coauthors[13] treated five patients with prednisone and betamethasone and reported an improvement in platelet count and liver enzymes.

Heyborne and coworkers[30] reported five cases in which temporary reversal of the HELLP syndrome was achieved using low-dose aspirin (81 mg/day) and corticosteroids. The average prolongation of pregnancy was 4 weeks; however, three pregnancies beginning at less than 25 weeks' gestation were prolonged for an average of 5.5 weeks. No long-term maternal morbidity occurred, although DIC and eclampsia developed in one patient. One criticism of the study was that three of five patients had platelet counts greater than 100,000 mm³ at initial diagnosis. Furthermore, hemolysis was not documented in three of five patients in this study.

Two reports by Magann and associates[31, 32] suggested that the use of corticosteroids either before or after delivery results in transient improvement in laboratory values and urine output in some patients diagnosed with HELLP syndrome. In the antepartum group, delivery was delayed by an average of 41 hours only, and the study was not placebo-controlled.[31]

Tompkins and Thiagarajah[33] also assessed the benefit of corticosteroids in HELLP syndrome. In their study, 93 patients between 24 and 34 weeks' gestation with HELLP syndrome were given intramuscular injections of either betamethasone or dexamethasone. Precorticosteroid and postcorticosteroid platelet counts and liver function tests results were compared. The authors noted that hematologic abnormalities improved after the administration of corticosteroids. The platelet count increased by $23.3 \times 10^3/\mu l$ ($P < .001$). A statistically significant decrease was seen in liver enzyme levels, with the ALT decreased by 31.6 IU/L and the AST decreased by 52.1 IU/L. Two doses of betamethasone given 12 hours apart was the most effective corticosteroid regimen.

O'Brien and coworkers[34] reviewed corticosteroid dosing and laboratory changes in patients with antepartum HELLP syndrome. Patients were classified on the basis of their exposure to steroid use and dosage. One control group did not receive glucocorticoids, whereas one treatment group received standard corticosteroid dosing for fetal lung maturity enhancement and a second treatment group received a higher-dosed steroid regimen (IV dexamethasone 10 mg q 6 h × 2 doses followed by 6 mg q 6 h × 2 to 4 doses). Liver function tests and platelet counts were analyzed in response to corticosteroid therapy. There was an improvement in the platelet count and liver function abnormalities with corticosteroids that was dose-dependent. These findings suggested that a higher dose of corticosteroids than standard regimens for fetal lung maturity enhancement might be needed for maximum resolution of abnormalities in HELLP syndrome.[34]

van Pampus and colleagues[35] described the clinical progress and maternal outcome of the HELLP and ELLP (findings of HELLP syndrome, but without evidence of hemolysis) syndrome in 127 patients with a live fetus in utero managed in the Academic Medical Center in Amsterdam between 1984 and 1996. Patients were treated by temporizing management, including the use of antihypertensive agents and magnesium sulfate ($MgSO_4$). The predominant indication for terminating pregnancy was fetal distress or fetal death, not maternal condition. All serious maternal complications occurred at the onset of the syndrome. Two mothers with HELLP syndrome died following a cerebral hemorrhage. Serious maternal morbidity occurred more often in cases of HELLP than in cases of ELLP syndrome (eclampsia 21% versus 8%, cerebral ischemic lesions 6% versus 21%, and serious complications 24% versus 10%). Seventy-nine (62%) of the women were not delivered after 3 days and 65 (51%) after 7 days. Although the authors noted it is unlikely that a more aggressive approach would have reduced maternal mortality or morbidity, their sample size was inadequate to evaluate rare serious maternal complications of HELLP or ELLP syndrome.

In a study by Visser and Wallenburg,[36] 128 consecutive preeclamptic patients with HELLP syndrome and a gestational age less than 34 weeks' gestation were matched for maternal and gestational age with 128 preeclamptic patients without HELLP syndrome. Both groups were treated with volume expansion and pharmacologic vasodilatation under invasive hemodynamic monitoring with the aim of prolonging gestation and enhancing fetal maturity. Except for variables pertaining to HELLP syndrome, clinical and laboratory data and median prolongation of pregnancy did not differ between the two groups. Complete reversal of HELLP occurred in 43% of patients. Perinatal mortality was 14.1% in HELLP syndrome patients and 14.8% in patients without HELLP. Inasmuch as the perinatal outcomes in this study are similar to those from studies performed in the United States where delivery was effected within 48 hours of the diagnosis of HELLP syndrome, the benefit of temporizing management of HELLP syndrome remains questionable. Ultimately, only a well-designed randomized trial should resolve this management issue.

The described conservative management techniques were often associated with the use of invasive procedures and medical and surgical treatments. These confounding variables make it difficult to evaluate any treatment modality proposed for this syndrome. Occasionally, some patients without the true HELLP syndrome may demonstrate antepartum reversal of hematologic abnormalities following bed rest, the use of steroids, or plasma volume expansion. In our experience, however, most of these patients demonstrate deterioration in either maternal or fetal condition within 1 to 10 days after conservative management.

Potential risks associated with conservative management of HELLP syndrome include:

- Abruptio placentae (placental abruption)
- Pulmonary edema
- Acute renal failure
- Eclampsia
- Perinatal death
- Maternal death

It is thus doubtful in our opinion that such a limited pregnancy prolongation would result in improved perinatal outcome, especially when maternal and fetal risks are substantial.

If the syndrome develops at or beyond 34 weeks' gestation or if fetal lung maturity or fetal or maternal jeopardy is evident before that time, delivery is the definitive therapy. Without laboratory evidence of DIC and in the absence of fetal lung maturity, the patient can be given two doses of steroids to accelerate fetal lung maturity with delivery to follow 48 hours later. Maternal and fetal conditions should be assessed continuously during this time.

The presence of this syndrome is not an indication for immediate delivery by cesarean section. Such an approach might prove detrimental for both mother and fetus. Patients presenting with well-established labor should be allowed to deliver vaginally in the absence of obstetric contraindications. Otherwise, labor may be initiated with oxytocin infusions as for routine induction in all patients with gestational age beyond 30 weeks, irrespective of the extent of cervical dilation or effacement.

A similar approach is used for patients at less than 30 weeks' gestation if the cervix is favorable for induction. In patients with an unfavorable cervix and gestational age less than 30 weeks, options for delivery management are an induction of labor with prostaglandins or elective cesarean section. A management protocol for the patient with HELLP syndrome requiring cesarean delivery is presented in Table 3–6.

Maternal analgesia during labor can be provided by intermittent use of small doses (25–50 mg) of IV meperidine. Local infiltration anesthesia can be used for all vaginal

---

TABLE 3–6. MANAGEMENT OF THE PATIENT WITH HELLP SYNDROME REQUIRING CESAREAN SECTION

1. General anesthesia for platelet count < 75,000/mm³
2. 10 units of platelets before surgery if platelet count < 40,000/mm³
3. Leave vesicouterine peritoneum (bladder flap) open
4. Subfascial drain
5. Secondary closure of skin incision or subcutaneous drain
6. Postoperative transfusions as needed
7. Intensive monitoring for 48 hours post partum
8. Consider dexamethasone therapy (10 mg IV q 12 h) until postpartum resolution of disease

IV, intravenously.

deliveries. The use of pudendal block is contraindicated in these patients because of the risk of bleeding into this area. Epidural anesthesia should be used with caution; however, many anesthesiologists are reluctant to place an epidural catheter in a patient with a platelet count below 75,000/mm³. Preliminary data indicate that administration of glucocorticoids for the benefit of fetal lung maturity enhancement may also improve thrombocytopenia such that an increased utilization of regional anesthesia may be possible. General anesthesia is the method of choice for cesarean sections in the presence of severe thrombocytopenia, coagulopathy, or hemodynamic instability. The anesthesiology service should be wary of laryngeal edema, which can occur as a consequence of HELLP syndrome and may complicate intubation or extubation.

Platelet transfusions are indicated either before or after delivery if the platelet count is less than 20,000/mm³. Correction of thrombocytopenia is particularly important before cesarean section, but repeated platelet transfusions are not necessary because consumption occurs rapidly and the effect is transient. Our policy is to administer 6 to 10 units of platelets in all patients with a platelet count below 40,000/mm³ prior to intubating the patient for cesarean section. Generalized oozing from the operative site is common, and to minimize the risk of hematoma formation, the bladder flap should be left open and a subfascial drain should be used for 24 to 48 hours.

COMPLICATIONS

Wounds

Briggs and associates[37] evaluated wound complications in patients with antepartum HELLP syndrome with primary closure versus delayed closure and Pfannenstiel versus midline skin incisions. A total of 104 patients were identified; 75 had a primary skin closure and 29 had a delayed closure 48 to 72 hours postoperatively. Immediate wound complications (wound infection, hematoma) occurred in 18 (26%) patients who had primary closure versus 8 (24%) who had a delayed closure, odds ratio 1.13 (95% confidence interval 0.39–3.27). A late wound breakdown was seen in only one patient with primary closure but in none with delayed closure. There were no fascial wound

dehiscences. No statistical difference in wound complication was found between midline (primary, delayed) and Pfannenstiel (primary, delayed) incisions, odds ratio 0.65 (95% confidence interval 0.23–1.88). The authors concluded that in women with antepartum HELLP syndrome delivered by cesarean section, the frequency of wound complications is not influenced by type of skin incision or time of skin closure (primary or delayed).[37]

Eclampsia

All patients with HELLP syndrome should receive IV infused $MgSO_4$ for prevention of eclampsia. Although IM $MgSO_4$ reduces the frequency of eclamptic seizures, this mode of administration may result in hematoma formation in patients with thrombocytopenia. IV loading doses of 4 to 6 g of $MgSO_4$ are utilized followed by a constant infusion of 1 to 3 g of $MgSO_4$/hour. Infusion dose should be adjusted based on patellar reflexes and urinary output. Serum magnesium levels should be followed closely in patients demonstrating renal dysfunction as a consequence of HELLP syndrome.

Hepatic Infarction/Hematoma

Radiologic Findings

We have reported hepatic imaging findings in selected patients with HELLP syndrome and correlated these findings with the severity of concurrent clinical and laboratory abnormalities.[38] Of the 34 patients evaluated in the study, 16 patients (47%) had abnormal hepatic imaging results. The most common CT abnormalities were subcapsular hematoma of the liver (n = 13) and intraparenchymal hemorrhage (n = 6). A magnetic resonance image (MRI) of an unruptured subcapsular hematoma of the liver is depicted in Figure 3–2. We compared the clinical characteristics and laboratory evaluations of patients with normal and abnormal hepatic imaging findings.

The results demonstrated a significant difference in platelet count nadir between the patients with normal and abnormal imaging findings but failed to show any statistically significant difference in gestational age, mean arterial pressure, or the other laboratory parameters studied. Of the 13 patients with severe thrombocytopenia (platelet

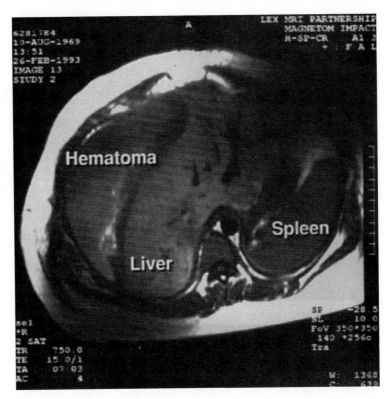

FIGURE 3–2. T1-weighted magnetic resonance axial image through the liver and spleen. (From Barton JR, Sibai B. Hepatic imaging in HELLP syndrome [hemolysis, elevated liver enzymes, and low platelet count]. Am J Obstet Gynecol 1996;174:1824.)

count $\leq$ 20,000/mm³), 10 (77%) showed abnormal hepatic imaging findings. A separate statistical analysis for patients with and without a subcapsular hematoma of the liver failed to demonstrate any statistical difference for gestational age, mean arterial pressure, or the other laboratory parameters studied. Emergency intervention was needed for six patients on the basis of these imaging findings. CT and MRI both have excellent sensitivity for detecting acute liver hemorrhage, but because CT was more available, faster, and safer for potentially unstable patients, it was the imaging modality of choice.

Liver Hematoma

The differential diagnosis of an unruptured subcapsular hematoma of the liver in pregnancy should include AFLP, abruptio placentae with DIC, ruptured uterus, acute cholecystitis with sepsis, and thrombotic thrombocytopenia purpura. Most patients with a subcapsular hematoma of the liver are seen in the late second or third trimester of pregnancy, although cases have been reported in the immediate postpartum period. In addition to the signs and symptoms of preeclampsia, physical examination findings consistent with peritoneal irritation

and hepatomegaly may be present. Stimulation of the phrenic nerve at the diaphragm can produce referred pain along the distribution of this nerve to its origin in the C4-C5 cervical plexus, including the pericardium, peritoneum, pleura, and shoulder. Because the gallbladder and esophagus share innervation by the phrenic nerve with the diaphragm, irritation of the diaphragm may produce sensations of pain in these organs.

Surgical repair has been recommended for hepatic hemorrhage without liver rupture. More recent experience suggests, however, that this complication can be managed conservatively in patients who remain hemodynamically stable.[39, 40] Management should include close monitoring of hemodynamics and coagulation status. Serial assessment of the subcapsular hematoma with ultrasound or CT is necessary, with immediate intervention for rupture or worsening of maternal status. It is important with conservative management to avoid exogenous sources of trauma to the liver such as abdominal palpation, convulsions, or emesis, and to use care in transportation of the patient. Indeed, any sudden increase in intra-abdominal pressure could potentially lead to rupture of the subcapsular hematoma.[41]

Rupture of a subcapsular hematoma of the

liver is a life-threatening complication of HELLP syndrome. In most instances, rupture involves the right lobe and is preceded by the development of a parenchymal hematoma. Patients frequently present with shoulder pain, shock, or evidence of massive ascites, respiratory difficulty, or pleural effusions, and often with a dead fetus. Ultrasonography or CT of the liver should be performed to rule out the presence of subcapsular hematoma of the liver and to assess for the presence of intraperitoneal bleeding. Paracentesis confirms the presence of intraperitoneal hemorrhage suspected by examination or radiographic imaging.

The presence of ruptured subcapsular liver hematoma resulting in shock is a surgical emergency requiring acute multidisciplinary treatment. Resuscitation should consist of massive transfusions of blood, correction of coagulopathy with fresh frozen plasma and platelets, and immediate laparotomy. Options at laparotomy include packing and drainage (preferred), surgical ligation of the hemorrhaging hepatic segments, embolization of the hepatic artery to the involved liver segment, and loosely suturing omentum or surgical mesh to the liver to improve integrity. Even with appropriate treatment, maternal and fetal mortality is over 50%. Maternal mortality is most commonly associated with exsanguination and coagulopathy. Initial survivors are at increased risk for developing adult respiratory distress syndrome, pulmonary edema,[42] and acute renal failure in the postoperative period.[43, 44]

Smith and associates[45] reviewed their management of seven patients with spontaneous rupture of the liver occurring during pregnancy. Of the four survivors, the mean gestational age was 32.8 weeks and the mean duration of hospitalization was 16 days. All the survivors were managed with packing and drainage of the liver, whereas the three patients treated with hepatic lobectomy died. The authors also extracted 28 cases from the literature reported since 1976. From a total of 35 cases analyzed, there was an 82% overall survival for the 27 cases managed by packing and drainage, whereas only 25% of eight patients undergoing hepatic lobectomy survived. The authors emphasized that hepatic hemorrhage with persistent hypotension unresponsive to transfusion of blood products may be managed surgically with laparotomy, evacuation of the hematoma, packing of the damaged liver, and draining of the operative site. If the patient is stable enough to undergo angiography, transcatheter embolotherapy is a reasonable alternative to surgery.[46]

At the University of Tennessee, Memphis, we have managed four patients with HELLP syndrome complicated by ruptured subcapsular hematoma in the last 18 years. Three patients required transfusion of 22 to 40 units of packed red blood cells and multiple units of platelets and fresh-frozen plasma. Two of these three patients had complications of pulmonary edema and acute renal failure, but all survived without any residual deficiency. The fourth patient presented in profound shock and with DIC. The patient subsequently died secondary to a ruptured pulmonary emphysematous bleb during management of adult respiratory distress syndrome (ARDS).[47]

On the basis of our experience and review of the literature, we have developed an algorithm for the management of hepatic complications of HELLP syndrome (Table 3–7).

TABLE 3–7. MANAGEMENT OF PATIENTS WITH DOCUMENTED SUBCAPSULAR HEMATOMA OF THE LIVER

GENERAL CONSIDERATIONS

1. Have the blood bank aware of the potential need for large amounts of packed red blood cells, fresh-frozen plasma, and platelet concentrate (i.e., 30 units of blood, 20 units of fresh-frozen plasma, 30–50 units of platelets)
2. Consult a general or vascular surgeon
3. Avoid direct and indirect manipulation of the liver
4. Closely monitor hemodynamic status
5. Give intravenous magnesium sulfate to prevent seizures

IF THE HEMATOMA IS UNRUPTURED

1. Manage conservatively with serial computed tomography scans or ultrasonography

IF THE HEMATOMA IS RUPTURED

1. Give massive transfusions
2. Perform immediate laparotomy
   a. If bleeding is minimal:
      1. Observe
      2. Drain area with closed suction
   b. If bleeding is severe:
      1. Apply laparotomy sponges as packs to provide pressure to the liver
      2. Perform surgical ligation of the hemorrhaging hepatic segment
      3. Embolize the hepatic artery to the involved liver segment
      4. Loose suture the omentum or apply surgical mesh to the liver to improve integrity

This algorithm emphasizes the potential for transfusion of large amounts of blood and blood products and the need for aggressive intervention if rupture of the hematoma is suspected. We recommend 30 units of packed red blood cells, 20 units of fresh frozen plasma, 30 to 50 units of platelets, and 20 to 30 units of cryoprecipitate be available if rupture of a subcapsular hematoma is suspected.

Our experience is in agreement with the recent observations of Smith and associates[45] in that a stable patient with an unruptured subcapsular hematoma should be conservatively managed. Constant monitoring must continue during this management, however, because patients can rapidly become unstable after rupture of the hematoma. Survival clearly is associated with rapid diagnosis and immediate medical or surgical stabilization. Coagulopathy must be aggressively managed, or the patient is at risk for renal failure. In addition, these patients should be managed in an intensive care unit facility with close monitoring of hemodynamic parameters and fluid status to avoid the potential for pulmonary edema or respiratory compromise.

Postpartum follow-up for patients with subcapsular hematoma of the liver should include serial CT, MRI, or ultrasonography until the defect resolves. For patients receiving numerous transfusions, the hepatitis and human immunodeficiency virus (HIV) status and isoantibody development should be assessed. Although the data on subsequent pregnancy outcome after a subcapsular hematoma of the liver in pregnancy are limited, we have managed two such patients who have had subsequent normal maternal and fetal outcomes.

Postpartum Management

HELLP syndrome may develop ante partum or post partum. An analysis of 442 cases studied by Sibai and associates[47] revealed that 309 (70%) had evidence of the syndrome ante partum and 133 (30%) post partum. There were four maternal deaths, and morbidity was frequent (Table 3–8). In the postpartum period, the time of onset of the manifestations ranged from a few hours to 7 days, with the majority developing within 48 hours post partum. Patients in this group

TABLE 3–8. SERIOUS MATERNAL COMPLICATIONS IN 442 PATIENTS WITH HELLP SYNDROME

COMPLICATION	NO. OF PATIENTS	%
Disseminated intravascular coagulopathy	92	21
Abruptio placentae	69	16
Acute renal failure	33	8
Severe ascites	32	8
Pulmonary edema	26	6
Pleural effusions	26	6
Cerebral edema	4	1
Retinal detachment	4	1
Laryngeal edema	4	1
Subcapsular liver hematoma	4	1
Adult respiratory distress syndrome	3	1
Death, maternal	4	1

From Sibai BM, Ramadan MK, Usta I, et al. Maternal morbidity and mortality in 442 pregnancies with hemolysis, elevated liver enzymes, and low platelets (HELLP syndrome). Am J Obstet Gynecol 1993;169:1000.

are at increased risk for development of pulmonary edema with acute renal failure.[42, 43]

Management is similar to that for the antepartum patient with HELLP syndrome, including the need for antiseizure prophylaxis. Hypertension control may be more aggressive, however, because there is no longer concern about compromising the uteroplacental circulation in the postpartum patient. The differential diagnosis in these cases should include TTP, HUS, and exacerbation of systemic lupus erythematosus.

After delivery, the patient should be monitored closely in an intensive care facility for at least 48 hours. Most patients show evidence of resolution of the disease process within 48 hours after delivery. Some patients, especially those with DIC, may demonstrate delayed resolution or even deterioration. Such patients may require intensive monitoring for several days. The patients are at risk for pulmonary edema from transfusions of blood and blood products, fluid mobilization, and compromised renal function.[42]

In a retrospective study, Martin and colleagues[48] reported the puerperal courses of 43 women with postpartum HELLP syndrome who were given dexamethasone and compared them with 237 similar patients not given corticosteroids. IV dexamethasone 10 mg at 12-hour intervals was given until disease remission was noted in treated patients, at which time up to two additional 5-

mg IV doses were given at 12-hour intervals. Patients who received dexamethasone for postpartum-onset HELLP syndrome experienced a shorter disease course, faster recovery, less morbidity, and less need for other interventionist therapy compared with patients with HELLP syndrome who did not receive dexamethasone.[24]

The authors concluded that the higher incidences of maternal complications in women with HELLP syndrome indicate strongly that (1) strict criteria for the definition of HELLP syndrome be used and (2) women with partial HELLP syndrome should be studied and managed separately from women with complete HELLP syndrome.

PERINATAL OUTCOMES

Patients with delayed resolution of HELLP syndrome (including persistent severe thrombocytopenia) represent a management dilemma. Exchange plasmapheresis with fresh-frozen plasma has been advocated as a treatment by some authors.[11, 49] Because in most instances disease will resolve spontaneously, early initiation of plasmapheresis may result in unnecessary treatment.

Schwartz[49] suggested that serial studies indicating a progressive elevation of bilirubin or creatinine associated with hemolysis and thrombocytopenia be considered an indication for plasmapheresis.

Martin and coworkers[11] reported on the use of plasma exchange with fresh-frozen plasma in seven women in the postpartum period with HELLP syndrome that persisted longer than 72 hours following delivery. All patients had persistent thrombocytopenia, rising LDH, and evidence of multiorgan dysfunction. Sustained increases in mean platelet count and reduction in LDH concentrations were associated with plasma exchange. The authors recommended that a trial of plasma exchange with fresh frozen plasma be considered in HELLP syndrome that persists past 72 hours from delivery and in which there is evidence of a life-threatening microangiopathy.

More recently, however, Martin and coworkers have reviewed 18 patients with HELLP syndrome at their institution who were treated post partum with single or multiple plasma exchange with fresh-frozen plasma.[50] Each patient was entered into the clinical trial either because of persistent evidence of atypical preeclampsia-eclampsia as HELLP syndrome longer than 72 hours after delivery (group 1) or with evidence of worsening HELLP syndrome at any time post partum in association with single-organ or multiple-organ injury (group 2). In the absence of other disease conditions, the nine patients in group 1 with persistent postpartum HELLP syndrome complicated only by severe clinical expressions of preeclampsia-eclampsia responded rapidly to one or two plasma exchange procedures with few complications and no maternal deaths. In contrast, in the nine patients of group 2 with HELLP syndrome presentations complicated by other organ disease, the response to plasma exchange was variable and there were two deaths in this group. This current series of patients details the successful postpartum application of plasma exchange therapy for unremitting HELLP syndrome but reveals that a uniformly positive response to this therapy will not always be observed where there is additional single- or multiple-organ injury.[50] Potential adverse effects of this plasma exchange include plasma-transmitted infections, anaphylaxis, volume overload, sepsis, and maternal death.

MATERNAL AND PERINATAL OUTCOMES

Pregnancies complicated by preeclampsia and the HELLP syndrome are associated with poor maternal and perinatal outcomes.[6, 31, 32, 47, 51, 52] The reported perinatal mortality has ranged from 7.7% to 60% and maternal mortality from 0% to 24%. Maternal morbidity is common. Most of these patients have required transfusions of blood and blood products and are at increased risk for development of acute renal failure, pulmonary edema, ascites, pleural effusions, and hepatic rupture.[43, 44, 47, 53, 54] Moreover, these pregnancies are associated with high incidences of abruptio placentae and DIC.

Abramovici and associates[52] compared the neonatal outcome after preterm delivery of infants whose gestation was complicated by HELLP syndrome, partial HELLP syndrome, or severe preeclampsia. There were no significant differences in complications among the 269 neonates studied in the three groups at each gestational age. These findings are summarized in Table 3–9. There was, as expected, a significant decrease in morbidity

TABLE 3–9. OUTCOMES FOR 269 PREGNANT WOMEN WITH HELLP SYNDROME, PARTIAL HELLP SYNDROME, AND SEVERE PREECLAMPSIA WITH NORMAL LABORATORY VALUES

	HELLP SYNDROME (n = 68)	PARTIAL HELLP SYNDROME (n = 65)	SEVERE PREECLAMPSIA (n = 138)
Latency (days, median)	0*†	1*	2
Gestational age at delivery (wk)‡	30.7 ± 3.2*	31.2 ± 3.3§	32.7 ± 2.8
Cesarean delivery			
Overall (%)	79†§	54	53
For fetal distress (%)	13	18	21
5-min Apgar score ≤ 6 (%)	29*	23*	13
Birth weight (g)‡	1340 ± 562*	1552 ± 731§	1795 ± 706
Intrauterine growth restriction (%)	28	31	22

*P < .005, compared with severe preeclampsia.
†P < .05, compared with partial HELLP syndrome.
‡Values are expressed as mean ± standard deviation.
§P < .05, compared with severe preeclampsia.
From Abramovici D, Friedman SA, Mercer BM, et al. Neonatal outcome in severe preeclampsia at 24 to 36 weeks' gestation: Does the HELLP (hemolysis, elevated liver enzymes, and low platelet count) syndrome matter? Am J Obstet Gynecol 1999;180:221–225.

and mortality rates with advanced gestational age. The authors concluded that in severe preeclampsia, neonatal morbidity and death are related to gestational age rather than to the presence or absence of HELLP syndrome.[50]

Inasmuch as it has been unclear whether women considered to have "partial" or "incomplete" or "impending" HELLP syndrome should be managed similarly to other women with severe preeclampsia, Audibert and coworkers[51] compared the incidence of maternal complications among women with HELLP syndrome, women with isolated laboratory abnormalities including one or two but not all three features of HELLP syndrome (partial HELLP syndrome), and women with severe preeclampsia and normal laboratory tests. Of the 316 women studied, 67 had HELLP syndrome, 71 had partial HELLP syndrome, and 178 had severe preeclampsia. Mean gestational ages at delivery in the HELLP, partial HELLP, and severe preeclampsia groups were, respectively, 31.7, 32.7, and 34.5 weeks (P < .001 between HELLP and severe preeclampsia). There was one maternal death from intracerebral hemorrhage in the HELLP group. In women with HELLP syndrome, there was a higher incidence of cesarean section (P < .001) than in the other two groups. Maternal complications noted in this study are summarized in Table 3–10.

Isler and colleagues[55] in a retrospective study reported information regarding 54 maternal deaths in patients with HELLP syndrome. According to Mississippi HELLP

syndrome[9] classification, 60.0% had class 1 disease, 35.6% had class 2 disease, and 4.4% had class 3 disease. Events associated with maternal deaths included cerebral hemorrhage (45%), cardiopulmonary arrest (40%), DIC (39%), ARDS (28%), renal failure (28%), sepsis (23%), hepatic hemorrhage (20%), and hypoxic-ischemic encephalopathy (16%). Delay in diagnosis of HELLP syndrome was implicated in 22 of 43 patient deaths (51.1%).

MATERNAL COUNSELING

In a retrospective review of patients with HELLP syndrome by Sullivan and associates,[10] a total of 195 subsequent gestations occurred in 122 of 481 patients identified. The authors concluded that in their patient population the overall recurrence risk for HELLP syndrome was 19% to 27%, with a total frequency of preeclampsia of 43%. The data also suggested that the severity in abnormality of laboratory parameters may positively correlate with the risk of recurrence of HELLP syndrome.

Sibai and coworkers,[56] however, reported a lower recurrence risk for HELLP syndrome. In their review of 341 cases of HELLP syndrome, 152 women subsequently became pregnant; 139 normotensive women had 192 subsequent pregnancies. Complications included preeclampsia (19%), preterm delivery (21%), intrauterine growth retardation (restriction) (12%), abruptio placentae (2%), perinatal death (4%), and HELLP syn-

TABLE 3–10. MATERNAL COMPLICATIONS IN 316 PREGNANCIES WITH HELLP SYNDROME, PARTIAL HELLP SYNDROME, OR SEVERE PREECLAMPSIA WITH NORMAL LABORATORY VALUES

	HELLP (n = 67)	PARTIAL HELLP (n = 71)	NORMAL LABORATORY VALUES (n = 178)
Blood products transfusion (%)	25*	4	3
Disseminated intravascular coagulation (%)	15*	0	0
Wound hematoma or infection (%)†	14‡	11§	2§
Pleural effusion (%)	6‡	0	1
Acute renal failure (%)	3‡	0	0
Eclampsia (%)	9	7	9
Abruptio placentae (%)	9	7	9
Pulmonary edema (%)	8	4	3
Subcapsular liver hematoma (%)	1.5	0	0
Intracerebral hemorrhage (%)	1.5	0	0
Death (%)	1.5	0	0

*$P < .001$, HELLP versus partial HELLP and normal laboratory values.
†Percentages of women who underwent cesarean delivery.
‡$P < .05$, HELLP versus normal laboratory values.
§$P < .05$, partial HELLP versus normal laboratory values.
From Audibert F, Friedman SA, Frangieh AY, Sibai BM. Clinical utility of strict diagnostic criteria for the HELLP (hemolysis, elevated liver enzymes, and low platelets) syndrome. Am J Obstet Gynecol 1996;175:460–464.

drome (3%). Thirteen women with preexisting chronic hypertension had 20 subsequent pregnancies, with a higher rate of preeclampsia (75%), preterm delivery (80%), intrauterine growth retardation (45%), abruptio placentae (20%), and perinatal death (40%) but a low rate of recurrent HELLP syndrome (5%).[55] Two patients with ruptured subcapsular liver hematomas had subsequent pregnancies without complications.

Liver function following pregnancy complicated by HELLP syndrome was reported by Knapen and associates.[57] In their study, serum levels of aminotransferases, LDH, γ-glutamyltransferase, alkaline phosphatase, albumin, and conjugated bilirubin were not elevated when measured in 54 women at a median of 31 months (range 3–101 months) after pregnancies complicated by HELLP syndrome. Total bilirubin levels, however, were elevated in 20% of these women, representing a significant difference from the prevalence in a control group of 151 women with a previous normal pregnancy ($\chi^2 = 12.23$, $P < .001$), or in the normal female population ($\chi^2 = 22.34$, $P < .00001$). The authors suggested that a dysfunction of the bilirubin-conjugating mechanism might represent a risk factor for development of HELLP syndrome.

CONCLUSION

Pregnancies complicated by HELLP syndrome require a well-formulated management plan. The development of this syndrome after 34 weeks' gestation or with documentation of fetal lung maturity is an indication for delivery. Vaginal delivery can be accomplished in most cases; however, if cesarean section is required, the use of general anesthesia, subfascial drains, and preoperative platelet transfusion for platelet counts less than 40,000/mm³ can help reduce the incidence of complications.

AFLP, TTP, or HUS may present with signs, symptoms, and laboratory abnormalities that may be confused with HELLP syndrome. Thorough investigation is warranted because of the variances in management of these complications of pregnancy. It is advisable that patients with complications of HELLP syndrome, such as pulmonary edema, acute renal failure, liver rupture, and extreme prematurity, be referred to a tertiary care center where maternal and neonatal facilities are available.

References

1. Chesley LC. Disseminated intravascular coagulation. *In* Chesley LC (ed). Hypertensive Disorders in Pregnancy. New York: Appleton-Century-Crofts, 1978, p 88.
2. Goodlin RC. Hemolysis, elevated liver enzymes, and low platelets syndrome. Obstet Gynecol 1984;64:449.
3. Killam AP, Dillard SH, Patton RC, Pederson PR. Pregnancy-induced hypertension complicated by

acute liver disease and disseminated intravascular coagulation. Am J Obstet Gynecol 1975;23:823–825.

4. McKay DG. Hematologic evidence of disseminated intravascular coagulation in eclampsia. Obstet Gynecol Surv 1972;27:399–417.

5. Weinstein L. Syndrome of hemolysis, elevated liver enzymes, and low platelet count: A severe consequence of hypertension in pregnancy. Am J Obstet Gynecol 1982;142:159–167.

6. Sibai BM, Taslimi MM, El-Nazer A, et al. Maternal-perinatal outcome associated with the syndrome of hemolysis, elevated liver enzymes, and low platelets in severe preeclampsia-eclampsia. Am J Obstet Gynecol 1986;155:501–509.

7. MacKenna J, Dover NL, Brame RG. Preeclampsia associated with hemolysis, elevated liver enzymes, and low platelets: An obstetric emergency? Obstet Gynecol 1983;62:751–754.

8. Weinstein L. Preeclampsia/eclampsia with hemolysis, elevated liver enzymes, and thrombocytopenia. Obstet Gynecol 1985;66:657–660.

9. Martin JN Jr, Blake PG, Lowry SL, et al. Pregnancy complicated by preeclampsia-eclampsia with the syndrome of hemolysis, elevated liver enzymes, and low platelet count: How rapid is postpartum recovery? Obstet Gynecol 1990;76:737–741.

10. Sullivan CA, Magann EF, Perry KG Jr, et al. The recurrence risk of the syndrome of hemolysis, elevated liver enzymes, and low platelets (HELLP) in subsequent gestations. Am J Obstet Gynecol 1994;171:940–943.

11. Martin JN Jr, Files JC, Blake PG, et al. Plasma exchange for preeclampsia: I. Postpartum use for persistently severe preeclampsia-eclampsia with HELLP syndrome. Am J Obstet Gynecol 1990;162:126–137.

12. Miles JF Jr, Martin JN Jr, Blake PG, et al. Postpartum eclampsia: A recurring perinatal dilemma. Obstet Gynecol 1990;76:328–331.

13. Thiagarajah S, Bourgeois FJ, Harbert GM, Caudle MR. Thrombocytopenia in preeclampsia: Associated abnormalities and management principles. Am J Obstet Gynecol 1984;150:1–7.

14. Sibai BM. The HELLP syndrome (hemolysis, elevated liver enzymes, and low platelets): Much ado about nothing? Am J Obstet Gynecol 1990;162:311–316.

15. Aarnoudse JG, Houthoff HF, Weits J, et al. A syndrome of liver damage and intravascular coagulation in the last trimester of normotensive pregnancy. A clinical and histopathological study. Br J Obstet Gynaecol 1986;93:145–155.

16. Mabie MC, Sibai BM. Transient diabetes insipidus in a patient with preeclampsia and HELLP syndrome. In Cefalo RC (ed). Clinical Decisions in Obstetrics and Gynecology. Rockville, MD: Aspen, 1990, pp 136–138.

17. Usta IM, Barton JR, Amon EA, et al. Acute fatty liver of pregnancy: An experience in the diagnosis and management of fourteen cases. Am J Obstet Gynecol 1994;171:1342–1347.

18. Treem WR, Shoup ME, Hale DE, et al. Acute fatty liver of pregnancy, hemolysis, elevated liver enzymes, and low platelets syndrome and long-chain 3-hydroxyacylcoenzyme A dehydrogenase deficiency. Am J Gastroenterol 1996;91:2293–2300.

19. Tyni T, Ekholm E, Pihko H. Pregnancy complications are frequent in long-chain 3-hydroxyacyl-coenzyme A dehydrogenase deficiency. Am J Obstet Gynecol 1998;178:603–608.

20. Ibdah JA, Bennett MJ, Rinaldo P, et al. A fetal fatty-acid oxidation disorder as a cause of liver disease in pregnant women. N Engl J Med 1999;340:1723–1731.

21. Ruggenenti P, Remuzzi G. The pathophysiology and management of thrombotic thrombocytopenic purpura. Eur J Haematol 1996;56:191–207.

22. Davies GE. Thrombotic thrombocytopenic purpura in pregnancy with maternal survival. Case report. Br J Obstet Gynecol 1984;91:396–398.

23. Martinez-Roman S, Gratacos E, Torne A, et al. Successful pregnancy in a patient with hemolytic-uremic syndrome during the second trimester of pregnancy. A case report. J Reprod Med 1996;41:211–214.

24. Brian MC, Pacie JV, Hourihane DOB. Microangiopathic hemolytic anemia: The possible role of vascular lesions in pathogenesis. Br J Haematol 1962;8:358.

25. Barton JR, Riely CA, Adamel TA, et al. Hepatic histopathologic condition does not correlate with laboratory abnormalities in HELLP syndrome (hemolysis, elevated liver enzymes, and low platelet count). Am J Obstet Gynecol 1992;167:1538–1543.

26. Hannah ME, Gonen R, Mocarski EJ, et al. Elevated liver enzymes and thrombocytopenia in the third trimester of pregnancy: An unusual case report and a review of the literature. Am J Obstet Gynecol 1989;161:322–323.

27. Arias F, Mancilla-Jimenez R. Hepatic fibrinogen deposits in preeclampsia-immunofluorescent evidence. N Engl J Med 1976;295:575–582.

28. Long RG, Scheuer PJ, Sherlock S. Preeclampsia presenting with deep jaundice. J Clin Pathol 1977;30:212–215.

29. Goodlin RC, Holdt D. Impending gestosis. Obstet Gynecol 1981;58:743–745.

30. Heyborne KD, Burke MS, Porreco RP. Prolongation of premature gestation in women with hemolysis, elevated liver enzyme, and low platelets: A report of 5 cases. J Reprod Med 1990;35:53–57.

31. Magann EF, Bass D, Chauhan SP, et al. Antepartum corticosteroids: Disease stabilization in patients with the syndrome of hemolysis, elevated liver enzymes, and low platelets (HELLP). Am J Obstet Gynecol 1994;171:1148–1153.

32. Magann EF, Perry KO Jr, Meydrech EF, et al. Postpartum corticosteroids: Accelerated recovery from the syndrome of hemolysis, elevated liver enzymes, and low platelets (HELLP). Am J Obstet Gynecol 1994;171:1154–1158.

33. Tompkins MJ, Thiagarajah S. HELLP (hemolysis, elevated liver enzymes, and low platelet count) syndrome: The benefit of corticosteroids. Am J Obstet Gynecol 1999;181:304–309.

34. O'Brien JM, Milligan DA, Barton JR. Impact of high-dose corticosteroid therapy for patients with HELLP (hemolysis, elevated liver enzymes, and low platelet count) syndrome. Am J Obstet Gynecol 2000;182 (Oct 2000).

35. van Pampus MG, Wolf H, Ilsen A, et al. Maternal outcome following temporizing management of the (H)ELLP syndrome. Hypertens Pregn 2000;19:211–220.

36. Visser W, Wallenburg HCS. Temporising management of severe pre-eclampsia with and without the HELLP syndrome. Br J Obstet Gynaecol 1995;102:111–117.

37. Briggs R, Chari RS, Mercer B, Sibai BM. Postoperative incision complications after cesarean section in patients with antepartum syndrome of hemolysis, elevated liver enzymes, and low platelets (HELLP): Does delayed primary closure make a difference? Am J Obstet Gynecol 1996;175:893–896.

38. Barton JR, Sibai BM. Hepatic imaging in HELLP syndrome (hemolysis, elevated liver enzymes, and low platelet count). Am J Obstet Gynecol 1996; 174:1820–1827.

39. Goodlin RC, Anderson JC, Hodgson PE. Conservative treatment of liver hematoma in the postpartum period. J Reprod Med 1985;30:368.

40. Manas KJ, Welsh JD, Rankin RA, Miller DD. Hepatic hemorrhage without rupture in preeclampsia. N Engl J Med 1985;312:424–426.

41. Neerhof MG, Zelman W, Sullivan T. Hepatic rupture in pregnancy: A review. Obstet Gynecol Surv 1989;44:407–409.

42. Sibai BM, Mabie BC, Harvey CJ. Pulmonary edema in severe preeclampsia-eclampsia: Analysis of 37 consecutive cases. Am J Obstet Gynecol 1987; 156:1174–1179.

43. Sibai BM, Ramadan MK. Acute renal failure in pregnancies complicated by hemolysis, elevated liver enzymes, and low platelets. Am J Obstet Gynecol 1993;168:1682.

44. Abroug F, Boujdaria R, Nouira S, et al. HELLP syndrome: Incidence and maternal-fetal outcome: A prospective study. Intensive Care Med 1992; 18:274.

45. Smith JG Jr, Moise KJ Jr, Dildy GA, et al. Spontaneous rupture of the liver during pregnancy: Current therapy. Obstet Gynecol 1991;77:171.

46. Lovinger EH, Lee WM, Anderson MC. Hepatic rupture associated with pregnancy: Treatment with transcatheter embolotherapy. Obstet Gynecol 1985;65:281.

47. Sibai BM, Ramadan MK, Usta I, et al. Maternal morbidity and mortality in 442 pregnancies with hemolysis, elevated liver enzymes, and low platelets (HELLP syndrome). Am J Obstet Gynecol 1993;169:1000.

48. Martin JN Jr, Perry KG Jr, Blake PG, et al. Better maternal outcomes are achieved with dexamethasone therapy for postpartum HELLP (hemolysis, elevated liver enzymes, and thrombocytopenia) syndrome. Am J Obstet Gynecol 1997;177:1011–1017.

49. Schwartz ML. Possible role for exchange plasmapheresis with fresh frozen plasma for maternal indications in selected cases of preeclampsia and eclampsia. Obstet Gynecol 1986;68:136–139.

50. Martin JN Jr, Files JC, Blake PG. Postpartum plasma exchange for atypical preeclampsia-eclampsia as HELLP (hemolysis, elevated liver enzymes, and low platelets) syndrome. Am J Obstet Gynecol 1995;172:1107–1127.

51. Audibert F, Friedman SA, Frangieh AY, Sibai BM. Clinical utility of strict diagnostic criteria for the HELLP (hemolysis, elevated liver enzymes, and low platelets) syndrome. Am J Obstet Gynecol 1996;175:460–464.

52. Abramovici D, Friedman SA, Mercer BM, et al. Neonatal outcome in severe preeclampsia at 24 to 36 weeks' gestation: Does the HELLP (hemolysis, elevated liver enzymes, and low platelet count) syndrome matter? Am J Obstet Gynecol 1999; 180:221–225.

53. Van Dam PA, Reiner M, Baeklandt M, et al. Disseminated intravascular coagulation and the syndrome of hemolysis, elevated liver enzymes, and low platelets in severe preeclampsia. Obstet Gynecol 1989;73:97.

54. Woods JB, Blake PG, Perry KG Jr, et al. Ascites: A portent of cardiopulmonary complications in the preeclamptic patient with the syndrome of hemolysis, elevated liver enzymes, and low platelets. Obstet Gynecol 1992;80:87.

55. Isler CM, Rinehart BK, Terrone DA, et al. Maternal mortality associated with HELLP (hemolysis, elevated liver enzymes, and low platelets) syndrome. Am J Obstet Gynecol 1999;181:924–928.

56. Sibai BM, Ramadan MK, Chari RS, et al. Pregnancies complicated by HELLP syndrome (hemolysis, elevated liver enzymes, and low platelets): Subsequent pregnancy outcome and long-term prognosis. Am J Obstet Gynecol 1995;172:125–129.

57. Knapen M, van Altena A, Peters W, et al. Liver function following pregnancy complicated by the HELLP syndrome. Br J Obstet Gynaecol 1998; 105:1208–1210.

4

SEVERE PREECLAMPSIA and ECLAMPSIA

Hein J. Odendaal

Preeclampsia is a common complication of pregnancy in both developed and developing countries. Although mild preeclampsia usually carries a good prognosis for both the mother and infant, severe preeclampsia and eclampsia may have grave consequences for the mother and fetus or newborn. These conditions represent a real problem in developing countries where sufficient numbers of trained personnel and adequate facilities are simply not available. These limited resources over many years have forced physicians to avoid unnecessary special investigations and use intensive care facilities as effectively as possible without unnecessarily endangering the lives of the mother or the baby. It is hoped that this chapter will be useful not only to obstetricians in developing countries but also in developed countries where active attempts are being made to curb the spiraling costs of medical care.

MANAGEMENT OF EARLY SEVERE PREECLAMPSIA

Preeclampsia is generally defined as *severe* under the following conditions[1, 2]:

- Systolic blood pressure at least 160 mmHg or diastolic pressure 110 mmHg
- Proteinuria of least 5 g/24 h
- Platelet count below 100,000/μL
- Elevated serum levels of transaminases
- Oliguria
- Pulmonary edema
- Epigastric pain
- Cerebral or visual disturbances

Management of the mother with early severe preeclampsia depends much on the availability of neonatal intensive care facilities and gestational age. If facilities are lacking, there is little chance for premature newborns to survive. It is therefore recom-

mended to give priority to the mother and to expedite delivery after her condition has been stabilized.

For the very preterm fetus, neonatal survival is dependent on gestational age at delivery (Fig. 4–1).[3, 4] Every week gained in gestational age from 26 to 33 weeks has a marked effect on the perinatal mortality (PNM) rate. If it is safe for the mother and if facilities are available, the physician might therefore try to prolong the pregnancy for 1 or 2 crucial weeks. Personnel in each unit treating patients with early severe preeclampsia should continuously assess its neonatal mortality rate to predict at which gestational age neonatal outcome is good. This should help in deciding whether *expectant* or *active* management should be followed.

"Expectant" or "Aggressive" Management

The first study of expectant management of severe preeclampsia from Tygerberg Hospi-

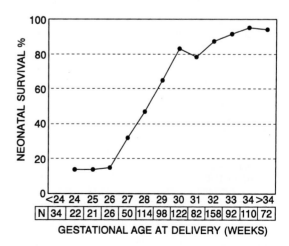

FIGURE 4–1. Neonatal survival rate depends much on gestational age at birth. A rapid improvement is noted from 26 to 30 weeks' gestation.

tal before 34 weeks' gestation was published in 1987.[5] Although delayed delivery demonstrated an improvement in PNM, when compared with other hospitals, the 36% intrauterine deaths due to abruptio placentae (placental abruption) was alarming and was the motivation for the first randomized controlled trial on expectant or aggressive management of patients with early severe preeclampsia.[6] In this small study, 20 patients were electively delivered 48 hours after admission and 18 when either maternal or fetal indications necessitated delivery (Table 4–1). The two groups of patients were comparable regarding severity of preeclampsia and results of special investigations. Pregnancy was prolonged with a mean of 7.1 days (range, 2–18 days). Gestational age at delivery was significantly higher, fewer babies received mechanical ventilation, and total neonatal mortality and morbidity rates were lower in the expectantly managed group. Abruptio placentae was found in three patients managed aggressively and in four managed expectantly.

In a subsequent, larger randomized controlled trial,[7] pregnancy was prolonged by a mean of 15.4 days (range, 4–36 days). No perinatal deaths were encountered in either group (see Table 4–1). Expectant management resulted in a significantly higher gestational age at delivery, higher birth weight, lower incidence of admission to the neonatal intensive care unit (NICU), lower mean days in the NICU, and lower incidence of neonatal complications. There were no cases of eclampsia, pulmonary edema, renal failure, or disseminated intravascular coagulation (DIC) in either group. Two cases of abruptio placentae occurred in each group.

Sibai and associates[8] also compared aggressive and expectant management between 24 and 28 weeks' gestation. Gestational age at entry to the two groups was similar, but the admission-to-delivery interval was 11 days longer in the expectantly managed group. This led to a reduction in the PNM rate from 76.4% to 35.5%. Maternal complications encountered were HELLP syndrome (*h*emolysis, *e*levated *l*iver enzymes, *l*ow *p*latelets, 20%), abruptio placentae (13.3%), and eclampsia (6.7%).

In another study of conservative management of severe early preeclampsia, Oláh and coworkers[9] compared women between 24 and 32 weeks' gestation at two centers. At

---

TABLE 4–1. EXPECTANT OR ACTIVE MANAGEMENT OF PATIENTS WITH EARLY SEVERE PREECLAMPSIA

AUTHOR	NO. OF PATIENTS	A-D INTERVAL	GESTATIONAL AGE AT DELIVERY	BIRTH WEIGHT	RDS OR NEONATAL VENTILATION	PERINATAL DEATHS
Odendaal et al (1990)[6]						
Aggressive management	20	1.3 days*	211 days*	1272 g	7*	5
Expectant management	18	7.1 days	223 days	1420 g	2	3
Oláh et al (1993)[9]						
Early intervention	28	1.4 days*	201 days*	1195 g*	9†	5
Conservative management	28	9.5 days	214 days	1480 g	3	2
Sibai et al (1994)[7]						
Aggressive management	46	—	30.8 wk‡	1233 g§	23¶	0
Expectant management	49	15.4 days	32.9 wk	1622 g	11	0
Visser et al (1994)[10]						
Hemodynamic temporizing	57	10 days	32.0 wk	1330 g	27‖	4
Conservative management	57	11 days	32.7 wk	1215 g	8	8

A-D, admission-delivery interval; RDS, respiratory distress syndrome.
*$P < .05$
†$P < .001$
‡$P < .0001$
§$P = .0004$
¶$P = .002$
‖$P < .01$.

Oxford, the women were managed conservatively; at Birmingham, the women were stabilized and early intervention was used. Only patients with a systolic blood pressure of above 170 mmHg or blood pressure above diastolic 110 mmHg with at least 1+ proteinuria and hyperuricemia were included in the study. There were 28 patients in each group. Patients managed conservatively gained a mean of 9.5 days (range, 2–26 days) (see Table 4–1). Infants of these women had greater birth weights, shorter stays in the NICU, and fewer neonatal complications. All women in the early intervention group recovered with no severe complications. In the group managed conservatively, however, there were two cases of HELLP syndrome and two of ELLP (elevated liver enzymes, low platelets) syndrome. In one case, temporary renal dialysis was required.

Visser and colleagues[10] compared two methods of delaying delivery in women with severe preeclampsia at or before 35 weeks' gestation (see Table 4–1). In Rotterdam, plasma value expansion was used with central hemodynamic monitoring control. If the cardiac index was still less than 3.5 after volume expansion, patients received an intravenous (IV) infusion of dihydralazine, starting at a rate of 1 mg/h. Methyldopa was given when the cardiac index and systemic vascular resistance had reached normal values but diastolic blood pressure remained 100 mmHg or higher.

In Amsterdam, the control group patients were prescribed absolute bed rest, no IV fluids, and a diet containing less than 400 mg sodium per 24 hours. Antihypertensive medication was given when diastolic blood pressure was 115 mmHg or higher. Methyldopa was the drug of choice. In both groups, pregnancy was prolonged by 10 to 11 days. A low maternal morbidity rate was seen in both groups, and there were no complications after hemodynamic monitoring. Gestational age at delivery was 32.9 weeks in the study group and 32.7 weeks in the control group. PNM was 7.1% in the study group and 14.3% in the control group, but the difference was not statistically significant. Neonatal ventilation and patent ductus arteriosus occurred significantly more in the study group, although fewer growth-retarded babies were born. It is uncertain whether either hospital used steroids to improve fetal lung maturity.

In a subsequent study, Visser and Wallenburg[11] reviewed their temporizing management in 254 consecutive patients with severe preeclampsia, remote from term, from 1985 to 1993. The median prolongation of pregnancy was 14 days (range, 0–62 days). The mean gestational age at delivery was 31.2 weeks. PNM was 20.5%, and complications of central hemodynamic monitoring were not observed. Hemodynamic monitoring was used to manage patients with HELLP syndrome.[12]

From these studies, it is clear that conservative management of severe early preeclampsia enables delivery to be postponed by 1 or 2 weeks with subsequent reduction in neonatal complications and improvement in the PNM rate. However, expectant therapy should be performed only in tertiary centers where obstetricians have adequate experience in obstetric intensive or high-risk care. One should be aware that deterioration of the maternal or fetal condition can occur rapidly. Careful monitoring of the condition of both mother and fetus is therefore absolutely essential. Maternal complications such as HELLP or ELLP syndromes are a possibility and should always be kept in mind. One must take into account the severity of the preeclampsia, the prevalence of underlying hypertension, patient compliance, and delay in referral to a tertiary center. The last item is of utmost importance because it is more difficult to treat patients with an advanced stage of severe preeclampsia expectantly.[13]

When to Start With Expectant Management

First, expectant management of patients with severe preeclampsia is recommended only in tertiary hospitals. Because maternal and fetal complications can develop very rapidly, good facilities for monitoring the mother and fetus should be available. Where such facilities do not exist and when the fetus is not yet viable, it may be safer for the mother to have the pregnancy terminated soon after the diagnosis of severe preeclampsia is certain. "Fetal viability" is a relative term because it also depends on NICU facilities, adequately trained personnel, and the financial resources to support these tertiary care facilities. At Tygerberg Hospital, a gestational age of 28 weeks or, rarely, 27 weeks is accepted for fetal viability. Although neonatal survival after delivery at 27 weeks' gestation is 32%,[4] the hospital does not have the facilities to care for fetuses at or below this gestational age. However, in developed countries fetal viability may start at 22 weeks or, in many developing countries, at 32 to 34 weeks.

As mentioned earlier, expectant management succeeded in prolonging the pregnancy with a mean of 7.1 to 15.4 days. It may therefore be unrealistic to introduce expectant management much longer than 2 weeks before fetal viability; yet, the upper range of the prolongation of pregnancy may be as high as 62 days.[11] A too early termination of pregnancy therefore sometimes deprives a patient of having a baby.

This very difficult decision—whether and when expectant management should be started—should always be individualized and discussed with the patient, her family, and the neonatologist. Care should be taken to explain all the advantages and disadvantages to the patient and involve her in the decision making.

The upper limit of gestational age at which a patient does not qualify for expectant management also differs. At Tygerberg Hospital, a gestational age of 34 weeks is recommended because the neonatal survival at later deliveries is not better and is worse when delivery is at 33 weeks or earlier.[4] Sibai and coworkers[7] used 32 weeks as the upper limit for entry in their study, but delivery was at 34 weeks. Thirty-two weeks was also accepted as the upper limit for entering to their study by Oláh and coworkers,[9] although Visser and colleagues[10] accepted 35 weeks. After a gestational age of 34 to 35 weeks has been reached, delivery is safer for both mother and fetus.

Specific Management

Hospitalization

Mothers with a diagnosis of preeclampsia should be hospitalized, mainly because her condition or the fetus's condition can change suddenly, necessitating speedy delivery. Exceptions may be made for the patient with mild preeclampsia who has transport readily available, who lives in close proximity to the hospital, who can take her own blood pressure and test her urine on a daily basis, and who can come for regular

non-stress testing.[14] Patients with mild preeclampsia can be admitted to an ordinary antenatal ward, but patients with severe preeclampsia should be admitted to either the labor ward or a special care unit where they can be observed more frequently by skilled nursing staff.

Initial Fetal Assessment

The fetal heart rate should be recorded as soon as possible after admission.[15, 16] Severe placental insufficiency and abruptio placentae are the two most common causes of intrauterine death in patients with severe preeclampsia, but they can be detected by the abnormal fetal heart rate (FHR) pattern they cause. It is also necessary to exclude fetal distress before any antihypertensive therapy is initiated, because drugs such as dihydralazine may cause sudden hypotension and therefore worsen the fetal distress.[17]

Antihypertensive Treatment

Inasmuch as hypertension is one of the most common causes of maternal death in several countries,[18–20] blood pressure of 160/110 mmHg or above should be treated. Parenterally administered drugs are commonly used, although oral nifedipine can also be used. Oral therapy is sufficient for the treatment of readings below 160/110 mmHg.

IV hydralazine is the parenteral drug of choice in many units. The advantages and disadvantages of hydralazine have been mentioned in many review articles,[21–24] and only specific remarks are made here. Because patients with severe preeclampsia are often hypovolemic, IV administration of hydralazine may occasionally cause severe hypotension with subsequent fetal distress.[17] To prevent this, 200 to 300 mL of fluid should be given intravenously before administration of this drug.

Regimens vary according to circumstances (Table 4–2). Midwives at rural clinics are advised to administer 5 mg hydralazine intramuscularly before transport of patients to hospital.[25] Nifedipine may also be used as an alternative to dihydralazine; an advantage is that it may be given orally.[26, 27] Although experience with nifedipine is less extensive than that with dihydralazine, disadvantages seem few. There is a real need to compare the efficiency and safety of these

TABLE 4–2. TREATMENT OF SEVERE ACUTE HYPERTENSION

I. Hydralazine
5–10 mg doses at 15–20 min intervals IV (initial dose 5 mg; maximum dose 25 mg)

II. Labetalol
20 mg IV initially, 40 mg after 10–20 min; 80 mg after another 10–20 min, maximum 300 mg
or
50 mg by slow IV bolus, followed by 60 mg/h infusion, doubling every 15 min until good control or a maximum of 480 mg/h is reached

III. Nifedipine
10–20 mg orally; repeat after 30 min; maximum 120 mg in 24 h

IV, intravenously.

two popular drugs in a large, randomized, controlled trial.

A third drug commonly used for the acute control of blood pressure is labetalol,[28–31] although it is seldom used at Tygerberg Hospital because many of the patients with severe preeclampsia have intrauterine growth retardation (IUGR). Labetalol possesses both α- and β-adrenoceptor blocking properties but appears to be a more potent inhibitor of β-adrenoceptors.[32] β-Blocking agents may inhibit the fetal adaptation to stress and cause neonatal hypoglycemia.[33] In addition, black patients do not respond well with β-adrenergic blocking agents.[34–37]

Magnesium Sulfate

Although magnesium sulfate (MgSO₄) is the drug of choice for prevention of further convulsions in eclampsia,[38–40] its use to prevent preeclampsia is still controversial. In an uncontrolled trial, Reti and associates[41] used MgSO₄ and hydralazine in 46 patients with severe preeclampsia. There were no cases of eclampsia and no maternal deaths. In a large study in 2138 women with hypertension during labor, 10 of the 1089 women, randomized to receive phenytoin, had eclamptic convulsions compared with none of the 1049 women who received MgSO₄.[42]

There are both supporters and critics of prophylactic use of MgSO₄. In a randomized, controlled trial in 64 patients with severe preeclampsia, 34 patients were given MgSO₄ and 30 were not.[43] No patient experienced eclampsia. It was concluded that

MgSO₄ is not necessary for prevention of eclampsia in patients with severe preeclampsia.

Our unit conducted a retrospective study of 1001 patients with severe early preeclampsia.[44] Although it was departmental policy to prescribe MgSO₄ to patients with severe preeclampsia or imminent eclampsia, many clinicians interpreted the symptoms of imminent eclampsia differently, and at the end of the study 510 patients received MgSO₄ and 491 did not. The two groups of patients did not differ significantly regarding the maximum height of blood pressure, amount of proteinuria, gestational age, results of special investigations, and perinatal outcome. Two patients, both receiving MgSO₄, had eclampsia before delivery. Three patients had postnatal convulsions, none of whom had received MgSO₄ prior to the eclampsia. Only one of the postnatal convulsions occurred within 24 hours of delivery.

The 0.5% prevalence of eclampsia in our study,[44] in which approximately half of the patients had not received prophylactic anticonvulsants, was almost the same as the 0.46% documented by Lucas and coworkers,[42] with both groups receiving prophylactic anticonvulsants but with hypertension and proteinuria less severe. The reason for this difference is speculative, but the more advanced gestational age of patients in the Lucas study, control of blood pressure by antihypertensive agents, and population differences may have played a role. Of note, eclampsia developed in only one patient in 254 after plasma volume expansion and antihypertensive therapy.[11] The prevalence of preeclampsia in the two aforementioned large studies was about 1 per 200 deliveries, whereas the national incidence in the United Kingdom was 1 per 2000.[45]

A survey in the United Kingdom[46] showed that 85% of consultants prescribe anticonvulsants to prevent convulsions. In the few small studies in which anticonvulsants were not administered to patients with severe preeclampsia, however, the incidence of eclampsia seems to be low. It is thus for the obstetrician to decide whether it is advisable to give MgSO₄ to about 200 patients to prevent one convulsion. More studies are necessary to conclude that prophylaxis is necessary, or is not cost effective, and that it is not acceptable to expose many patients to the risk of a drug that is potentially dangerous in order to prevent a disease that occurs in about 1 of 200 patients.

For a detailed analysis regarding MgSO$_4$, see Chapter 13.

Corticosteroids

Since the double-blind study of Liggins and Howie,[47] in which the improvement of fetal lung maturity by antenatal administration of corticosteroids was described for the first time, this form of therapy has become mandatory in the management of patients in whom preterm delivery is a risk. Although there was initial concern regarding its safety for the fetus when administered to patients with severe preeclampsia, later studies failed to confirm these observed risks for fetal death. Administration of glucocorticosteroids to patients with pregnancy-induced hypertension also did not have an worsening effect on maternal blood pressure.[48]

Because the stress of maternal hypertension during pregnancy may reduce the incidence of respiratory distress syndrome (RDS), Bowen and colleagues[49] investigated the incidence of RDS in newborns of mothers with hypertension. RDS occurred in 60% of newborns of the 40 hypertensive mothers in contrast to 33% in the 223 control patients. The increased rate of RDS related to the severity of hypertension but not to the duration of the hypertension. Twenty-eight per cent of the babies in the hypertension group were growth retarded in contrast to 4% in the control group, suggesting that the fetuses were indeed subjected to some form of intrauterine stress.

In another study, Schiff and associates[50] compared fetal lung maturity tests in 127 patients with preeclampsia and matched controls and the occurrence of RDS in 69 of these pairs. No significant differences were found. The prevalence of IUGR in the preeclampsia group was 20%, in contrast to 8% in the control group. These studies therefore excluded the beneficial effects of preeclampsia on fetal lung maturity and stressed the necessity of corticosteroid therapy for patients with early severe preeclampsia when imminent delivery is always a strong possibility.

Kirsten[51] monitored 242 neonates born to mothers with early-onset severe preeclampsia. A total of 146 (60%) had some form of RDS. No differences were noted between the clinical characteristics of women with and without infants with RDS. The mean gestational age of 29.6 weeks in those with RDS was significantly shorter than the 31.2 weeks of those in whom RDS did not develop. Antenatal betamethasone was administered to 85% of mothers. When betamethasone was not given, 68% of infants developed RDS in contrast to 43% to whom the drug was given ($P = .01$). Grade 3 or grade 4 RDS developed in 44% of infants when steroids were not given in contrast to 11% when it was given ($P = .006$). Multiple logistic regression to determine the association between RDS and various categories of the umbilical artery flow velocity waveforms, adjusting for many confounding variables, showed that only birth weight above 1250 g, gestational age above 30 weeks, and antenatal steroids reduced the likelihood of RDS. These findings once again support the beneficial effects of antenatal steroid therapy for fetal lung maturity.

Recently, Amorim and associates reported a double-blind randomized trial in 218 women with severe preeclampsia and gestational age between 26 and 34 weeks. The women were randomized to either betamethasone or placebo. The overall incidence of RDS was significantly lower in the steroid group (23% versus 43%; risk ratio [RR] .53; 95th confidence interval [CI] 0.35–0.82). In addition, the rates of intraventricular hemorrhage and perinatal infection were also reduced in the steroid group.[52]

Sedation

There is no role for sedation with diazepam or phenobarbitone in patients with preeclampsia, since there is no evidence that either drug improves maternal outcome. In contrast, the drugs may hamper the interpretation of FHR patterns because they both cause reduced accelerations and baseline variability,[53, 54] making it difficult to distinguish from poor variability due to asphyxia.[55]

Maternal Assessment

On admission, patients with mild preeclampsia should have blood taken for baseline values of packed cell volume, platelet count, serum urea and creatinine levels, urine culture, and a 24-hour urine specimen for proteinuria. In addition, patients with severe preeclampsia or with a low platelet count should undergo liver function tests. An abnormal platelet count is also an indication for coagulation studies. Further special investigations depend on specific clinical findings.

Mothers should be informed about the importance of symptoms such as headache, epigastric pain, and uterine contractions as well as vaginal bleeding and a decreased fetal movement. These abnormalities should immediately be reported to the nursing staff.

Blood Pressure. Blood pressure should be recorded every 15 minutes or continuously during treatment of acute hypertension; thereafter, it should be taken every 4 to 6 hours. Levels above 170/110 mmHg, despite adequate antihypertensive therapy, are an indication for delivery.

Urine Testing for Protein. Chua and Redman[56] studied 42 women with preeclampsia and proteinuria of 5 g or higher in a 24-hour period. In 88% of cases, delivery was necessary within 2 weeks of the onset of severe proteinuria. In some very preterm pregnancies, however, delivery was able to be deferred for 3 weeks or more. The authors concluded that in some cases pregnancy can be prolonged for significant periods of time, thereby improving the chances of better neonatal outcome without apparent risk to the mother.

Schiff and associates[57] conservatively managed 66 women with severe preeclampsia before 32 weeks' gestation. The increase in median protein excretion from admission was 660 mg/24 h. When comparing patients with an increase of more than 2 g with those of less than 2 g, they found no significant differences in maternal or fetal outcome.

Kirsten[51] analyzed the neonatal outcome of 242 babies born to mothers with severe preeclampsia and compared the maternal parameters of the 49 who died neonatally with those of the 193 who survived. The grade of proteinuria, blood pressure, parity, and umbilical artery flow velocity waveforms did not differ between the two groups. However, outcomes were significantly better in newborns with greater gestational age at delivery.

It thus appears that severe proteinuria per se is not an indication for delivery but does signify severe disease with a high PNM rate. Daily testing of urine with dipsticks is probably sufficient, with 24 hours' quantification once weekly. Because proteinuria, as such, does not seem to influence maternal outcome, precise quantification is probably not necessary for clinical practice. However, because dipstick findings may vary much from test to test, more precise measurements are necessary for research purposes.

Uric Acid Measurements. Redman and coworkers[58] studied 332 pregnant women with hypertension. PNM was markedly increased when maternal plasma urate levels were elevated. Maternal hypertension, even severe but without hyperuricemia, was associated with excellent fetal prognosis; mild maternal hypertension with severe hyperuricemia was associated with poor fetal prognosis.

Schuster and Weppelmann[59] found an association between low birth weight and increased maternal plasma urate levels. Sagen and associates[60] also found an association between serum urate levels and growth retardation; in addition, they were also associated with perinatal distress. They concluded that a rapidly rising urate level reliably predicted perinatal distress.

Yoshimura and colleagues[61] also found increased uric acid levels in patients with preeclampsia, but there was a great overlap with normal patients. Sibai and coworkers[62] found increased uric acid levels in 67 patients with eclampsia in comparison with a control group. However, they did not prove that serum uric acid could be used as a predictor for maternal or fetal outcome.

To study the effect of uric acid levels on perinatal outcome in patients with severe preeclampsia, Odendaal and Pienaar[63] compared the PNM rate of 25 patients with a uric acid level of more than 1 standard deviation (SD) above the mean with mean ±1 SD values in 184 patients and lower than 1 SD below the mean values in 20 patients. Mean gestational age at delivery in the high and normal uric acid groups were 30.8 and 31.1 weeks, respectively, and mean birth weights 1400 g and 1357 g, respectively. Of the women with normal uric acid levels, 55% had small-for-gestational-age newborns; in the group with high uric acid levels, the rate was 38%. For babies weighing 1000 g or more, the PNM rate in the high uric acid group was 40/1000; for the low uric acid group, 50/1000; and for the normal group, 11/1000. Inasmuch as there was no clear indication of increased PNM in patients with high uric acid values, the authors did not recommend using high uric acid values per se as an indication for delivery.

Platelet Count. There is a risk of HELLP syndrome in patients with severe preeclampsia, and platelet counts should be performed at least twice weekly or more often when initial or subsequent values are low. Although the incidence of DIC is low, even in patients with eclampsia,[8] coagulation studies are indicated for patients with platelet counts below $100 \times 10^3/mm^3$.

Liver Function Tests. Liver function tests are warranted in all patients with a platelet count below $100 \times 10^3/mm^3$ or when severe disease is indicated. Tests should be repeated at least twice weekly or more often when platelet counts remain low. Abnormal liver functions per se in patients with severe preeclampsia are usually not an indication for immediate delivery because therapy may improve liver function.[11] Decision to deliver is also influenced by other aspects of the maternal or fetal condition and, especially, gestational age.

Fetal Assessment

The prevalence of IUGR in patients with early severe preeclampsia may be as high as 51%,[63] and the frequency of abruptio placentae 12% to 18%[6, 64] or even as high as 22% in patients with preeclampsia in the second trimester.[65] Abruptio placentae is responsible for 36% of intrauterine deaths in patients with severe preeclampsia.[68] For these reasons, accurate fetal monitoring is an essential part of the management of patients with severe preeclampsia.

Fetal Heart Rate Monitoring. In many cases of abruptio placentae, the FHR pattern becomes abnormal before the mother perceives any abdominal pain or vaginal bleeding.[66] Therefore, at Tygerberg Hospital it is recommended that the FHR be monitored every 6 hours. Because the baseline variability of the FHR is a reliable method of fetal assessment,[66, 67] we use it for the management of our patients. A nonreactive FHR pattern with good baseline variability is not associated with fetal asphyxia at birth, provided that the FHR is monitored four times a day (Fig. 4–2).[68] The baseline variability can usually be assessed within 5 to 10 minutes, and therefore monitoring of the FHR every 6 hours does not place a heavy workload on the staff. A variability of less than 5 beats/min is a cause for concern (Fig. 4–3). In these cases, monitoring is continued for 1 hour. Poor variability lasting longer than an hour, in the absence of any sedation, warrants immediate repetition of non-stress testing. Poor variability for longer than 2 hours warrants delivery.

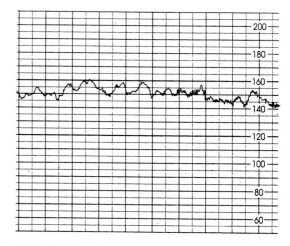

FIGURE 4–2. Good baseline variability of the fetal heart rate is demonstrated. In most cases, it can easily be observed within 10 minutes of monitoring.

Acceleration patterns occur less frequently in growth-retarded babies. Waiting for accelerations to occur in preterm pregnancies with a high prevalence of IUGR prolongs the monitoring time unnecessarily, placing an extra workload on the nursing staff. Since the introduction of frequent monitoring in the conservative management of patients with severe preeclampsia, the PNM rate has decreased to 24/1000 during the last part of the study of 1001 patients with severe preeclampsia.[4] No intrauterine deaths occurred in the last 108 patients.

Steyn and Odendaal[69] used the Sonicaid system 8000 to monitor the FHR in 110 consecutive women hospitalized for severe preeclampsia. Abruptio placentae developed in 20 (18%) patients. On the basis of the mean-minute range of successive recordings, three distinctive FHR patterns preceding the abruptio placentae emerged. Five patients had a constant low mean-minute range and were subsequently delivered. Six patients initially had a good mean-minute range, which decreased to less than 20 milliseconds. In the remaining nine patients, the mean-minute range remained normal within 6 hours before delivery, indicating that the FHR variability was abnormal in more than half of the patients.

In units where the prevalence of abruptio placentae is low, less frequent monitoring is adequate. Chari and coworkers[70] encountered no stillbirths in 68 women where the fetus was assessed daily. Their assessment

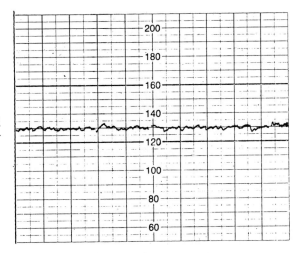

FIGURE 4–3. Poor baseline variability of the fetal heart rate is of concern. Monitoring should be continued for at least 1 hour unless the pattern improves.

included non-stress testing, biophysical profile, and amniotic fluid volume assessment.

Doppler Flow Velocity Waveforms of the Umbilical Artery. Although use of the umbilical artery flow velocity waveform (FVW) technique can reduce PNM in high-risk cases,[71] routine use of this modality in low-risk patients is questionable.[72, 73] It has neither clinical value in the prediction of fetal compromise during labor[74] nor a significant effect on the perinatal outcome in hypertensive patients.[75]

Absent end-diastolic FVW before 34 weeks' gestation is not an indication for delivery when the baseline FHR variability is still normal. Depending on the resistance index, FVWs are instituted every week or two. Reverse flow during diastole is an indication for delivery, but these cases usually also have an abnormal FHR pattern. Absent end-diastolic FVW (Fig. 4–4) in patients with severe preeclampsia before 28 weeks' gestation is indicative of a poor fetal or neonatal prognosis. In such situations, the obstetrician should consider termination of pregnancy rather than subject the mother to prolonged expectant management.

Ultrasonography. Ultrasonography is important early in pregnancy to confirm the gestational age and, at 20 weeks' gestation, to exclude congenital abnormalities in mothers at risk for preeclampsia. Depending on the department policy, ultrasonography may be performed later in pregnancy to assess fetal growth or as part of the biophysical profile.[76] However, we believe that frequent FHR monitoring gives a better overall assessment of the condition of the fetus. In addition, it can clearly indicate when to deliver. Ultrasonography is essential in pa-

tients with absent end-diastolic flow velocity who have not had early ultrasonography in order to exclude congenital abnormalities.

Cordocentesis. Cordocentesis is indicated only in patients where there is an urgent need to exclude a chromosomal abnormality, since one would not wish to continue with conservative therapy when the fetus is severely abnormal.

Amniocentesis. Amniocentesis is controversial. Some physicians prefer to perform an amniocentesis to confirm lung maturity, since one would not like to continue with expectant therapy if the lungs are mature; however, with good fetal monitoring the chances of intrauterine death are very low indeed. Therefore, the decision for delivery should not be based on lung maturity alone, because other organs may still be immature and it may be safe for the fetus to remain in

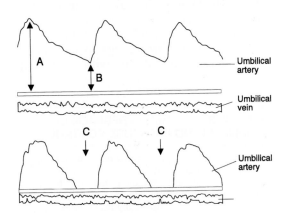

FIGURE 4–4. Flow velocity of the umbilical artery. "A" indicates flow velocity during systole; "B," during diastole; and "C," absent end-diastolic velocity.

the uterus. In our unit, only specific maternal or fetal reasons are indications for delivery or when a gestational age of 34 weeks has been reached.

Control of Blood Pressure During Expectant Management

Methyldopa is the drug most widely used because it has been shown to be safe,[24, 77] even after prolonged follow-up.[78] As an alternative, nifedipine or labetalol would be the drug of choice.[1, 7] If single-drug therapy is insufficient to control the blood pressure, a combination of drugs should be used. When a combination is used, it is difficult to know which combination is most effective. Walker[79] recommends 10 mg oral nifedipine retard to start with, increasing it to 30 mg twice a day in addition to 300 mg labetalol four times daily. Sibai and colleagues[7] recommend oral nifedipine 10 mg every 6 hours for a maximum of 120 mg/day and labetalol up to a maximum of 2400 mg/day.

Oláh and coworkers[9] used methyldopa as the first drug, adding slow-release nifedipine when the maximum dose of methyldopa was reached. Moodley and associates[108] add 75 to 200 mg monohydralazine per day if 2 g of methyldopa/24 hr is insufficient.

At Tygerberg Hospital, the regimen is to start with methyldopa 1 g immediately and 500 mg three times daily, increasing to 500 mg every 6 hours. Nifedipine is added as the second drug, starting at 10 mg/day and increasing gradually to 60 mg/day. If these two drugs are insufficient to control the blood pressure below 160/110 mmHg, prazosin is added. One starts with 1 mg three times daily and increases it by 3 mg/day to 21 mg/day. One randomized controlled trial has shown that nifedipine is preferable to prazosin as the second drug[79a] (Table 4–3). Failure of these three drugs to control the blood pressure in patients with preeclamp-

TABLE 4–3. TYGERBERG REGIMEN OF CHRONIC BLOOD PRESSURE CONTROL

First drug—methyldopa—1 g stat and 500 mg every 6–8 h; maximum 2 g/day
Add second drug—nifedipine—10 mg three times daily; increase to 60 mg/day
Add third drug—prazosin—1 mg three times daily; increase by 3 mg/day; maximum 21 mg/day
Aim: To keep blood pressure below 160/100 mmHg but not lower than 130/80 mmHg

TABLE 4–4. COMMON INDICATIONS FOR DELIVERY BEFORE 34–35 WEEKS' GESTATION

MATERNAL
Uncontrollable blood pressure
Deteriorating renal functions
Pulmonary edema
Persistent HELLP syndrome
Severe ascites
Imminent eclampsia

FETAL
Fetal distress
Abruptio placentae
Absent end-diastolic flow velocity of umbilical artery before 28 weeks' gestation

HELLP, hemolysis, elevated liver enzymes, low platelets.

sia is an indication for delivery.[4] In patients with chronic hypertension, we would add a diuretic in the form of amiloride/hydrochlorothiazide.[80, 81]

Delivery: When and How

Although the aim of expectant management is to reach a gestational age of 34 to 35 weeks and to have an elective delivery, maternal or fetal complications frequently necessitate earlier delivery (Table 4–4). Because these complications, especially fetal distress and abruptio placentae, may arise very suddenly, patients and staff should be informed about these possibilities, should be on the alert to recognize them early, and should know what to do if they occur (Table 4–5).

The method of delivery depends on various circumstances, such as fetal distress, or on an underlying obstetric factors, such as two previous cesarean sections, breech presentation, or an unfavorable cervix. If circumstances are favorable, membranes may be ruptured for surgical induction, or the cervix may be ripened by the local administration of prostaglandin E_2 (PGE$_2$). However, if there is fetal distress or an urgent maternal indication for delivery, cesarean section is preferred. As might be expected, the cesarean section rate is high. Sibai and colleagues[7] performed surgical deliveries in 73% of cases, a rate almost near the 68% rate of Odendaal's group.[4]

MANAGEMENT OF LATER SEVERE PREECLAMPSIA (AFTER 34 TO 35 WEEKS)

Although controversy remains regarding expectant management of patients with early

TABLE 4–5. COMPLICATIONS OF SEVERE PREECLAMPSIA

FETOPLACENTAL

Poor fetal growth
Abruptio placentae
Intrauterine death
Complications related to prematurity
Neonatal death

MATERNAL

Uncontrollable hypertension
Renal failure
Ascites
Pulmonary edema
HELLP syndrome
Eclampsia
Cerebral edema
Intracranial hemorrhage
Subcapsular hematoma
Laryngeal edema
Transient blindness
Intravascular coagulation
Maternal death

COMPLICATIONS OF TREATMENT

Fluid overload
Hypotension caused by antihypertensive drugs
Neonatal complications due to unnecessary early
  delivery
Complications of operative delivery

HELLP, *h*emolysis, *e*levated *l*iver enzymes, *l*ow *p*latelets.

severe preeclampsia, most obstetricians readily agree that delivery should be initiated in patients with severe preeclampsia at a gestational age of 34 weeks or, at the most, 35 weeks.

Specific Management

Generally, management is similar to that of patients with early severe preeclampsia. As-pects in which management differs are presented here.

Magnesium Sulfate

As mentioned earlier, the prophylactic use of $MgSO_4$ in the expectant management of early severe preeclampsia is still controversial. After 34 to 35 weeks' gestation, however, when there is the greater risk that patients might be in labor or that labor will be induced, administration of $MgSO_4$ is recommended until it can be shown that its use is not necessary.

There are two reasons for its prophylactic use. First, in the study on 1001 patients with early severe preeclampsia, all five episodes of eclampsia occurred during or after labor.[44] Second, in a large study, Lucas and coworkers[42] found that $MgSO_4$ to be superior to phenytoin in prevention of eclampsia. Furthermore, none of the 1049 women assigned to $MgSO_4$ therapy experienced convulsions (Table 4–6).

Corticosteroids

Because steroids have no effect in enhancing lung maturity after 34 weeks' gestation[47] and because delivery usually occurs within 24 hours, steroids are not used for these patients.

Maternal Assessment

Blood Pressure. During labor or induction, blood pressure should be recorded at least hourly and more frequently during acute control of hypertension. One should try to maintain values below 160/110 mmHg but not below 140/90 mmHg.

Urine Testing. Regular testing of urine for protein during labor is usually done but is of little clinical value in patients in whom

TABLE 4–6. TRIALS ON THE PREVENTION OF ECLAMPSIA WITH MAGNESIUM SULFATE (MgSO₄)

AUTHOR	TYPE OF STUDY	DRUGS	NO.	GESTATIONAL AGE AT DELIVERY	ECLAMPSIA	PNM
Lucas et al (1995)[42]	Randomized	MgSO₄	1049	226 Preterm	0*	12.2
		Phenytoin	1089	216 Preterm	10	14.5
Chen et al (1995)[43]	Randomized	MgSO₄	34	10 Preterm	0	0
		No MgSO₄	30	12 Preterm	0	0
Odendaal and Hall (1996)[44]	Retrospective	MgSO₄	510	30.2 wk	2	47
		No MgSO₄	491	30.6 wk	3	41

PNM, perinatal mortality rate per 1000 total births.
*$P = .004$.

labor is induced for other reasons. Charts of hourly urinary output or urinary output over 4 hours are essential for diagnosis of oliguria or anuria in time.

Uric Acid Measurements. Because patients usually deliver after 34 to 35 weeks' gestation, routine testing for uric acid levels is of little clinical value and, therefore, is not recommended.

Platelet Count and Liver Function Tests. These tests are indicated at the beginning of labor induction. When low values are found, the tests should be repeated during labor and after delivery for prompt diagnosis of HELLP syndrome.

Fetal Assessment

Fetal Heart Rate Monitoring. Continuous FHR monitoring is essential because there are many potential causes of fetal distress. Depending on the cervical dilation and specific heart rate pattern, one should always try to determine the degree of fetal acidemia by determining scalp blood pH because unnecessary cesarean section for minor or no distress should be avoided in these ill mothers.

Ultrasonography. Routine ultrasound examinations during labor are not indicated unless the fetal position or size is known.

Other Methods of Fetal Assessment. Amniocentesis, cordocentesis, and umbilical artery Doppler studies have little place in the assessment of the fetus after 34 weeks' gestation because the main aim is to deliver. Rarely do the results of one of these tests lead to alternative management.

MATERNAL FOLLOW-UP

Women who have had preeclampsia are at greater risk for having underlying medical disease than women who have been normotensive during pregnancy.[2, 82–87] In addition, women with chronic hypertension have a high risk of perinatal death and small-for-gestational-age newborns.

Selvaggi and coworkers[86] found that 57% of women who have had hypertension in pregnancy develop hypertension in successive pregnancies. Dekker and associates[82] tested 101 patients with a history of early-onset severe preeclampsia. Chronic hypertension was found in 39% of these women. Of the 85 women treated for coagulation disturbances, 25% had protein S deficiency.

Tests for activated protein C resistance had positive results in 16%, hyperhomocystinemia was found in 18%, and anticardiolipin antibodies in 29%.

Nisell and colleagues[87] found that 37% of women with a history of pregnancy-induced hypertension and 20% with a history of preeclampsia were hypertensive when followed up 7 years later. Black patients show a high prevalence of hypertension, inasmuch as 41% of them were found to be hypertensive during labor or during the first 24 hours after delivery.[88] Therefore, long-term follow-up is essential in patients who have had early severe preeclampsia.

NEONATAL FOLLOW-UP

In a matched control study, 223 infants born to mothers with preeclampsia before 35 weeks' gestation were compared with a control group. Maternal preeclampsia alone did not affect the postnatal course.[89]

Ounsted and coworkers[90] studied the intellectual abilities of 242 children, born to women who had been hypertensive during pregnancy, at the age of 7½ years. Children whose mothers had had superimposed preeclampsia had higher scores than those whose mothers had not had preeclampsia. In a small subgroup of particularly high-risk pregnancies in which the PNM rate was 10 times greater than the rest of the sample, intellectual ability did not differ from that of the rest.

In another study, however, children born to mothers with preeclampsia had a significantly lower mean mental developmental index, and significantly more of these children had one or more impairments compared with the control group at 2 years of age.[91]

Kirsten[51] followed up 126 newborns at 24 months, when a Griffiths developmental quotient was done. A corrected score of 80 or more was noted in 96% of newborns. No difference was found between those who had a resistance index below the 95th percentile, those with a resistance index between the 95th and 99th percentile, and those whose mothers had absent end-diastolic flow velocity during pregnancy. Cognitive impairment was associated with poor socioeconomic factors only and not with any abnormal FHR patterns or neonatal complications. Neurodevelopmental outcome was assessed for 157 children at 48 months. Motor development was normal in 97% of children born to mothers with early severe preeclampsia; 3% had cerebral palsy.

FUTURE DEVELOPMENTS

Although it has not been proven that antihypertensive therapy restores endothelial function in patients with essential hypertension, chronic lipid-lowering therapy is effective in restoring endothelial function in patients with hypercholesterolemia.[92] Aiming therapy to specific underlying causes of hypertensive diseases may therefore be beneficial, especially if such therapy is started early. More studies are also needed to determine whether strict control of blood pressure can improve perinatal outcome and which combination of drugs is best for this control.

The use of ketanserin and aspirin for mild hypertension in early pregnancy has resulted in an encouraging reduction in PNM and preeclampsia as well as an increase in birth weight and gestational age.[93] However, it remains uncertain whether this is due to the antihypertensive or antiserotonin effect of ketanserin or whether a synergistic effect of this drug and aspirin played a role. Although aspirin is not recommended for the prevention of preeclampsia, it may be justified in women at risk for early-onset preeclampsia, severe enough to need very preterm delivery. More studies are therefore needed.

ECLAMPSIA

The maternal mortality of eclampsia ranges from very high in developing countries to 1 in 245[94] or 1 in 254[8] cases in developed countries. An accurate general maternal mortality is probably 4.2%, derived from the 70 maternal deaths in the 1680 cases in the eclampsia trial (Table 4–7).[38] The PNM rate is much higher. In the eclampsia trial, the PNM rate ranged between 22.4% and 30.7% in the different arms of the study. In contrast, Sibai and colleagues[95] found a PNM rate of 13.3% in 1981, which was lowered to 11.8% in their 1990 study.[94] Generally, the range may be between 13% and 30%.[96]

Inasmuch as there are excellent reviews on the management of patients,[26, 97–100] many of these aspects will not be mentioned again, but some clinical problems or controversies will be addressed.

Epidemiology

Saftlas and associates[101] studied the incidence of eclampsia in the United States from the National Hospital Discharge Survey during 1979 to 1986. The rate of mild or unspecified preeclampsia remained constant, between 21.4 and 25.6 per 1000 deliveries. In contrast, the rate of severe eclampsia increased from 2.4 per 1000 deliveries in 1979 to 4.7 in 1985 and 5.2 in 1986. Eclampsia was found in 0.56 per 1000 deliveries, which is higher than the rate of 0.29 per 1000 deliveries for Sweden between 1976 and 1980.[102]

Douglas and Redman,[45] examining the oc-

TABLE 4–7. MATERNAL MORTALITY AND MORBIDITY OF ECLAMPSIA

AUTHOR	DELIVERIES	ECLAMPSIA CASES	INCIDENCE RATE PER 1000 DELIVERIES	MATERNAL MORTALITY	MAJOR MORBIDITY
Pritchard et al (1984)[94]	Not stated	245	—	0.4%	Not studied
Saftlas et al (1990)[101]	Not stated	±16,000	0.56	Not studied	Not studied
Sibai (1990)[105]	83,720	254	3.03	0.4%	120*
Douglas and Redman (1994)[45]	774,436	383	0.49	1.8%	35%
Eclampsia trial (1995)[38]	MgSO$_4$	453	—	3.8%	12.4%
	Diazepam	452	—	5.1%	13.1%
	MgSO$_4$	388	—	2.6%	23.7%
	Phenytoin	387	—	5.2%	25.3%

*More than one complication may have occurred in the same patient.
MgSO$_4$, magnesium sulfate.

currence of eclampsia at all 279 hospitals in the United Kingdom with a consultant obstetric unit during 1992, found a national incidence of 0.49 per 1000 deliveries, almost exactly that of the United States. Of interest is that the incidence of eclampsia is similar in the United States and United Kingdom, where 85% of consultants in the United Kingdom used anticonvulsants to prevent convulsions[45] and 99% in the United States did so.[103]

In Canada, Burrows and Burrows[104] conducted an 8-year cross-sectional study at one institution where 467 patients with preeclampsia or superimposed preeclampsia were managed without seizure prophylaxis. Convulsions occurred in 3.9% of patients. There was no seizure-related maternal mortality or morbidity.

Odendaal and Hall[44] managed 1001 patients with early severe preeclampsia with $MgSO_4$ prophylaxis for half of them but with strict hypertension control for all. Eclampsia developed in only 0.5% of patients.

Perinatal Mortality Rate

The decline in maternal mortality due to eclampsia has not been followed by a reduction in perinatal mortality. In the United Kingdom, the PNM rate is 56.3/1000.[45] In a large study in the United States, the PNM was 118/1000 at a tertiary referral hospital.[105] PNM is even higher when only antepartum eclampsia is included.[100] In the Collaborative Eclampsia Trial,[38] the overall PNM rate was 266/1000. In 1982 the PNM rate was 218/1000.[106]

Despite improved techniques of fetal diagnosis and monitoring and NICUs, the improvement in perinatal outcome has been very modest indeed. The main reason probably is that obstetricians, rightly so, put a high priority on the condition of the mother and therefore always induced labor or delivery operatively once her condition was stable. This directly led to the delivery of many preterm infants and, therefore, more neonatal deaths. It is still uncertain whether administration of corticosteroids with delivery 24 hours later improves fetal outcome without endangering the maternal condition by delaying delivery.

Magnesium Sulfate Administration

It is now certain that $MgSO_4$ is superior to phenytoin and diazepam in the management of eclampsia (Table 4–8).[38] Either the intramuscular (IM) regimen or the IV 1 g/h regimen is used (Table 4–9). However, Sibai and coworkers[99] have found that the 1 g/h regimen produced serum magnesium levels that were much lower than those achieved by the IM regimen. The latter regimen also produced higher mean magnesium levels during the first 3 hours of therapy than the 2 g/h IV regimen. After 3 hours, there was no significant difference between the IM and 2 g/h IV regimens. Using the IM regimen to prevent seizures, Lucas and coworkers[42] found no convulsions in 1049 patients in contrast to 10 in the 1089 patients who received phenytoin.

There seems to be little difference between the two regimens. The greatest disadvantage of the IM regimen is the painful injection and the occasional gluteal abscess, although it is safer because it is unlikely that a patient would receive an overdose of $MgSO_4$, which is possible with the IV route.

TABLE 4–8. EFFICACY OF MAGNESIUM SULFATE ($MgSO_4$) TO ARREST FURTHER CONVULSIONS

AUTHOR	DRUG	ECLAMPSIA CASES	RECURRENCE	PNM
Dommisse (1990)[110]	$MgSO_4$	11	0	2 intrauterine deaths
	Phenytoin	11	4	2 intrauterine deaths
Eclampsia trial (1995)[38]	$MgSO_4$	453	13.2%*	24.8
	Diazepam	452	27.9%	22.4
	$MgSO_4$	388	5.7%†	26.1
	Phenytoin	387	17.1%	30.7

*52% lower risk of further convulsions (95% confidence interval [CI], 64%–37% reduction).
†67% lower risk of further convulsions (95% CI, 79%–47% reduction).
PNM, perinatal mortality rate.

TABLE 4–9. MAGNESIUM SULFATE (MgSO₄) ADMINISTRATION FOR ARREST AND PREVENTION OF ECLAMPSIA

IM ROUTE

Loading dose	4 g MgSO$_4$ 20% solution, IV over 4 min, and 5 g MgSO$_4$, 50% solution in each buttock
	Use 3-inch-long 20-gauge needle
	Add 1 ml 2% lignocaine (lidocaine) to reduce pain
	Add 2–4 g MgSO$_4$ after 15 min if convulsions persist
Maintenance dose	5 g IM q 4 h

IV ROUTE

Loading dose	6 g over 20 min
Maintenance dose	2 g/h

DISCONTINUE

24 h after delivery

IV, intravenously; IM, intramuscularly.

The lack of availability of infusion pumps in rural areas may be another disadvantage of the continuous infusion method.

At Tygerberg Hospital, the IM method is used because it is safer and less time-consuming in our situation. In developing countries, facilities for assessing blood magnesium levels are available at only a few hospitals. We have found it unnecessary to assess magnesium levels regularly, provided that the standard precautions in its administration are precisely taken (Table 4–10).

Induction of Labor

Induction of labor should be seriously considered in eclampsia patients unless there is an obstetric indication for cesarean section. Eclampsia as such is not an indication for operative delivery.

In the case of an unfavorable cervix, intravaginal or intracervical prostaglandins are recommended with rupture of the mem-

TABLE 4–10. MANDATORY OBSERVATIONS BEFORE NEXT INTRAMUSCULAR MAGNESIUM SULFATE INJECTION

Present patellar reflex
Urinary output more than 100 mL during previous 4 h
Respiratory rate > 14/min

branes when the cervix is favorable. Oxytocin is used to stimulate contractions if amniotomy has not resulted in adequate contractions. Continuous electronic monitoring of the FHR is essential because several factors, such as placental insufficiency, excessive uterine contractions following prostaglandin administration, further convulsions, and antihypertensive therapy, all may cause fetal distress.

Method of Delivery

As stated earlier, vaginal delivery is preferable unless induction is unsuccessful or fetal or maternal indications for cesarean section develop during induction. However, little information is available concerning the duration of time during which labor should be induced. At Tygerberg Hospital, a second prostaglandin dose, 4 to 6 hours after the first, or occasionally a third dose, 4 to 6 hours later, has been used to induce labor. If the cervix still does not allow easy amniotomy, a cesarean section is performed.

However, more difficult problems are encountered in Durban, where the King Edward VIII Hospital receives referrals from a large rural area.[108] There, long delays are encountered, from the initial eclamptic convulsion to eventual admission to the teaching hospital. During this delay, many patients have more than four convulsions. Inasmuch as a further delay in delivery may increase maternal mortality, the hospital's management policy is for a cesarean section if delivery is unlikely within 6 hours. It is essential to control convulsions and blood pressure, obtain results of special examinations, and correct abnormalities such as hypovolemia and metabolic acidosis before a cesarean section is performed.

The First 24 Hours After Delivery

Careful monitoring of the eclamptic patient for the first 24 hours after delivery is crucial because many complications may occur during this period. In particular, one should be watchful for pulmonary edema. Not all units follow a policy in which fluid administration is limited to 60 to 125 mL/h.[96] In addition, colloids are sometimes used freely to correct the hypovolemia. All these steps increase the risk of pulmonary edema when mobilization of the accumulated fluid in the interstitial space increases the intravascular volume. On the other hand, hypovolemic patients tolerate hemorrhage poorly. One should therefore replace blood loss during postpartum hemorrhage carefully.

In the management of patients with severe preeclampsia, it is important to know that eclampsia can occur more than 48 hours after delivery. This late postpartum eclampsia constitutes 56% of cases.[109]

CONCLUSION

Although MgSO$_4$ appears to be the best drug to arrest convulsions in cases of eclampsia, many aspects of treatment of the disease are less certain. Until larger studies present clear solutions, these uncertainties will remain for years to come.

We should also remember that populations and circumstances differ. Unrealistic global standardization of treatment should therefore not be pursued. An adaptive policy, which best maximizes economic limitations but is safe for the mother and fetus, should be sought.

Management of patients with preeclampsia and eclampsia is only symptomatic. Blood pressure is controlled; convulsions are treated or prevented. As a last resort, the fetus and placenta are delivered because delivery is the only real effective way of reversing the preeclampsia. Until we know what causes the disease, treatment will remain basically symptomatic.

References

1. Schiff E, Friedman SA, Sibai BM. Conservative management of severe preeclampsia remote from term. Obstet Gynecol 1994;84:626.
2. Sibai BM, Mercer B, Sarinoglu C. Severe preeclampsia in the second trimester: Recurrence risk and long-term prognosis. Am J Obstet Gynecol 1991;165:1408.
3. Derham RJ, Hawkins DF, De Vries LS, et al. Outcome of pregnancies complicated by severe hypertension and delivered before 34 weeks, stepwise logistic regression analysis of prognostic factors. Br J Obstet Gynaecol 1989;96:1173.
4. Odendaal HJ, Steyn DW, Norman K, et al. Improved perinatal mortality rates in 1001 patients with severe preeclampsia. S Afr Med J 1995; 85:1071.
5. Odendaal HJ, Pattinson RC, Du Toit R. Fetal and neonatal outcome in patients with severe preeclampsia before 34 weeks. S Afr Med J 1987;71:555.
6. Odendaal HJ, Pattinson RC, Bam R, et al. Aggressive or expectant management for patients with severe preeclampsia between 28–34 weeks' gesta-tion: A randomized controlled trial. Obstet Gynecol 1990;76:1070.
7. Sibai BM, Mercer BM, Schiff E, et al. Aggressive versus expectant management of severe preeclampsia at 28 to 32 weeks' gestation: A randomized controlled trial. Am J Obstet Gynecol 1994;171:818.
8. Sibai BM, Sherif A, Fairlie F, et al. A protocol for managing severe preeclampsia in the second trimester. Am J Obstet Gynecol 1990;163:733.
9. Oláh KS, Redman CWG, Gee H. Management of severe, early preeclampsia: Is conservative management justified? Eur J Obstet Gynecol Reprod Biol 1993;51:175.
10. Visser W, Van Pampus MG, Treffers PE, et al. Perinatal results of hemodynamic and conservative temporizing treatment in severe preeclampsia. Eur J Obstet Gynecol Reprod Biol 1994; 53:175.
11. Visser W, Wallenburg HCS. Maternal and perinatal outcome of temporizing management in 254 consecutive patients with severe preeclampsia remote from term. Eur J Obstet Gynecol Reprod Biol 1995;63:147.
12. Visser W, Wallenburg HCS. Temporising management of severe preeclampsia with and without the HELLP syndrome. Br J Obstet Gynaecol 1995;102:111.
13. Sibai BM, Graham JM, McCubbin JH. A comparison of intravenous and intramuscular magnesium sulfate regimens in preeclampsia. Am J Obstet Gynecol 1984;150:728.
14. Twaddle S. Day care for women with high-risk pregnancies. Nurse Times 1995;91:46.
15. Odendaal HJ. Fetal heart rate patterns in patients with intrauterine growth retardation. Obstet Gynecol 1976;48:187.
16. Odendaal HJ, Burchell H. Raised uterine resting tone in patients with abruptio placentae. Int J Gynecol Obstet 1985;23:121.
17. Vink GJ, Moodley J, Philpott RH. Effect of dihydralazine on the fetus in the treatment of maternal hypertension. Obstet Gynecol 1980;55:519.
18. Report on confidential enquiries into maternal deaths in the United Kingdom 1991–1993. London: Her Majesty's Stationery Office.
19. Schuitemaker NWE, Bennebroek K, Gravenhorst J, et al. Maternal mortality and its prevention. Eur J Obstet Gynecol Reprod Biol 1991;42(Suppl):531.
20. Theron GB. Maternal mortality in the Cape Province, 1990–1992. S Afr Med J 1996;86:412.
21. Chari RS, Friedman SA, Sibai BM. Antihypertensive therapy during pregnancy. Fetal Matern Med Rev 1995;7:61.
22. Dekker GA, Van Geijn HP. Hypertensive disease in pregnancy. Curr Opin Obstet Gynecol 1992;4:10.
23. Lowe SA, Rubin PC. The pharmacological management of hypertension in pregnancy. J Hypertens 1992;10:201.
24. Redman CWG. Hypertension in pregnancy. In Turnbull AC, Chamberlain G (eds). Obstetrics. London: Churchill Livingstone, 1989, p 515.
25. Theron GB. Perinatal Education Programme. Manual I, Maternal Care. Cape Town: University of Cape Town Press, 1993.
26. Sibai BM, Barton JR, Akl S, et al. A randomized prospective comparison of nifedipine and bed rest versus bed rest alone in the management of pre-

eclampsia remote from term. Am J Obstet Gynecol 1992;167:879.

27. Seabe SJ, Moodley J, Becker P. Nifedipine in acute hypertensive emergencies in pregnancy. S Afr Med J 1989;76:248.

28. Mabie WC, Gonzalez AR, Sibai BM, et al. A comparative trial of labetalol and hydralazine in the acute management of severe hypertension complicating pregnancy. Obstet Gynecol 1987;70:328.

29. Lamming GD, Symonds EM. Use of labetalol and methyldopa in pregnancy-induced hypertension. Br J Clin Pharmacol 1979;8(Suppl 2):217S.

30. Mahmoud TZK, Bjornsson S, Calder AA. Labetalol therapy in pregnancy induced hypertension: The effects on fetoplacental circulation and fetal outcome. Eur J Obstet Gynecol Reprod Biol 1993;50:109.

31. Ashe RG, Moodley J, Richards AM, et al. Comparison of labetalol and dihydrallazine in hypertensive emergencies of pregnancy. S Afr Med J 1987;71:354.

32. MacCarthy EP, Bloomfield SS. Labetalol: A review of its pharmacology, pharmacokinetics, clinical uses and adverse effects. Pharmacotherapy 1983;3:193.

33. Lunell NO, Hjemdahl P, Fredholm BB, et al. Acute effects of labetalol on maternal metabolism and uteroplacental circulation in hypertension of pregnancy. In Riley A, Symonds EM (eds). The Investigation of Labetalol in the Management of Hypertension in Pregnancy (International Congress Series, No. 591). Amsterdam: Excerpta Medica, 1981, p 152.

34. Humphreys GS, Deboin DG. Ineffectiveness of propranolol in hypertensive Jamaicans. Br Med J 1968;2:601.

35. Seedat YK. Perspectives in hypertension. S Afr Med J 1992;81:1.

36. Seedat YK. Race, environment and blood pressure: The South African experience. J Hypertens 1983;1:7.

37. Hypertension—in black and white [editorial]. Lancet 1992;339:28.

38. Eclampsia Trial Collaborative Group. Which anticonvulsant for women with eclampsia? Evidence from the Collaborative Eclampsia Trial. Lancet 1995;345:1455.

39. Chien PF, Khan KS, Arnot N. Magnesium sulphate in the treatment of eclampsia and preeclampsia: An overview of the evidence from randomised trials. Br J Obstet Gynaecol 1996;103:1085.

40. Anthony J, Johanson RB, Duley L. Role of magnesium sulfate in seizure prevention in patients with eclampsia and preeclampsia. Drug Safety 1996;15:188.

41. Reti LL, Ross A, Kloss M, et al. The management of severe preeclampsia with intravenous magnesium sulphate, hydralazine and central venous catheterization. Aust N Z J Obstet Gynaecol 1987;27:102.

42. Lucas MJ, Leveno KJ, Cunningham FG. A comparison of magnesium sulfate with phenytoin for the prevention of eclampsia. N Engl J Med 1995;333:201.

43. Chen F-P, Chang S-D, Chu K-K. Expectant management in severe preeclampsia: Does magnesium sulfate prevent the development of eclampsia? Acta Obstet Gynecol Scand 1995;74:181.

44. Odendaal HJ, Hall DR. Is magnesium sulfate prophylaxis really necessary in patients with severe preeclampsia? J Matern Fetal Invest 1996;6:14.

45. Douglas KA, Redman CWG. Eclampsia in the United Kingdom. BMJ 1994;309:1395.

46. Hutton JD, James DK, Stirrat GM, et al. Management of severe preeclampsia and eclampsia by UK consultants. Br J Obstet Gynaecol 1992;99:554.

47. Liggins GC, Howie RN. A controlled trial of antepartum glucocorticoid treatment for prevention of the respiratory distress syndrome in premature infants. Pediatrics 1972;50:515.

48. Semchyshyn S, Zuspan FP, Cordero L. Cardiovascular response and complications of glucocorticoid therapy in hypertensive pregnancies. Am J Obstet Gynecol 1983;145:530.

49. Bowen JR, Leslie GI, Arnold JD, et al. Increased incidence of respiratory distress syndrome in infants following pregnancies complicated by hypertension. Aust N Z J Obstet Gynaecol 1988;28:109.

50. Schiff E, Friedman SA, Mercer BM, et al. Fetal lung maturity is not accelerated in preeclamptic pregnancies. Am J Obstet Gynecol 1993;169:1096.

51. Kirsten GF. The long term neurodevelopmental outcome of infants born to mothers with severe preeclampsia and absent enddiastolic umbilical artery flow velocity waveforms. MD dissertation, promotor HJ Odendaal, University of Stellenbosch, 1996.

52. Amorim MMR, Santos LC, Faundes A. Corticosteroid therapy for prevention of respiratory distress syndrome in severe preeclampsia. Am J Obstet Gynecol 1999;180:1283.

53. Yeh SY, Paul RH, Cordero L, et al. A study of diazepam during labor. Obstet Gynecol 1974;43:363.

54. De Haan J, Van Bemmel JH, Stolle LAM, et al. Trend detection in the fetal condition. Int J Gynaecol Obstet 1972;10:202.

55. Cetrulo CL, Schifrin BS. FHR patterns preceding death in utero. Obstet Gynecol 1976;48:521.

56. Chua S, Redman CWG. Prognosis for preeclampsia complicated by 5 g or more of proteinuria in 24 hours. Eur J Obstet Gynecol Reprod Biol 1992;43:9.

57. Schiff E, Friedman SA, Lu Kao RN, et al. The importance of urinary protein excretion during conservative management of severe preeclampsia. Am J Obstet Gynecol 1996;175:1313.

58. Redman CWG, Beilin LJ, Bonnar J, et al. Plasma-urate measurements in predicting fetal death in hypertensive pregnancy. Lancet 1976;i:1370.

59. Schuster E, Weppelmann B. Plasma urate measurements and fetal outcome in preeclampsia. Gynecol Obstet Invest 1981;12:162.

60. Sagen N, Haram K, Nilsen ST. Serum urate as a predictor of fetal outcome in severe preeclampsia. Acta Obstet Gynecol Scand 1984;63:71.

61. Yoshimura A, Ideura T, Iwasaki S, et al. Significance of uric acid clearance in preeclampsia. Am J Obstet Gynecol 1990;162:1639.

62. Sibai BM, Garland D, Anderson GD, et al. Eclampsia II. Clinical significance of laboratory findings. Obstet Gynecol 1982;59:153.

63. Odendaal HJ, Pienaar ME. Are high uric acid levels in patients with early preeclampsia an indication for delivery? S Afr Med J 1997;87:213.

64. Brink AL, Odendaal HJ. Risk factors for abruptio placentae. S Afr Med J 1987;72:250.

65. Sibai BM, Taslimi M, Abdella TN, et al. Maternal and perinatal outcome of conservative management of severe preeclampsia in midtrimester. Am J Obstet Gynecol 1985;152:32.

66. Odendaal HJ, Pattinson RC, Du Toit R, et al. Frequent fetal heart-rate monitoring for early detection of abruptio placentae in severe proteinuric hypertension. S Afr Med J 1988;74:19.

67. Smith JH, Anand KJS, Cotes PM, et al. Antenatal fetal heart variation in relation to the respiratory and metabolic status of the compromised human fetus. Br J Obstet Gynaecol 1988;95:980.

68. Odendaal HJ, Steyn W, Theron GB, et al. Does a nonreactive fetal heart rate pattern really mean fetal distress? Am J Perinatol 1994;11:194.

69. Steyn DW, Odendaal HJ. Fetal heart rate variability prior to delivery in women with severe hypertension who developed placental abruption. Br J Obstet Gynaecol 1994;101:1005.

70. Chari RS, Friedman SA, O'Brien JM, et al. Daily antenatal testing in women with severe preeclampsia. Am J Obstet Gynecol 1995;173:1207.

71. Alfirevic Z, Neilson JP. Doppler ultrasonography in high-risk pregnancies: Systematic review with meta-analysis. Am J Obstet Gynecol 1995;172:1379.

72. Pattinson RC, Norman K, Odendaal HJ. The use of Doppler velocimetry of the umbilical artery before 24 weeks' gestation to screen for high-risk pregnancies. S Afr Med J 1993;83:734.

73. Goffinet F, Paris J, Heim N, et al. Predictive value of Doppler umbilical artery velocimetry in a low risk population with normal fetal biometry. A prospective study of 2016 women. Eur J Obstet Gynecol Reprod Biol 1997;71:11.

74. Howarth GR, Pattinson RC, Kirsten G, et al. Umbilical artery Doppler velocimetry in the prediction of intrapartum fetal compromise. S Afr Med J 1992;81:248.

75. Pattinson RC, Norman K, Odendaal HJ. The role of Doppler velocimetry in the management of high risk pregnancies. Br J Obstet Gynaecol 1994;101:114.

76. Manning FA, Morrison I, Lange IR, et al. Antepartum determination of fetal health: Composite biophysical profile scoring. Clin Perinatol 1982;9:285.

77. Redman CWG, Beilin LJ, Bonnar J, et al. Fetal outcome in trial of antihypertensive treatment in pregnancy. Lancet 1976;ii:753.

78. Cockburn J, Ounsted M, Moar VA, et al. Final report of study on hypertension during pregnancy: The effects of specific treatment on the growth and development of the children. Lancet 1982;i:647.

79. Walker JJ. Care of the patient with severe pregnancy induced hypertension. Eur J Obstet Gynecol Reprod Biol 1996;65:127.

79a. Hall DR, Odendaal HJ, Steyn DW, Smith M. Nifedipine or prazosin as a second agent to control early severe hypertension in pregnancy: A randomised controlled trial. Br J Obstet Gynaecol 2000;107:759.

80. Rienhardt GW, Steyn PS, Odendaal HJ. Conservative management of severe chronic hypertension in pregnancy. Eur J Obstet Gynecol Reprod Biol 1994;57:215.

81. Hall DR, Odendaal HJ. Addition of a diuretic to antihypertensive therapy for early severe hypertension in pregnancy. Int J Gynaecol Obstet 1998;60:63.

82. Dekker GA, De Vries JIP, Doelitzsch MS, et al. Underlying disorders associated with severe early-onset preeclampsia. Am J Obstet Gynecol 1995;173:1042.

83. Pattinson RC, Odendaal HJ, Du Toit R. Conservative management of severe proteinuric hypertension before 28 weeks' gestation. S Afr Med J 1988;73:516.

84. Sibai BM, El-Nazer A, Gonzalez-Ruiz A. Severe preeclampsia-eclampsia in young primigravid women: Subsequent pregnancy outcome and remote prognosis. Am J Obstet Gynecol 1986;155:1011.

85. Rey E, Couturier A. The prognosis of pregnancy in women with chronic hypertension. Am J Obstet Gynecol 1994;171:410.

86. Selvaggi L, Loverro G, Schena FP, et al. Long term follow-up of women with hypertension in pregnancy. Int J Gynaecol Obstet 1988;27:45.

87. Nisell H, Lintu H, Lunell NO, et al. Blood pressure and renal function seven years after pregnancy complicated by hypertension. Br J Obstet Gynaecol 1995;102:876.

88. Cronjé HS, Bam RH, Muir AR, et al. The prevalence of postpartum hypertension in black women. J Obstet Gynaecol 1996;16:331.

89. Friedman SA, Schiff E, Kao L. Neonatal outcome after preterm delivery for preeclampsia. Am J Obstet Gynecol 1995;172:1785.

90. Ounsted M, Moar VA, Cockburn J, et al. Factors associated with the intellectual ability of children born to women with high risk pregnancies. Br Med J 1984;288:1038.

91. Szymonowicz W, Yu VYH. Severe preeclampsia and infants of very low birth weight. Arch Dis Child 1987;62:712.

92. Schmieder RE, Schobel HP. Is endothelial dysfunction reversible? Am J Cardiol 1995;76:117A.

93. Steyn DW, Odendaal HJ. Ketanserin and aspirin in the prevention of pre-eclampsia—a randomised controlled trial. Lancet 1997;350:1267.

94. Pritchard JA, Cunningham FG, Pritchard SA. The Parkland Memorial Hospital protocol for treatment of eclampsia: Evaluation of 245 cases. Am J Obstet Gynecol 1984;148:951.

95. Sibai BM, McCubbin JH, Anderson GD, et al. Eclampsia. I. Observations from 67 recent cases. Obstet Gynecol 1981;58:609.

96. Cunningham FG, MacDonald PC, Gant NF, et al (eds). Williams Obstetrics, 20th ed. Upper Saddle River, NJ: Prentice Hall International, 1997, p 693.

97. Cunningham FG, Gant NF. Management of eclampsia. Semin Perinatol 1994;18:103.

98. Magann EF, Martin JN. Complicated postpartum preeclampsia-eclampsia. Obstet Gynecol Clin North Am 1995;22:337.

99. Sibai BM, Lipshitz J, Anderson GD, et al. Reassessment of intravenous $MgSO_4$ therapy in preeclampsia-eclampsia. Obstet Gynecol 1981;57:199.

100. Sibai BM, McCubbin JH, Anderson GD, et al. Eclampsia: Treatment and referral. South Med J 1982;75:267.

101. Saftlas AF, Olson DR, Franks AL, et al. Epidemiology of preeclampsia and eclampsia in the United

States, 1979–1986. Am J Obstet Gynecol 1990; 163:460.

102. Moller B, Lindmark G. Eclampsia in Sweden, 1976–1980. Acta Obstet Gynecol Scand 1986; 65:307.

103. Catanzarite V, Quirk JG, Aisenbrey G. How do perinatologists manage preeclampsia? Am J Perinatol 1991;8:7.

104. Burrows RF, Burrows EA. The feasibility of a control population for a randomized control trial of seizure prophylaxis in the hypertensive disorders of pregnancy. Am J Obstet Gynecol 1995;173:929.

105. Sibai BM. Eclampsia. VI. Maternal-perinatal outcome in 254 consecutive cases. Am J Obstet Gynecol 1990;163:1049.

106. López-Llera M. Complicated eclampsia. Fifteen years experience in a referral medical center. Am J Obstet Gynecol 1982;142:28.

107. Moodley J, Naicker RS, Mankowitz E. Eclampsia—a method of management: A preliminary report. S Afr Med J 1983;63:530.

108. Moodley J, Koranteng SA, Rout C. Expectant management of early onset of severe preeclampsia in Durban. S Afr Med J 1993;83:584.

109. Lubarsky SL, Barton JR, Friedman SA, et al. Late postpartum eclampsia revisited. Obstet Gynecol 1994;83:502.

110. Dommisse J. Phenytoin sodium and magnesium sulphate in the management of eclampsia. Br J Obstet Gynaecol 1990;97:104.

5 PREVENTION of PREECLAMPSIA

Gustaaf A. Dekker

Hypertension occurs in approximately 6% to 10% of all pregnancies, and hypertensive disorders of pregnancy and especially preeclampsia are the leading causes of maternal and perinatal mortality and morbidity in developing and developed countries.[1, 2] Until recently, it has always been assumed that pregnancy-induced hypertensive disorders are a pathologic response. In developed countries, however, nonproteinuric hypertension arising late in pregnancy is associated with neither an increase in perinatal mortality or morbidity nor decreased birth weight.[3, 4] In this chapter these cases are designated *gestational hypertension*. In the rarer, severe form of the disease, usually arising in the late second or early third trimester and usually accompanied by significant proteinuria, there is a marked increase in perinatal mortality and morbidity[5, 6]; these cases are designated *preeclampsia*. The term *pregnancy-induced hypertensive disorders* is used as a denomination for all hypertensive disorders, with or without proteinuria, induced by the pregnant state.

Prevention of preeclampsia would mean a significant step forward in prenatal care. In preventive medicine, the general term *prevention* may have three different connotations:

- Primary—averting the occurrence of a disease
- Secondary—breaking off the disease process before the emergence of clinically recognizable disease
- Tertiary—prevention of complications caused by the disease process, somewhat synonymous to treating a disease

Hospitalization and strict bed rest are the most common methods used for tertiary prevention of preeclampsia. This policy was introduced by Hamlin[7] in 1952 as part of a management scheme (high-protein/low-salt diets and complete bed rest) that aimed to reduce the incidence of severe preeclampsia and abolish eclampsia. The Hamlin protocol was not directed specifically at improving perinatal outcome.[7] In Hamlin's original study, the introduction of this policy was associated with a significant fall in the rate of serious complications associated with preeclampsia and the incidence of eclampsia, and consequently became adopted by others.

Crowther and Chalmers[8] reviewed the literature on the effects of hospitalization and bed rest. They concluded that hospitalization of women with nonproteinuric hypertension may reduce the incidence of severe hypertension (diastolic blood pressure ≥ 110 mmHg). Bed rest also appeared to be associated with diuresis and resolution of edema, but the effect on the development of proteinuria was inconsistent; no evidence was documented for a beneficial effect on perinatal outcome.

In conclusion, the main reason to hospitalize women with pregnancy-induced hypertensive disorders is the need for thorough evaluation and frequent maternal and fetal surveillance to detect any deterioration as soon as possible. Whether the hospitalization should be linked with strict rest in bed is less clear.[8] Patients with an established pregnancy-induced hypertensive disorder may be hospitalized for an initial evaluation of the maternal and fetal condition. Outpatient management may be considered in a select group of patients with an apparently mild and stable course of the disease. Outpatient management can be a substitute for hospitalization only if it includes blood pressure monitoring along with patient instruction, restricted activity, urine dipstick measurements of proteinuria, and fetal monitoring.

More specific aspects of tertiary prevention (management of preeclampsia) are detailed in other chapters throughout this book. Following a short paragraph on primary prevention of preeclampsia, this chapter focuses on secondary prevention.

PRIMARY PREVENTION

The most preferable modus operandi to cope with human disease, primary prevention, is achievable only if the etiology mechanism of the disease is understood and if it is feasible to avoid or manipulate the determinants that are involved in the etiology of that particular disease.

Shallow, endovascular cytotrophoblast invasion in the spiral arteries and endothelial cell dysfunction are two key features in the pathophysiology of preeclampsia.[9] However, because the cause of these two key features remains unknown, the only way to prevent preeclampsia is by preventing pregnancy. Dekker and van Geijn[10] reviewed, in some detail, the perspectives for primary prevention of preeclampsia in the coming decade, as related to the three major current hypotheses on the etiology of preeclampsia:

1. *Placental ischemia hypothesis:* According to this hypothesis, placental ischemia results in an increased release of syncytiotrophoblast microvillous membranes, which may be the cause of the generalized endothelial cell dysfunction.[11]

2. *Immune maladaptation hypothesis:* According to this hypothesis, immune mechanisms are involved in the pathogenesis of preeclampsia. Immune maladaptation provides an attractive explanation for the disturbed endovascular trophoblast invasion, and abnormal activation of decidual lymphoid cells may explain the increased levels of free radical species, neutrophil elastase, and cytokines, such as tumor necrosis factor (TNF) and interleukin-1 (IL-1), which have been found to exist in preeclampsia.[12, 13]

3. *Preeclampsia as a genetic disease:* Severe preeclampsia and eclampsia have a familial tendency. The development of preeclampsia-eclampsia may be based on a single recessive gene or a dominant gene with incomplete penetrance. Penetrance may be dependent on the fetal genotype. Multifactorial inheritance is another possibility.[14]

At the moment, there are no therapeutic possibilities to prevent placental ischemia,

and the preeclampsia gene, if it exists, has yet to be discovered. The therapeutic potential of immunotherapy in preventing preeclampsia is controversial, to say the least. However, epidemiologic studies strongly suggest that exposure to sperm provides at least a partial protection against the development of preeclampsia.[15–20] The conclusions derived from these studies, although not directly useful for implementation in daily practice, may have practical consequences for practicing physicians, even if the exact etiology of preeclampsia remains unresolved:

1. According to the *primipaternity* concept, a multiparous woman with a new partner should be approached as being a primigravid woman.

2. Artificial donor insemination and oocyte donation are associated with an increased risk for development of pregnancy-induced hypertensive disorders.

3. A more or less prolonged period of sperm exposure provides a partial protection against pregnancy-induced hypertensive disorders. Currently, all women with changing partners are strongly advised to use condoms in order to prevent sexually transmitted diseases. However, a certain period of sperm exposure within a stable relationship, when the couple is aiming for pregnancy, is associated with a partial protection against preeclampsia.

Reducing the production of free radical species is an attractive approach, but specific and potent inhibitors of oxygen free radical production are not yet available. The beneficial effects of low-dose aspirin, if any, may be, at least partially, related to its effects on placental lipid peroxide production.[21] Increasing the levels of scavengers may be more attainable than inhibiting the production of free radical species. However, antioxidants are not without risk. Many homeostatic functions depend on them, and certain antioxidants in specific settings may act as pro-oxidants.[22] Nor is it immediately evident which antioxidant would be the most appropriate.

Administration of *N*-acetylcysteine, as glutathione precursor, may in the future turn out to be an attractive approach in this respect.[10] Glutathione peroxidase is an important cytosolic antioxidant peroxide-removing enzyme and is of utmost importance in protecting the mitochondrial housekeeping against cytokines and free radicals. Endogenous glutathione is of pivotal importance in protection of tissues from injury after ischemia-reperfusion. Glutathione peroxidase and the closely related phospholipid hydroperoxide glutathione peroxidase are both selenium-dependent enzymes.

An interesting support for the importance of an equilibrium between oxygen free radicals and scavengers comes from women suffering as a result of a geochemical lack of selenium in the Heilongjiang province of China.[23] Selenium deficiency may lead to reduced concentrations of selenium-containing enzymes such as glutathione peroxidase. In this region in China, there is a high incidence of preeclampsia.

Oxidative disequilibrium in preeclampsia is probably closely linked with cytokine activity, particularly TNF.[24] Bioactive TNF-α levels are increased in preeclampsia.[13] Antioxidants selectively inhibit the release of TNF because they control the oxidation-reduction status of glutathione, which is of major importance as an endogenous modulator of TNF production. Mitochondria are a major target for oxygen free radical attack. In mitochondria, TNF subverts part of the electron flow to release oxygen free radicals and lipid peroxides. If these are not removed with subsequent efficient reduction of the oxidized glutathione, serious toxic effects ensue because of the persisting toxic lipid peroxides, the oxidized glutathione, and consequently the further production of TNF.

In morphologic studies, the first detectable intracellular effects of TNF are swelling and malfunction of mitochondria. Shanklin and Sibai[25, 26] demonstrated that preeclampsia is associated with disseminated mitochondrial damage that is similar to oxygen free radical–induced mitochondrial damage.

Stark[24] reviewed the evidence that preeclampsia might be caused by a genetic TNF-mediated mitochondrial dysfunction. *N*-acetylcysteine is a well-known glutathione precursor. Thus, the use of *N*-acetylcysteine is an attractive option because it may protect endothelial cells and their mitochondria from TNF-α–mediated toxicity.[10]

SECONDARY PREVENTION

Secondary prevention, which implies breaking off the disease process before the emergence of clinically recognizable disease, is the focus of this chapter. Secondary prevention of a disease is possible only if the following three basic requirements are met:

- Knowledge of pathophysiologic mechanisms
- Availability of methods of early detection
- Means of intervention and correction of pathophysiologic changes

Knowledge of Pathophysiologic Mechanisms

Current concepts on the pathophysiology of hypertensive disorders are discussed in detail in recent reviews.

Availability of Methods of Early Detection

The signs and symptoms of preeclampsia are generally apparent at a relatively late stage in pregnancy, usually in the third trimester. However, the disorder results from abnormal interaction between the mother and the invading endovascular trophoblast much earlier in pregnancy. For that reason, it seems logical to search for earlier indicators of this disorder; indeed a multitude of tests have been proposed, especially during the past two decades, as a means of predicting the later development of the disease. A detailed discussion on methods used for early detection of preeclampsia is not within the scope of this chapter; see detailed reviews elsewhere.[27–29] This section briefly discusses those methods for early detection of preeclampsia that are currently available or feasible in most hospitals in developed countries.

Clinical Assessment

Blood Pressure. Hypertension is the most common sign and potentially the most dangerous clinical manifestation of pregnancy-induced hypertensive disorders. The increase in blood pressure in these disorders is caused by an increase in systemic peripheral resistance and is a rather early feature of the disease. Measuring blood pressure or second-trimester mean arterial pressure (MAP) is not useful for the early diagnosis of preeclampsia. If an increased diastolic blood pressure, MAP, or second-trimester MAP predicts anything, it is transient hypertension but not the real disease preeclampsia-eclampsia, with its associated perinatal morbidity and mortality. The evaluation of incremental changes in blood pressure is not a useful method of screening outpatient pregnant women for impending preeclampsia.[30–32]

Edema and Weight Gain. The one visible sign of pregnancy-induced hypertensive disorders is swelling, but this is not a reliable sign. Moderate edema can be detected in 60% to 80% of normotensive pregnancies, and pedal edema, even extending to the lower tibia, is a common finding in normal pregnant women. Edema affects 85% of women with a pregnancy-induced hypertensive disorder. The diagnostic signs of pregnancy-induced hypertensive disorders usually antedate symptoms. The classic sequence of the signs is edema, increased blood pressure, and proteinuria. However, any order of appearance may occur, and edema is not a prerequisite for diagnosing pregnancy-induced hypertensive disorders. Weight gain cannot be used to predict the development of pregnancy-induced hypertensive disorders, and excess weight gain alone imparts no adverse prognosis to perinatal outcome.[28]

Roll-over Test. The roll-over test has gained some popularity because of its simplicity, and the good results that were reported in the initial studies. Later studies have demonstrated that (1) a major part of the pressor response in this test is caused by the relative change in the position of the cuff in relation to the level of the heart when turning supine, and (2) the roll-over test is of no use in predicting preeclampsia.[28, 33]

Biochemical Markers

It is important to emphasize that most women with a pregnancy-induced hypertensive disorder are asymptomatic. This lack of symptoms is, in fact, an important part of the rationale for the frequent antenatal care visits in late pregnancy. Laboratory tests have been used for prediction, diagnosis, and monitoring of disease progress. The diagnosis of "preeclampsia" is even based on a laboratory test.

Uric Acid. Preeclamptic hyperuricemia is caused by a decreased urate clearance by the kidneys, and uric acid clearance drops disproportionally in preeclampsia as compared with creatinine and urea clearance.

The pathophysiologic explanation for this specific decrease in urate clearance is based on the biphasic pattern of renal involvement in preeclampsia. Impairment of tubular physiology, an early feature of renal involvement in preeclampsia, results in a reduced renal clearance of uric acid and thus an increase of plasma uric acid levels. Later on in the development of the disease, about the time proteinuria appears, glomerular function—along with urea and creatinine clearance—becomes impaired.

Preeclamptic hyperuricemia is correlated more or less with the decrease in plasma volume and plasma renin activity.[28, 29] Preeclamptic hyperuricemia is probably caused by a combination of intrarenal (peritubular) vasoconstriction and hypovolemia. Increments in urate levels are correlated with the severity of the preeclamptic lesion in renal biopsies, the degree of uteroplacental vascular pathology, and poor fetal outcome.[34]

Hyperuricemia has been reported to be a better predictor than blood pressure of adverse perinatal outcome. In most patients, the increase in urate levels appears to coincide with the increase in blood pressure and precedes the development of the proteinuric stage of the disease. Uric acid levels have been used for the early diagnosis of preeclampsia but not for hypertension itself.[32]

On the whole, the value of uric acid in the prediction of preeclampsia appears to be limited. Serial measurements of uric acid levels (establish first-trimester baseline level) in patients at a high risk (e.g., chronic hypertension) for development of preeclampsia are useful in the early diagnosis of (superimposed) preeclampsia and the identification of hypertensive patients with an increased risk for adverse perinatal outcome. In addition, uric acid may be used as an indicator of disease severity in established preeclampsia.[34]

Proteinuria. The presence of significant proteinuria is obligatory for the classic diagnosis of preeclampsia. Proteinuria is a late sign of pregnancy-induced hypertensive disorders and is a reflection of advanced disease. HELLP (*h*emolysis, *e*levated *l*iver enzymes, *l*ow *p*latelets) syndrome and eclampsia (prior to seizures) may occur in the absence of proteinuria.[6] The occurrence of proteinuria is an expression of glomerular dysfunction and generally coincides with a decrease in creatinine clearance. Hypertension plus proteinuria is associated with a twofold increased risk of perinatal death, compared with normotensive pregnancy and hypertension without proteinuria.

Because the development of proteinuria is a late feature of the disease, routine use of dipsticks in a normotensive low-risk population is probably just as ineffective as measurement of maternal weight gain. Microalbuminuria tests have been tried in order to predict preeclampsia. On the whole, there appears to be little value in using precise techniques of detecting proteinuria in the early diagnosis of preeclampsia. Other signs, such as an increase in blood pressure, a fall in the number of platelets, and a rise in plasma uric acid levels, appear to antedate the occurrence of detectable microalbuminuria.[28, 32]

Urinary Calcium Excretion. Hypocalciuria is present in most patients with severe stage of the disease. Preeclamptic hypocalciuria (like a decreased urate clearance) is an expression of tubular dysfunction. Sanchez-Ramos and associates[35] studied the value of urinary calcium as an early marker for preeclampsia in 103 consecutive nulliparous women. At 10 to 24 weeks' gestation, patients who later developed preeclampsia excreted significantly less urinary calcium than patients who remained normotensive. This reduction persisted throughout gestation. The difference in the incidence (87%) of preeclampsia between pregnant women with calcium excretion values at or below the threshold of 195 mg/24 h and those with values above that level (2%) was highly significant.

Because tubular function is impaired at an earlier stage of the preeclamptic disease process than glomerular function, the urinary calcium:creatinine (U_{ca}/U_{cr}) ratio has been used for the early diagnosis of preeclampsia. Rodriguez and colleagues[36] assessed the value of the U_{ca}/U_{cr} ratio between 24 and 34 weeks' gestation. A U_{ca}/U_{cr} ratio of 0.04 or less was reported to have a sensitivity of 70%, a specificity of 95%, a positive predictive value of 64%, and a negative predictive value of 96% (11.4% incidence of preeclampsia). In contrast, Hutchesson and coworkers[37] and several other investigators[28] were unable to demonstrate a reduction in urinary calcium excretion in preeclamptic women prior to the onset of hypertension and renal involvement. Masse and colleagues[32] found no difference in urinary cal-

cium excretion between preeclamptic and normotensive patients.

On the whole, measuring urinary calcium excretion appears to be of little or no value in the early diagnosis or prediction of preeclampsia.

Human Chorionic Gonadotropin (hCG). Some studies found elevated levels of β-hCG in pregnancy-induced hypertensive disorders, and it has been suggested that β-hCG determination may have value for the early diagnosis of preeclampsia.[38, 39]

The results of a large study were published by Muller and associates.[40] In a prospective trisomy 21 hCG screening program, data from 5776 patients were examined to assess the relationship between hCG and pregnancy-induced hypertension (PIH; n = 234), preeclampsia (n = 34), and small-for-gestational-age (SGA) neonates (n = 236); hCG levels (multiples of the median) were higher in the three populations with pathologic disorders. This difference was statistically significant in patients with SGA neonates and preeclampsia but not in those with PIH. The authors do not provide data to calculate the positive predictive value, but their data do show that with an hCG cut-off value of 2 multiples of the median, 10% of the population would be considered at risk and 30% of preeclampsia cases would be identified. With an hCG cut-off value of 1 multiple of the median, 50% of the population would be considered at risk and 100% of preeclampsia cases would be identified.

Overall, most studies have found a large scatter and a considerable overlap between β-hCG levels in normotensive and hypertensive pregnancies. Thus, the clinical value of β-hCG measurements for predicting or monitoring pregnancy-induced hypertensive disorders seems limited at the most.[28]

Hematologic Markers

Factor VIII–Related Antigen/Factor VIIIc. The ratio of factor VIII–related antigen to factor VIIIc (fVIIIrag/fVIIIc ratio) in healthy subjects is 1.0 by definition. An increase in the numerator of this ratio, the fVIIIrag, is associated with endothelial release of this antigen. Several authors have demonstrated an early rise of the fVIIIrag/fVIIIc ratio in pregnancy-induced hypertensive disease and a positive correlation between the magnitude of increase of the ratio and the severity of the disease, the degree of hyperuricemia, placental infarcts, adverse perinatal outcome, and a strong negative correlation between this ratio and platelet life span. The increase in fVIIIrag, and thereby the ratio, is most pronounced in preeclampsia associated with fetal growth retardation. Endothelial release of fVIIIrag is not increased in chronic hypertension.

Measuring fVIIIrag or the fVIIIrag/fVIIIc ratio is a useful and quite sensitive indicator of both the severity and the degree of endothelial cell damage and the extent of placental insufficiency in pregnancy-induced hypertensive disorders. The ratio correlates with fetal growth retardation and perinatal morbidity and mortality. In time, the increase in fVIIIrag runs parallel with the increase in serum uric acid levels and the increase in blood pressure.[28, 41]

Fibronectin. Fibronectin is a major cell-surface glycoprotein. The soluble form in plasma is mainly synthesized by endothelial cells and hepatocytes. Plasma levels of fibronectin are similar to or just slightly increased in normal pregnancy compared with levels in nonpregnant individuals. Because pregnant women with chronic hypertension have normal fibronectin levels, the increase in plasma fibronectin is not simply a consequence of hypertension. In established preeclampsia, most studies show consistently an approximately twofold to threefold increase in plasma fibronectin levels.[28, 41] The exact source of the increased fibronectin levels is uncertain; it may reflect (1) endothelial cell damage or activation in the uteroplacental or systemic circulation, or in both or (2) increased hepatocyte production, or it may be a sign of placental damage.

Ballegeer and coworkers[42] compared plasma fibronectin, plasminogen activator inhibitor–1 (PAI-1), fVIIIrag, and uric acid and concluded that fibronectin is the best predictor of preeclampsia. Evaluating the presence of increased fibronectin levels at 25 to 32 weeks' gestation in the early diagnosis of preeclampsia, they found a sensitivity of 96% and a specificity of 94%. According to these authors,[42] the increase in plasma fibronectin antedates the increase in blood pressure by 4 to 6 weeks on average.

Previously, we found that elevated fibronectin precedes the increase in blood pressure by about 4 weeks in patients with gestational hypertension and about 12 weeks in patients with subsequent preeclampsia. Measuring fibronectin levels is feasible with immunochemistry techniques that are available in most hospitals and may be helpful in the early diagnosis of preeclampsia, especially the severe early-onset type.[28, 32, 43]

Platelet Count. Platelet life span is significantly shorter in pregnancy-induced hypertensive disorders, in particular when complicated by fetal growth retardation, than in uncomplicated pregnancies. In preeclamptic women, the fall in the platelet count coincides more or less with the increase in uric acid levels, and both precede the development of proteinuria by about 3 weeks. The standard deviations in the number of circulating platelets in normotensive and hypertensive pregnant women preclude the use of platelet counts as an effective method for early detection in low-risk nulliparous women.[28, 41]

Hemoglobin Level, Hematocrit, Mean Corpuscular Volume. Abnormally high hemoglobin and hematocrit (Hb/Hct) levels are a better predictor of adverse perinatal outcome than abnormally low estriol or human placental lactogen (hPL) levels. High maternal Hb/Hct levels are associated with low birth weight and placental weight, increased incidence of prematurity and perinatal mortality, and increased peripheral vascular resistance, and the degree of maternal hypertension. Serial measurements of Hb/Hct are definitely useful in monitoring pregnancies at high risk for uteroplacental insufficiency and in monitoring the course of disease in established pregnancy-induced hypertensive disorders or pregnancies complicated by fetal growth retardation, or both. Marked elevation of hemoglobin levels in the second trimester precedes the development of pregnancy-induced hypertensive disorders and is useful as a predictor. The predictive value of less pronounced hemoglobin levels is low.[32, 44]

Doppler Ultrasound Assessment of the Uteroplacental Circulation

The absence or presence of physiologic changes in the uteroplacental vessels is the pathophysiologic basis for the use of Doppler flow studies in the early diagnosis of preeclampsia. The increase of the uteroplacental flow velocity waveform resistance indices correlates with the results of pathologic examination of the placental bed and placentas. These pathologic vascular changes exist in a significant proportion of normotensive pregnancies complicated by fetal growth retardation.

Indices (resistance index = RI) of uteroplacental blood flow velocity waveforms (FVWs) decrease in early pregnancy until 20 to 26 weeks' gestation and then remain stable to term. The high end-diastolic blood flow velocity and low ratios during the last half of pregnancy reflect the low peripheral resistance of the uteroplacental vascular bed. There is no standard method of reporting uteroplacental FVWs.

Pearce and McParland[45] suggested that both sides of the uterus should be examined and the FVWs reported as follows:

1. Uniform low resistance: FVWs from both sides of the uterus have a RI less than 0.58.
2. Uniform high resistance: FVWs from both sides of the uterus have a RI greater than 0.58.
3. Mixed resistance pattern: One waveform (almost invariably that from the placental side) is of low resistance (RI < 0.58); the waveform from the other side is of high resistance.

There is more information in the waveform shape than just an FVW index. The presence or absence of a notch is especially important in this respect. The early diastolic notch of uteroplacental FVWs has been reported in normal pregnancy until approximately 26 weeks' gestation.[45] On the placental side of the uterus, it is rarely found after 20 weeks' gestation.

In 1986, Campbell and colleagues[46] were the first to report on the use of uteroplacental Doppler velocimetry as a screening test in early pregnancy for hypertension, fetal growth retardation, and fetal asphyxia. This first study yielded extremely promising results. The excellent predictive value found in this study was caused by a complication rate of 25% in the study group.

The studies currently reported in the literature concerning the clinical value of Doppler ultrasound evaluation of the uteroplacental circulation have resulted in widely varying results. These variations may be related to wide differences in technique as well as to different definitions of pregnancy-induced hypertensive disorders, fetal growth retardation, fetal distress, and adverse perinatal outcome. However, the major reason for the various conclusions concerning the value of Doppler FVWs of the utero-

placental vessels is probably that investigators used different selection processes in dividing populations with a normal or abnormal uteroplacental Doppler flow pattern. Abnormality was sometimes based on the worst FVW, an average, the four-site averaged RI, or even the best FVW. The scattered occurrence of "preeclamptic lesions" in the spiral arteries suggests that it is more logical to look for the worst Doppler flow patterns, and indeed investigators using the worst FVW have consistently reported the best results with uteroplacental Doppler in the early detection of preeclampsia.

The results of Doppler ultrasound examination of the uteroplacental circulation as a screening test for any degree of hypertension are disappointing, but in the early detection of severe preeclampsia associated with adverse perinatal outcome, uteroplacental Doppler has had a high sensitivity.[47] Other advantages are that it is relatively easy to use, inexpensive, and noninvasive. Doppler flow studies can be done in early pregnancy and are suitable for therapeutic intervention in an attempt to reduce the incidence of preeclampsia and its complications.

The results of several studies with color Doppler flow velocimetry in the early diagnosis of preeclampsia have been promising. Harrington and associates[48] found that bilateral notching at 19 to 21 weeks' gestation had a sensitivity of more than 70% and a positive predictive value of 27%, 31.2%, and 37.5%, respectively, for preeclampsia, SGA babies, and any complication. In another study of 652 women with singleton pregnancies, Harrington and colleagues[49] demonstrated that the presence of bilateral notching at the end of the first trimester (12–16 weeks' gestation) was associated with a typical odds ratio of 42 (95% confidence interval [CI] 5.66–312) for developing preeclampsia later in pregnancy.

Thus, at the moment no good tests are available for predicting preeclampsia. Doppler ultrasound evaluation of the uteroplacental circulation as an overall screening method and (serial) measurement of fibronectin levels in high-risk patients are probably the best tests available at the moment.

Intervention and Correction of Pathophysiologic Changes

To date, strategies aimed at secondary prevention of pregnancy-induced hypertensive disorders have all focused on mechanisms thought to be involved in the disease process.

Sodium Restriction and Diuretics

The use of prophylactic sodium restriction or administration of diuretics, or both, in an attempt to prevent pregnancy-induced hypertensive disorders was based on the hypothesis that sodium retention was an etiologic factor. Possibly the most ardent advocate of the view that salt plays a crucial role in eclampsia was De Snoo (1877–1949), a Dutch obstetrician. By the late 1940s, it was considered daring to allow pregnant women, especially those with "toxemia," to eat a diet containing a normal amount of salt. Despite many enthusiastic clinical reports, no convincing evidence has ever been produced that salt restriction helps to prevent hypertension during pregnancy.[50]

In a controlled, albeit poorly, study of more than 2000 women, preeclampsia occurred twice as often in women advised to take less salt compared with women told to take salt supplementation.[51] Van Buul and coworkers,[52] studying the effects of long-term sodium restriction on pregnancy outcome in healthy nulliparous pregnant women, found no differences in the incidence of hypertension or in birth weight. Excessive water and salt retention is a secondary feature of preeclampsia, caused by a shift in the renal pressure–natriuresis curve as well as by endothelial cell damage with subsequent vasoconstriction and increased microvascular permeability.[34] Strict sodium restriction decreases blood pressure, probably by decreasing intracellular free calcium in the vascular smooth muscle cells,[53] but also results in a decrease in the circulating plasma volume. Actually, no attempts by the medical profession to prescribe dietary restriction of weight gain (e.g., by a low-calorie, low-carbohydrate, and low-salt diet) have ever been demonstrated to have a beneficial effect with respect to prevention of preeclampsia.[53, 54]

In the 1960s, interest in dietary salt restriction waned somewhat as a result of the introduction of diuretic drugs. During that decade, prophylactic administration of diuretics was actively investigated. Collins and coworkers[55] analyzed 10 prospective, randomized trials of diuretic therapy administered primarily for edema or rapid weight gain, or for both. The analysis of these studies, involving 7000 women, appeared to indicate a significant reduction in the incidence of "preeclampsia." As noted by these authors, at least two major methodologic difficulties precluded a firm conclusion. First, the criteria used for the diagnosis "preeclampsia" were unreliable or even not stated. Second, because diuretics can be expected to decrease blood pressure and reduce edema, such therapy may simply mask two of the diagnostic signs of pregnancy-induced hypertensive disorders without altering the presence and course of the underlying disease and its adverse impact.

Consequently, Collins and coworkers[55] used a more direct method of assessment of the potential benefits of diuretic therapy by analyzing perinatal outcome and the incidence of preeclampsia. Perinatal death rates were 1.9% in the control group and 1.7% in the diuretic-treated women. Administration of diuretics had no effect on the incidence of preeclampsia. Further evaluation of potential adverse drug effects did not reveal significant differences between treated and control subjects. In the diuretic therapy group, several cases of neonatal thrombocytopenia and jaundice as well as maternal electrolyte imbalance and pancreatitis (including four fatal cases) were reported. Thus, the balance of risk-benefit considerations contraindicates the use of prophylactic diuretic treatment during pregnancy.[56]

Magnesium Supplementation

The use of magnesium sulfate in the prevention or treatment of convulsions in severe preeclampsia-eclampsia has led to the hypothesis that antepartum magnesium supplementation might have beneficial effects on the incidence of preeclampsia. However, magnesium intake does not appear to influence the incidence of preeclampsia or fetal growth retardation,[57] and randomized, placebo-controlled studies[58] have not shown any reduction in the incidence of preeclampsia.

Zinc Supplementation

Zinc is an essential element in oxidative metabolism, deoxyribonucleic acid (DNA) and ribonucleic acid (RNA) synthesis, immunocompetence, and membrane stabilization. Placental and plasma zinc levels have been reported to be reduced in preeclampsia (but not in pregnant women with chronic hypertension), and maternal plasma zinc levels have been reported to correlate with birth weight.[59] Other investigators found no significant changes in serum and erythrocyte zinc concentrations in women with pregnancy-induced hypertensive disorders.

Results from two zinc supplementation trials for prevention of pregnancy-induced hypertensive disorders are inconsistent. Hunt and colleagues[60] reported that zinc supplementation reduced the occurrence of "pregnancy-induced hypertension" (2.3% versus 15.5%) in Mexican-American women. These results must be viewed with some caution as far as preeclampsia is concerned; women with "pregnancy-induced hypertension" did not all necessarily have true preeclampsia. Moreover, the occurrence of hypertension was not related to serum zinc concentrations.

Mahomed and associates[61] found no significant difference in the incidence of pregnancy-induced hypertensive disorders between mothers given zinc supplementation (4.6%) and those given a placebo (1.3%). Even if further studies provide definite proof that severe preeclampsia is associated with lower plasma zinc levels, this decrease is probably just a consequence of the concurrent hypoalbuminemia.

Zinc supplementation appears to be of no use in preventing pregnancy-induced hypertensive disorders, and because zinc deficiency is extremely rare in the diet of women in developed countries, routine supplementation beyond 15 mg/day (the recommended daily allowance) is not warranted at this time.[59]

Protein Supplementation

Until the 1930s, the fashion was to restrict dietary proteins in "toxemia," presumably to avoid metabolic "toxins." After the 1930s, a new hypothesis emerged in which a lack of dietary protein was held responsible for causing pregnancy-induced hypertensive disorders. This concept seems to have arisen from observations of hypoproteinemia in preeclamptic women. However, several surveys have found no relation between daily protein intake and the incidence of pregnancy-induced hypertensive disorders (reviewed by Green[54]). Controlled studies have not revealed any convincing benefit of protein supplementation in the prevention of pregnancy-induced hypertensive disorders.

Calcium Supplementation

In the 1930s, Theobald stated that toxemia was the result of "an absolute or relative insufficiency of some substance or substances in the diet, the most important of which is calcium" (reviewed by Green[54]). Epidemiologic studies suggested that the incidence of eclampsia is inversely proportional to nutritional calcium intake.[59] However, most studies on calcium-deficient pregnant women come from developing countries, where overall nutrition is deficient or inadequate in a significant percentage of the population. Also, in the majority of these countries, the prenatal care system is not optimal, and this may be a confounding factor in the epidemiologic analysis of the impact of nutritional calcium intake on the incidence of eclampsia.

Data from several studies provide evidence against the hypothesis of nutritional deficiencies, including a deficient calcium intake, as a specific etiologic or pathogenetic factor. No consistent differences in vitamin or mineral content between the diets of preeclamptic and nonpreeclamptic women have emerged from the more convincing dietary surveys.

Thomson[62] found that the diets of women with preeclampsia tended to contain less vitamin C than diets of normotensive or hypertensive women and more of other vitamins and calcium. In addition, it has been argued that the substantially lower incidence of pregnancy-induced hypertensive disorders in second and subsequent pregnancies is difficult to reconcile with nutritional deficiencies. In the Dutch "hunger winter" of 1944–1945, when overall nutritional intake and calcium intake were less than minimal, the incidence of eclampsia decreased.

In 1991, Repke[59] reviewed the results of four calcium supplementation studies available at that time. He concluded that calcium supplementation results in a significant reduction in blood pressure, preterm delivery, and preeclampsia. However, most of these studies were too small to draw any definite conclusions, and most studies focused on a decrease in blood pressure and the incidence of gestational hypertension, not on prevention of genuine preeclampsia.

In 1991, Belizan and coworkers[63] reported on the largest calcium supplementation trial completed so far. They studied 1194 nulliparous women who were in the 20th week of gestation at the beginning of the study. The women were randomly allocated to receive 2 g/day of elemental calcium (n = 593, calcium carbonate) or placebo (n = 601). The rates of hypertensive disorders were lower in the calcium group than in the placebo group (9.8% versus 14.8%; odds ratio [OR] 0.63; 95% CI 0.44–0.90). The risk of hypertensive disorders was lower at all times during gestation, particularly after the 28th week of gestation. According to the authors, the incidence of both gestational hypertension and preeclampsia was reduced. The incidence of preeclampsia in the calcium group was 2.6%, and in the placebo group 3.9%, a minor difference with a 95% CI of 0.35 to 1.25 for the OR. Perinatal death rate was similar in the calcium group (n = 6), compared with the placebo group (n = 7). Birth weight and length in both groups were identical. The incidence of preterm delivery was similar.

In a meta-analysis, Bucher and associates[64] reviewed the effect of calcium supplementation during pregnancy on blood pressure, preeclampsia, and adverse outcomes of pregnancy. The authors searched MEDLINE and EMBASE for 1966 to May 1994 and contacted authors of eligible trials to ensure accuracy and completeness of data and to identify unpublished trials. Fourteen randomized trials involving 2459 women were eligible. The pooled analysis showed a reduction in systolic blood pressure of 5.40 mmHg (95% CI −7.81 to −3.00 mmHg; P < .001) and in diastolic blood pressure of 3.44 mmHg (95% CI −5.20 to −1.68 mmHg; P < .001). The OR for preeclampsia in women with calcium supplementation compared with placebo was 0.38 (95% CI 0.22–0.65). Thus, it was concluded that calcium supplementation during pregnancy leads to an important reduction in systolic and diastolic blood pressure and preeclampsia.

However, a large case-control study on 172 women with preeclampsia, 251 women with gestational hypertension, and 505 controls, all primiparae who delivered in Quebec or Montreal,[65] demonstrated no correlation between calcium intake and the incidence of preeclampsia. For gestational hypertension, adjusted ORs in successive quartiles gradually decreased from 1.00 in the lowest quartile to 0.81, 0.66, and 0.60 in the highest quartile. Thus, the authors concluded that their data provided strong support for the view that calcium intake is inversely related to the risk of gestational hypertension but not to the incidence of preeclampsia.

The definitive answer on the effects of calcium supplementation was published by Levine and coworkers in 1997.[66] Their work concerned the results of the National Institutes of Health (NIH) Calcium for Preeclampsia Prevention (CPEP) trial conducted in five large medical centers. The decision to embark on this large trial was based partly on the fact that most trials so far had been conducted in countries where, unlike in the United States, the usual diet contains little calcium. The investigators randomized 4589 patients who were 13 to 21 weeks' pregnant to receive daily treatment with either 2 g of elemental calcium or placebo for the remainder of their pregnancies. Calcium supplementation did not significantly reduce the incidence or severity of preeclampsia or delay its onset. Preeclampsia occurred in 6.9% of the women in the calcium group and in 7.3% in the placebo group. In addition, there was no significant difference between the two groups in the prevalence of pregnancy-associated hypertension without preeclampsia or of all hypertensive disorders. Calcium did not reduce the numbers of preterm deliveries, SGA infants, or fetal and neonatal deaths. They also detected no benefit in women with low baseline 24-hour calcium excretion levels, nor was there any benefit among women whose baseline dietary calcium intake was in the lowest quintile and whose median daily intake of 422 mg was similar to or less than that reported for women in many developing countries.

Table 5–1 represents the data on the effects of calcium supplementation as published in the meta-analysis by Bucher's group[64] and in the NIH trial.[66]

The most recent update of the Cochrane Library[66a] on preventative effects of calcium supplementation includes nine studies and more than 6000 women. The data show a modest reduction in the risk of preeclampsia (relative risk [RR] 0.72; 95% CI, 0.60–0.86). The effect was greatest for women at high risk for hypertension (RR, 0.22; 95% CI, 0.11–0.43) and those with low baseline calcium intake (RR 0.32; 95% CI, 0.21–0.49). The results for high-risk subjects remain equivocal, since only 225 women have been analyzed so far.[66b] The idea that calcium dietary intake is the most important con-

TABLE 5-1. EFFECT OF CALCIUM SUPPLEMENTATION ON PREECLAMPSIA

PREECLAMPSIA	CALCIUM	PLACEBO	ODDS RATIO	95% CI
Small studies[64]*	35/1099	88/1176	0.40	0.27–0.60
NIH trial[66]†	158/2295	168/2294	0.94	0.76–1.16
All studies	193/3394	256/3475	0.76	0.62–0.92

*Meta-analysis of small trials.
†NIH Calcium for Preeclampsia Prevention (CPEP) trial.
CI, confidence interval; NIH, National Institutes of Health.

founder in assessing the effects of calcium supplementation is supported by the significant protective effects of calcium supplementation in developed countries with a low calcium intake, such as Australia,[66c] versus complete absence of any beneficial effect of calcium supplementation in developed countries with a high calcium intake.[35] Two important (related) facts have to be emphasized:

1. Countries with a high calcium intake (United States, The Netherlands) still have their share of preeclampsia, especially that type of preeclampsia that kills babies and mothers.
2. Preventing a definition (i.e., hypertension and proteinuria) is not the same as improving perinatal outcome.

The Cochrane review[66a] shows that calcium supplementation does not improve perinatal outcome. Is there a place for calcium supplementation? Calcium supplementation does not improve perinatal outcome but may, by reducing the prevalence of near term preeclampsia, result in cost savings, a relevant benefit in countries with limited health care budgets.

Antihypertensive Drugs
The effects of antihypertensive drugs have been assessed by studying the effect on development of severe preeclampsia in women presenting with mild or moderate hypertensive disease. This approach is based on the premise that early treatment of hypertension may forestall the appearance of other manifestations of preeclampsia. However, the placental, renal, hepatic, and hemostatic features of preeclampsia do not appear to be a direct consequence of elevated blood pressure. Although it is clear that the use of antihypertensive drugs in women with mild to moderate hypertension reduces the incidence of severe hypertension, these drugs have no beneficial effect on the incidence of preeclampsia or perinatal death.[56]

Anticoagulants
Because excessive thrombin action and intravascular fibrin deposition were once thought to be the primary mechanism in the pathogenesis of preeclampsia, women with established pregnancy-induced hypertensive disorders have been treated with anticoagulants in an attempt to improve clinical course and perinatal outcome. Heparin used in uncontrolled studies involving single cases, or small series of patients, has been demonstrated to be of no use in secondary or tertiary prevention. Anecdotal reports on the use of coumarins to prevent recurrent preeclampsia in multiparous women have not demonstrated any beneficial maternal or perinatal effect. In addition, the use of anticoagulants may be dangerous in cases of severe hypertension, especially if associated with thrombocytopenia.[56, 67]

Low-Dose Aspirin for Correction of Prostacyclin/Thromboxane A_2 Imbalance
Whether the endothelial cell injury in preeclampsia causes primarily a decrease in prostacyclin (PGI_2) synthesis or a decrease in, for example, nitric oxide (NO), platelets play a central role in the disease process. Redman[68] stated "preeclampsia is a trophoblast-dependent process mediated by platelet dysfunction and prevented at least in part by antiplatelet agents." On the virtually nonendothelialized surface of the spiral arteries in the absence of an adequate production of antiaggregatory PGI_2 or nitric oxide by the uteroplacental vasculature or endovascular trophoblast, surface-mediated platelet activation may be expected to occur. Platelets adhere and release alpha-granule and dense granule constituents. Thromboxane A_2 (TXA_2) and serotonin are generated,[69]

contributing to platelet aggregation and inducing the formation of fibrin to stabilize the platelet thrombus that may occlude maternal blood flow to a placental cotyledon, thus leading to placental infarction. The absence of the normal stimulation of the renin-angiotensin system, despite significant hypovolemia, and the increased vascular sensitivity to angiotensin II and norepinephrine[70] can be explained by a single mechanism: endothelial cell injury causing a deficiency in production or activity of vasodilator prostaglandins, in particular PGI_2, or in both. The increased TXA_2/PGI_2 ratio may be the cause of the selective platelet destruction, sometimes accompanied by microangiopathic hemolysis, and the reduced uteroplacental blood flow with spiral artery thrombosis and placental infarction. Because the PGI_2/TXA_2 imbalance provides an explanation for many of the clinical manifestations of preeclampsia, several attempts have been made to correct this imbalance or to diminish its consequences.[71–74]

Aspirin induces a long-lasting functional defect in platelets, which is primarily, if not exclusively, related to the permanent inactivation of platelet cyclooxygenase activity and inhibition of the resultant platelet secretory reaction. Aspirin acetylates the hydroxyl group of a single serine residue at the active site of the cyclooxygenase enzyme. Because the acetyl group of aspirin is covalently bound to the active site of cyclooxygenase, inhibition of the enzyme is irreversible. The aspirin metabolite salicylate binds reversibly at or close to the active site in a way that prevents enzyme acetylation by aspirin. However, the concentration effects profiles of aspirin and salicylate in vivo suggest that salicylate protection of cyclooxygenase is an improbable pharmacodynamic interaction following oral aspirin in humans.[75] TXA_2 is synthesized and released by platelets in response to a variety of stimuli (e.g., thrombin, collagen, adenosine diphosphate) and in turn induces irreversible platelet aggregation. Thus, it provides a mechanism for amplifying the platelet response to such diverse agonists.

The anucleate platelet is a unique cellular target for the action of aspirin. Platelets cannot resynthesize cyclooxygenase because they lack nuclei. Thus, because of the irreversible nature of the aspirin-induced enzyme inhibition, doses that incompletely inhibit TXA_2, when given acutely, cumulate to complete inhibition during chronic drug administration. Thus, the daily administration of 30 to 50 mg of aspirin results in virtually complete suppression of platelet TXA_2 biosynthesis after 7 to 10 days in nonpregnant patients.

Several studies have demonstrated that 60 to 80 mg of aspirin is also enough to inhibit cyclooxygenase-dependent platelet aggregation, release reaction, and serum TXA_2 production in normal pregnancy and in gestational hypertension.[76–78] Recovery of the ability to generate TXA_2 depends on the synthesis of new platelets, taking 10 to 12 days for a complete turnover.[75] The optimal antithrombotic dose of aspirin remains disputed. Doses as high as 3.5 g/day and as low as 20 to 40 mg/day have been reported to be effective in preventing thrombotic events. In the case of aspirin, it is of particular importance to use the lowest effective dose because of its concomitant effect on vessel wall cyclooxygenase and the relation between the aspirin dose and especially gastrointestinal side effects.[75] Aspirin also inhibits endothelial cyclooxygenase; however, the vessel wall may be less sensitive and has the capacity to synthesize new cyclooxygenase when aspirin is removed from the system.

Another mechanism involved in the causation of the "paradoxical" selectivity of low-dose aspirin on platelet cyclooxygenase is based on the pharmacokinetic characteristics of this drug. Absorption of a low oral dose of aspirin causes relatively high concentrations in the portal circulation, leading to a cumulative inhibition of cyclooxygenase in platelets passing through the gut capillaries, whereas the concentration in the peripheral circulation (after deacetylation of aspirin in the liver) remains too low to affect endothelial cyclooxygenase.[79] Actually, the inhibition of cyclooxygenase is rapid, occurring even before the appearance of aspirin in the systemic circulation, which demonstrates the importance of the inactivation of platelet cyclooxygenase in the portal circulation.[78]

Thus, the antiplatelet effect of aspirin is unrelated to its systemic bioavailability. Increasing the dose of aspirin may influence other components of interactions between platelets and endothelium that might help prevent or limit thrombus formation, but larger doses have other potentially deleterious effects.[78] Analgesic doses of aspirin may exert some fibrinolytic effects, but low-dose aspirin has no demonstrable effect in this respect.[78, 80] Aspirin does not inhibit adenosine diphosphate–induced platelet alpha-granule release.[81]

Aspirin exerts more effects that are of potential therapeutic value in preventing preeclampsia. In a clinical study of pregnant women at risk of preeclampsia, Walsh and associates[82] demonstrated that low-dose aspirin resulted in significant reductions in the maternal plasma concentrations of both TXA_2 and lipid peroxides. The inhibitory effect was much greater on TXA_2 levels than on lipid peroxide levels because sources other than cyclooxygenase contribute to lipid peroxide formation. This study provided evidence that lipid peroxide formation is at least partially coupled to TXA_2 production by the enzyme cyclooxygenase. Low-dose aspirin therapy for preeclampsia may exert beneficial effects because of this dual inhibitory action.[21]

Considering the potential involvement of abnormal leukocyte-endothelium interaction in the pathogenesis of preeclampsia,[12] another effect of aspirin on platelet-induced endothelial release of IL-8 deserves special notion. Kaplanski and colleagues[83] demonstrated that platelets induce IL-8 secretion by endothelial cells via membrane-associated IL-1 activity. Aspirin was found to inhibit platelet-induced endothelial release of IL-8 by 90%.

Low-Dose Aspirin in the Prevention of Pregnancy-Induced Hypertensive Disorders. In 1979, the results of a retrospective study suggested that preeclampsia occurred less frequently in regular aspirin users than in non–aspirin-using pregnant women.[84] Low-dose aspirin has been demonstrated to restore, at least partially, vascular refractoriness in angiotensin II–sensitive pregnant women.[85, 86]

In 1985, Beaufils and coworkers[87] published the first preliminary results of a prospective study on the effects of low-dose aspirin in preventing preeclampsia. The conclusion of a review of the first seven low-dose aspirin trials in identified high-risk patients[88] was that low-dose aspirin appeared to be effective in reducing the incidence of gestational hypertension (−30%), preeclampsia (−85%), and fetal growth retardation (−50%). Most of these studies used the obstetric history to identify high-risk patients; other studies used Doppler velo-

cimetry of the uteroplacental circulation, the angiotensin II infusion test, and even the roll-over test for this purpose. Although the results of these randomized trials were very promising, evidence of a beneficial effect of low-dose aspirin was inconclusive because of the limited size of these earlier studies. Thus, a whole series of larger trials was initiated in order to confirm or refute the very promising results found by the small trials in high-risk patients. The subsequent paragraphs review these larger trials in some detail.

Italian Low-Dose Aspirin Trial. Parazzini and associates[89] reported on the results of the multicenter Italian low-dose aspirin trial in women judged to be at moderate risk for preeclampsia. Women were included according to prophylactic criteria—age under 18 or over 40 years, chronic hypertension, nephropathy, history of pregnancy-induced hypertensive disorders or fetal growth retardation, and twin pregnancy—or therapeutic criteria—elevated blood pressure or early signs of fetal growth retardation in current pregnancy; 583 women were randomized for low-dose aspirin (50 mg) treatment, and the other 523 women in this trial received *no* treatment. The authors found no significant differences between the no-treatment and aspirin groups in numbers of stillbirths, perinatal mortality, birth weight, or births before 37 weeks' gestation, and the groups did not differ in the frequency of pregnancy-induced hypertensive disorders with or without proteinuria (51 [15.2%] versus 81 [19.3%]). Because the trial was not double-blinded or placebo-controlled, bias may have been introduced. Actually, this was the first study that reported negative findings regarding low-dose aspirin. The number of patients lost to follow-up in the no-treatment group (46/523; 8.8%) was significantly greater than those in the aspirin-treated group (18/583; 3.1%). The investigators state that "this difference suggests that clinicians followed women randomized to the active group more carefully."

Louden[90] stated that the difference may be attributable to some patients allocated to the no-treatment group electing to leave the study, either because they wanted to take aspirin or to seek antenatal care from a physician willing to prescribe active treatment. The fact that patients with the strongest motivation for such behavior would be those at the highest risk introduces a serious bias.

Another explanation for the discrepancy between the earlier studies and this study—and this is also true for the majority of the other large trials—is that trials that showed reduced incidence of preeclampsia covered women at higher average risk than the women in the Italian study; in earlier trials, rates of preeclampsia among controls ranged form 11% to 35%, compared with 2.7% reported by Parazzini and associates.[89] An additional problem with this Italian study might be the dose of aspirin that was used, namely 50 mg/day. According to Walsh,[21] this dose of aspirin may have been insufficient to reach the placenta to inhibit placental TXA_2 and lipid peroxide biosynthesis, which may account for its lack of effect in this study. If the placental production of lipid peroxides is not sufficiently inhibited, these lipid peroxides might act as a continuing and powerful stimulus for further placental TXA_2 synthesis.

Birmingham Study. The Birmingham Study reported by Hauth and coworkers[91] was initiated to assess the effect of low-dose aspirin in preventing preeclampsia in 600 healthy nulliparous women with a singleton gestation between 20 and 22 weeks' gestation. Compliance was checked by measuring serum TXB_2 levels. At randomization, serum TXB_2 level medians were similar in both groups. TXB_2 levels in the aspirin group decreased significantly from baseline level at 29 to 31 weeks, 34 to 36 weeks, and at delivery as compared with an overall increase in the placebo group. The overall incidence of hypertension was similar in all three groups: the aspirin group, the placebo group, and the noncompliant group. However, preeclampsia developed in five of 302 women (1.7%) who received aspirin versus 17 of 302 (5.6%) who received the placebo ($P = .009$). Preeclampsia was severe in one aspirin and in six placebo recipients ($P = .06$).

National Institute of Child Health and Human Development (NICHD) Maternal-Fetal Medicine Network Study. This study assessed the effects of low-dose aspirin in low-risk nulliparous pregnant women.[92] A total of 4241 eligible women were assigned to a single-blind compliance test. Each woman was given 10 placebo tablets with instructions to take one tablet daily and to return 10 days later. A woman was considered compliant if she had ingested at least *half* the tablets. A total of 3135 women found to be compliant in this test were randomly assigned to receive aspirin (60 mg) or placebo.

The incidence of preeclampsia was lower in the aspirin group (4.6%) than in the placebo group (6.3%) (relative risk 0.7; 95% CI 0.6 to 1.0; $P = .05$), whereas the incidence of gestational hypertension was 6.7% and 5.9%, respectively. Aspirin appeared to have a greater prophylactic effect in the subgroup of 519 women with higher systolic blood pressure (120–134 mmHg) and little effect with baseline blood pressure below 120 mmHg. The incidence among the women with initially higher systolic blood pressures was 5.6% in the aspirin group versus 11.9% in the placebo group ($P = .01$).

The incidence of severe preeclampsia was lower (n = 29; 2%) in the aspirin group than in the placebo group (n = 45; 3%). Eight women had eclampsia (three in the aspirin group and 5 in the placebo group), and six had HELLP syndrome (one in the aspirin group and five in the placebo group). If severe preeclampsia, HELLP syndrome, and eclampsia are counted as serious maternal morbidity, 33 (2.2%) patients in the aspirin group versus 55 (3.7%) in the placebo group had complicated or severe disease.

This has been the only study so far that found an increased incidence of abruptio placentae (placental abruption) among women receiving aspirin (11 women, versus two in the placebo group; $P = .01$).

The CLASP Trial. In the Collaborative Low-Dose Aspirin Study in Pregnancy (CLASP) study,[93] 9364 women were randomly assigned 60 mg of aspirin daily or matching placebo; 74% were entered for prophylaxis of preeclampsia, 12% for prophylaxis of fetal growth retardation, 12% for treatment of preeclampsia, and 3% for treatment of fetal growth retardation. In this study, women were eligible if they were between 12 and 32 weeks' gestation and if there were *no* clear indications *for* or *against* the use of aspirin. For the purposes of analysis, women remained in the treatment group to which they had been originally allocated; that is, intention-to-treat analyses were reported.

Overall, the use of aspirin was associated with a reduction of only 12% in the incidence of preeclampsia, which was not significant. In the women entered for prophylactic reasons at 20 weeks' gestation or earlier, the use of aspirin was associated with a reduction of 22%. The use of aspirin after 20 weeks' gestation in the CLASP study was, if anything, associated with increased perinatal mortality.[93] The incidence of eclampsia was similar in both groups; the incidence of HELLP syndrome was not mentioned. There was no significant effect of aspirin use on the incidence of fetal growth retardation or stillbirth and neonatal death. Aspirin did, however, significantly reduce the likelihood of preterm delivery (19.7% aspirin group versus 22.2% control group; absolute reduction of 2.5 ± 0.9 per 100 women treated; $P = .003$). There was a significant trend ($P = .004$) toward progressively greater reductions in preeclamspia the more preterm the delivery. There were similar significant trends to less use of antihypertensive and anticonvulsant therapy among aspirin-treated women who delivered early. In an analysis of patients entered for prophylaxis of preeclampsia, the rates of stillbirth or neonatal death attributed to preeclampsia, hypertension, or fetal growth retardation that occurred before 32 weeks' gestation, when the effect of preventing early-onset disease should be the greatest, were 5.3% among women allocated aspirin compared with 10.6% among those allocated placebo.

Not shown in the original paper[93] but revealed to the Working Group[94] was another post hoc analysis showing that the protective effects of aspirin were associated with gestational age at entry; the earlier the treatment was started, the greater was the observed protection. These data are inconsistent with the results of Wallenburg's trial,[95] which showed large protective effects after 28 weeks' gestation, or with those of McParland and colleagues,[96] which showed a protective effect of aspirin given after 24 weeks' gestation. The CLASP results, in contrast, suggest that if there is any benefit, it may be prophylactic rather than therapeutic.

The ECPPA Trial. The ECPPA[97] study group initiated a large multicenter study (12 teaching maternity hospitals and 182 obstetricians' offices) in Latin America in order to determine the effectiveness of aspirin in women at high risk of adverse outcomes associated with preeclampsia. One thousand nine women considered to be at high risk for the development of preeclampsia, or its complications, entered the study between 12 and 32 weeks' gestation. Women were randomly allocated to receive aspirin (498

women) or placebo (511 women) until delivery, and follow-up was obtained for 96%.

There were no significant differences between the treatment groups in the incidence of preeclampsia (6.7% aspirin-allocated compared with 6.0% placebo-allocated women), of intrauterine growth retardation (8.5% versus 10.1%), or of stillbirth and neonatal death (7.3% versus 6.0%). In addition, there were no significant differences in the incidence of preeclampsia in any subgroup of women studied, including those with systolic blood pressures of 120 mmHg or above at entry (8.5% versus 7.3%) or those with chronic hypertension (10.0% versus 7.1%). It was concluded that the results of the ECPPA study do not support the routine prophylactic administration of low-dose aspirin in pregnancy to any category of high-risk women, even those who have chronic hypertension or who are considered to be especially at risk for early-onset preeclampsia.

In their paper, the ECPPA group[97] also presented a meta-analysis of all trials. These results are reassuring with regard to maternal and neonatal complications, with no significant excesses of abruptio placentae, other antepartum hemorrhage, transfusion, or mortality due to bleeding. Prior to ECPPA, a systematic overview of the available results from all randomized trials of antiplatelet therapy indicated a 25% reduction in the incidence of preeclampsia, in contrast with the reduction of about 75% suggested by the first small trials.[88] The addition of ECPPA results reduces still further the apparent size of the benefit, and if the "hypothesis-generating" trials are excluded, the apparent reduction in the larger trials is only 17%. In absolute terms, these more modest proportional reductions imply that antiplatelet therapy would typically prevent preeclampsia in about one woman per 100 treated, with CI ranging from about zero to two per 100. In addition, there is no evidence of an effect of aspirin on the incidence of stillbirths and neonatal deaths.

The recently published second NIH trial[98] is the largest trial on the effects of low-dose aspirin in identified high-risk women. This multicenter, randomized, placebo-controlled, double-blind trial included 471 women with insulin-dependent diabetes, 747 with chronic hypertension, 688 with multifetal gestation, and 606 with preclampsia in a previous pregnancy. The patients were randomized between 13 and 26 weeks' gestation (mean, 20 weeks), and the primary outcome was preeclampsia. Comparing aspirin with placebo, the following results were obtained in the subgroups: for diabetes, 18.3% versus 21.6%; for multifetal pregnancies, 11.5% versus 15.9%; for women with a history of preclampsia, 16.7% versus 19%, and for patients with chronic hypertension, 26% versus 24.6%.

Thus, for all subgroups, there is a nonsignificant trend toward slightly better results with low-dose aspirin, except for patients with chronic hypertension. As a result, it was concluded that aspirin did not reduce the incidence of preeclampsia (relative risk 0.91, 95% CI 0.78–1.07) in the aggregate group or in any of the individual risk groups. Also, findings of the Barbados Low-dose Aspirin Study in Pregnancy (BLASP study)[99] and the Jamaica low-dose aspirin study[100] were negative.

Table 5–2 summarizes the low-dose aspirin trials. In essence, 20 trials, both large and small, have been unable to establish aspirin as a drug that eradicates preeclampsia, but the issue is still not totally settled.

PROBLEMS WITH THE EARLIER SMALLER TRIALS. The CLASP Collaborative Group[93] rightly raises some doubt about conclusions based on the earlier smaller trials, because in the same time period during which these smaller trials were published, about 300 versus 220 women have been randomized in other small but unpublished trials, and it may be that some small trials with unpromising results have not been published because their results were less remarkable.

According to a MRCOG (Member of the Royal College of Obstetricians and Gynaecologists) Workshop,[94] the differences in rates of preeclampsia of the smaller trials are distributed asymmetrically around those of the largest trials, with an excess of strongly positive results among the smaller studies. This suggests bias (e.g., publication bias) among the smaller studies. If this is true, the available results from small trials would give a biased estimate of the positive effects of antiplatelet therapy. However, some negative bias, as far as major international journals are concerned, may have also been operative after the publication of the negative large trials.

Several studies have since been reported in selected groups[101] or in developing countries showing good results associated with low-dose aspirin. Most of these studies have been published in regional medical journals instead of the well-known international journals. One of the more interesting trials is reported by Ramaiya and Mgaya,[102] who used samples of urine for detection of aspirin in order to check patient compliance. They conducted a double-blind prospective randomized study; 201 primigravidae at 20 weeks' gestation and above were screened using the roll-over test. Of the 127 women with an increase in blood pressure during the roll-over test, 126 women entered the study and were treated with a daily dose of either aspirin (80 mg) or placebo. The incidence of PIH in the aspirin-treated group was significantly lower than in the placebo-treated group: 3.17% versus 15.9% ($P = .02$). The authors concluded that low daily doses of aspirin taken from 20 weeks' gestation significantly reduce the incidence of PIH.

This is the third trial in which compliance was tested for by biochemical methods, and all three of these trials have provided data strongly in favor of the use of aspirin.[91, 95] Other trials conducted in countries outside the United States or Europe with results in favor of aspirin have been reported from China by Wang and Li[103] and from Pakistan by Gilani and Khan.[104] Thus, the specter of

TABLE 5–2. EFFECT OF LOW-DOSE ASPIRIN ON PREECLAMPSIA

PREECLAMPSIA	ASPIRIN	PLACEBO	ODDS RATIO	95% CI
Small studies[93]*	10/319	50/284	0.18	0.09–0.36
Large studies	949/13,928	1032/13,765	0.90	0.83–0.99
All studies	2404/13,729	1082/14,049	0.87	0.80–0.96

*Details of the trials included are given in CLASP; see Lancet 1994;343:619–629.[93]
CI, confidence interval.
Adapted from data published by Caritis S, Sibai BM, Hauth J, et al. Low-dose aspirin for the prevention of preeclampsia in high-risk women. N Engl J Med 1998;338:701–705.

publication bias may also exert its effect in the opposite direction.

An editorial in the *British Journal of Obstetrics and Gynaecology*[105] suggested another explanation for the negative results in the major trials. The large low-dose aspirin trials were pragmatic trials in which the results may have been influenced by the dilution of the trials by many women at low risk for genuine preeclampsia. According to Grant,[105] the magnitude of the treatment effect in the small trials is genuine, and the reason for the difference between the large trials and the smaller trials is the entry criteria. Women in the smaller trials were at a high risk for preeclampsia, with an incidence range from 13% to 40%.[105] According to Grant,[105] the apparently negative results of the large trials are misleading because the trials have been swamped by women at low risk for preeclampsia. The only large high-risk study is the second NIH study.[98] Unfortunately, in this study, mean gestational age at randomization was 20 weeks.

PROBLEMS WITH THE LARGE TRIALS. Compliance is the most important problem associated with the large trials. Pregnant women are known to be noncompliant in ingesting prescribed drugs, and, despite the randomization of more than 25,000 women, analyses that take into account compliance are scanty.[106] In an Australian study in *high-risk* patients,[107] 15% of the aspirin group and 20% of the placebo-treated patients were noncompliant. In the CLASP study,[93] 96% started the study medication, and 66% and 88% continued study treatment for at least 95% and 80%, respectively, of the time between randomization and delivery. In the CLASP[93] trial, noncompliance figures resulted from compliance questionnaires sent about 3 months after delivery to approximately 10% of the patients; this 10% sample consisted of women whose infants were believed to be alive and well. Although this is probably the only way to set up such a gigantic study, it implies that the potential risk of noncompliance is not excluded, especially among women with adverse perinatal outcome.

As mentioned earlier, the only three trials using biochemical tests to check for compliance reported that women assigned to aspirin had a significantly decreased incidence of preeclampsia.[91, 95, 102]

The other problem with the large trials is the time of randomization. For instance, the ECPPA trial[97] was set up similarly to the CLASP[93] study; patients were randomized between 12 and 32 weeks' gestation. A closer look reveals that only 8% of the women started with low-dose aspirin at 12 weeks' gestation, and only about one third of all patients were randomized before 20 weeks' gestation.[97]

The same problem is encountered in the second NIH study[98]—the mean time at randomization is about 20 weeks' gestation. However, neither trial,[97, 98] when one analyzes the data of the subgroups of women recruited before 20 weeks' gestation, suggested that aspirin had any beneficial effects.

A word of caution should be raised against those studies in which aspirin was not stored in airtight containers, especially if these studies were conducted in (sub)tropical areas. Aspirin is stable in dry air but gradually hydrolyzes in contact with moisture, especially in warm environments, to acetic and salicylic acids. If aspirin is not stored correctly in warm and moist environments, it may lose its efficacy over time.[108] In addition, caution is indicated in interpreting the results of studies that used protein-stick testing to define significant proteinuria, because it is a poor predictor of absent or severe proteinuria.[109]

The Cochrane Collaboration has now updated the systematic review of the effectiveness and safety of antiplatelet agents (predominantly aspirin) for the prevention of preeclampsia[110] and showed that use of aspirin is associated with:

1. A 15% reduction in the risk of preeclampsia (32 trials with 29,331 women; RR, 0.85; 95% CI, 0.78–0.92). This reduction exists regardless of risk status but appears to be greater when a placebo is not used, when the dose of aspirin is greater or gestation at randomization earlier.

2. A 7% reduction in the risk of delivery before 37 completed weeks (23 trials with 28,268 women; RR, 0.92; 95% CI, 0.88–0.97).

3. A 14% reduction in fetal and/or neonatal death (30 trials with 30,093 women; RR, 0.86; 95% CI, 0.75–0.99). This reduction in death was the greatest among high-risk women (4134 women; RR, 0.73; 95% CI, 0.56–0.96). There were no significant differences between treatment and control groups in the incidence of SGA infants (25 trials

with 20,235 women; RR, 0.91; 95% CI, 0.83–1.00), abruptio placentae, and induction of labor or cesarean section.

The Cochrane reviewers conclude it is not possible to make clear recommendations despite the potential benefits overall.

Low-dose aspirin does correct the PGI_2/TXA_2 imbalance, so why is it that it is not the wonder drug we all hoped for?

1. The most probable explanation for this apparent discrepancy is that the PGI_2/TXA_2 imbalance is not the only, and certainly not the major, involved pathogenic biochemical pathway. Endothelial-derived relaxation factor (nitric oxide) may turn out to be the major physiologic vasodilator and platelet inhibitor during pregnancy. If PGI_2 is "only" a local rescue hormone in case of an endangered microcirculation, we can hope to see some impact of low-dose aspirin only on the incidence of severe or early-onset preeclampsia, or both, and especially on the incidence of HELLP syndrome. In addition, TXA_2 is certainly not the only platelet-derived factor that is of pathophysiologic importance; for example, Middelkoop and colleagues[69] demonstrated the presence of a marked increase in free-circulating platelet-derived serotonin in established preeclampsia.[69]

2. Acute atherosis is similar to the atheromatous lesion in atherosclerosis. Thrombin is the major platelet agonist in case of disrupted atheromatous lesions. Because thrombin is an aspirin-independent agonist,[74, 111] it is to be expected that aspirin would not influence local arterial thrombosis in a spiral artery endangered by acute atherosis.

3. According to Walsh,[21, 82] the dose of aspirin should be high enough to inhibit placental prostaglandin H synthase, and thus placental lipid peroxide production. If the placental production of lipid peroxides is not sufficiently inhibited, these lipid peroxides might act as a continuing and powerful stimulus for further placental TXA_2 synthesis.

If aspirin works independently of its influence on platelets, such as by reducing (placental) lipid peroxide production, a higher dose might possibly be effective. Some support for this idea comes from the two studies, one nonrandomized[87] but the other randomized,[112] that used a larger dose (150 mg) of aspirin. Both studies showed a reduction in the incidence of both preeclampsia and fetal risk.

4. Fetal platelet consumption is a feature of placental insufficiency[113] that is probably related to fetal endothelial cell activation.[114] Following maternal oral intake of aspirin, only a very small dose eventually reaches the placenta. Fetal platelet behavior is not or is only mildly influenced by low-dose aspirin therapy. The fact that fetal platelets are not affected by low-dose aspirin, as a consequence of the characteristic pharmacokinetics of aspirin, may be another explanation for the modest effects of low-dose aspirin.

5. It is noteworthy that there was no reduction in perinatal mortality overall in any of the major trials. This may reflect inadequate power; alternatively, aspirin may not have a real effect on uteroplacental vessels but may simply prevent maternal manifestations such as proteinuria.[94]

The safety aspects of aspirin are described in other detailed reviews.[88, 115–117]

Overall, the large trials have demonstrated that aspirin is safe for the fetus and newborn infant, with no evidence of an increased likelihood of neonatal bleeding. Low-dose aspirin is safe for the mother, and epidural anesthesia is safe when the pregnant woman uses low-dose aspirin.[92, 93, 118]

Other Attempts to Correct the PGI_2-TXA_2 Imbalance: Omega-3 Long-Chain Polyunsaturated Fatty Acids

Although earlier studies suggested that dietary fish had some properties that could potentially prevent coronary artery disease, it was not until the epidemiologic studies of Dyerberg and Bang in 1975[119] that the association became noteworthy. Daviglus and colleagues[120] provided epidemiologic data from a group of 1822 men that showed an inverse relationship between fish consumption and death from coronary heart disease. When ω-3 fatty acids are included in the diet, eicosapentaenoic acid and docosahexaenoic acid compete with arachidonic acid in several ways:

1. They inhibit the synthesis of arachidonic acid from linoleic acid.
2. They compete with arachidonic acid for the 2-position in membrane phospholipids, thereby reducing plasma and cellular levels of arachidonic acid.

3. Eicosapentaenoic acid competes with arachidonic acid as the substrate for cyclooxygenase, inhibiting the production of TXA_2 by platelets, and produces only small amounts of a physiologically inactive TXA_3.

In endothelial cells, the production of PGI_2 is not markedly inhibited, and the physiologic activity of PGI_3, which is synthesized from eicosapentaenoic acid, is added to that of PGI_2. The net result is a change in the hemostatic balance toward a vasodilatory state, with less platelet aggregation.[121] Dietary ω-3 fatty acids also reduce experimental vascular proliferative lesion formation in primates, an effect that is probably at least partially mediated by defective thrombin production.[74, 111] Adair and associates[122] evaluated the effects of ω-3 fatty acid supplementation on vascular reactivity as measured by the angiotensin II sensitivity test. Ten subjects with uneventful pregnancies who were free of any chronic medical illnesses and between 24 and 34 weeks' gestation participated. Each subject was provided with capsules containing 3.6 g of eicosapentaenoic acid per day. The angiotensin II sensitivity test was performed before and 28 days after supplementation. The effective pressor dose before treatment (13.6 $\pm$ 6.3 ng/kg/min) was significantly less ($P = .001$) than after supplementation (35.8 $\pm$ 15.9 ng/kg/min), demonstrating that high-dose ω-3 fatty acid supplementation results in an enhancement of the pregnancy-acquired refractoriness to angiotensin II.

The largest study on the effects of fish oil supplementation, composed of more than 5000 pregnant women, was reported in 1946 by the People's League of Health. Although this study had methodologic limitations, the incidence of preeclampsia was reported to be reduced in this study.[123] In a questionnaire study of more than 6500 pregnant women in Denmark who did not smoke during pregnancy, Olsen and coworkers[124] showed a significant positive association between fish consumption and placental weight, birth weight, and neonatal head circumference. Fish oil administration in late pregnancy results in increased TXB_3 and PGI_3 levels and reduced TXB_2 levels.[125, 126]

Because of these potentially beneficial effects several trials have been initiated to assess the preventative effects of fish oil. Olsen et al[127] have published the results of the largest trial so far, the European Multicentre Fish Oil Supplementation trial (FOTIP trial). In six trials, women with high-risk pregnancies were randomly assigned to receive fish oil or olive oil from around 20 weeks' gestation (Table 5–3). Four of these trials were prophylactic, enrolling 232, 280, and 386 women who had experienced previous preterm delivery, IUGR, or pregnancy-induced hypertension and preeclampsia, respectively and 579 women with twin pregnancies. Fish oil reduced risk of preterm delivery from 33% to 21% (OR, 0.54; 95% CI, 0.30–0.98) but did not affect any other outcomes. In twin pregnancies, the risks for all three outcomes were similar to the two intervention arms. Again, fish oil does not appear to be the solution.

Modulation of the L-Arginine– Nitric Oxide–Cyclic Guanosine 3',5'-Monophosphate (cGMP) Pathway

One of the most exciting discoveries in recent years has been the finding of nitric oxide plus L-citrulline synthesis from L-arginine in many cell types, including endothelial cells, platelets, and macrophages. In theory, nitric oxide donors form an exciting novel approach to prevent preeclampsia.[128]

TABLE 5–3. EFFECTS OF FISH OIL ON PREGNANCY-INDUCED HYPERTENSIVE DISORDER: EUROPEAN MULTICENTER FISH OIL TRIAL

PIH	FISH OIL	OLIVE OIL	ODDS RATIO	95% CI
Recurrence of PIH*	55/167	61/183	0.98	0.63–1.53
Twin pregnancy	38/274	38/279	1.39	0.83–2.32

*Recurrence of a pregnancy-induced hypertensive disorder in patients with a history of previous preeclampsia and/or pregnancy-induced hypertension.

CI, confidence interval; PIH, pregnancy-induced hypertension.

Adapted from Olsen S, Secher W, Tabor A, et al. Randomised clinical trials of fish oil supplementation in high risk pregnancies. Br J Obstet Gynaecol 2000;107:382–399. Courtesy of Blackwell Science, Ltd.

Although nitrates have been described to treat angina pectoris for more than a century, only recently has the mechanism of action become clarified. Nitrates form nitric oxide, which causes direct vasodilatation of the coronary arteries. The term *nitrovasodilators* has been coined for all agents that can lead to the formation of the reactive nitric oxide–free radical in incubations and increase cGMP synthesis.

The first studies with nitroglycerin in pregnancy have been done in patients with established severe preeclampsia.[129-131] Cotton and associates[129] demonstrated that intravenous nitroglycerin is a potent, rapidly acting agent with a hemodynamic half-life measured in minutes. Nitroglycerin alone reduced mean arterial pressure by 27.5% without any significant changes in heart rate, central venous pressure, or stroke volume in six patients with severe "pregnancy-induced hypertension." The pulmonary capillary wedge pressure fell from 9 ± 3 to 4 ± 2 mmHg, while the cardiac index decreased from 3.51 ± 0.67 to 2.87 ± 0.76 L/min/m². Oxygen delivery fell significantly, from 617 ± 78 to 491 ± 106 mL/min/m². Although volume expansion alone had no effect on mean arterial pressure, the combination of blood volume expansion and nitroglycerin resulted in a marked resistance to the hypotensive effect of nitroglycerin. Cardiac index, pulmonary capillary wedge pressure, and oxygen utilization were not significantly different from baseline values when volume expansion preceded nitroglycerin.

Grunewald and colleagues[132] studied 12 patients with severe preeclampsia (diastolic blood pressure of 110 mmHg or higher). All received intravenous nitroglycerin with step-wise dosage increases beginning at 0.25 µg/kg/min until diastolic blood pressure had decreased below 100 mmHg. During infusion, blood pressure decreased significantly. The Doppler flow patterns of the uterine artery did not change significantly, whereas the pulsatility indices in the umbilical artery decreased significantly from 1.41 $\pm$ 0.14 to 1.23 $\pm$ 0.08, with more pronounced decreases in patients with high basal values. Blood levels of cGMP remained essentially unchanged.

Similar effects have been reported by Giles and coworkers.[133] Ramsay and colleagues[134] demonstrated that intravenous glyceryl trinitrate given in the first trimester can mimic the physiologic alterations of the uterine artery FVW patterns seen with advancing gestation and also causes a significant fall in uterine artery resistance in patients at high risk for preeclampsia because of a markedly abnormal uterine artery resistance index.

De Belder and associates[135] reported a case of HELLP syndrome, which was successfully managed with S-nitrosoglutathione, a nitric oxide donor donor, and Lees and colleagues[136] reported that S-nitrosoglutathione infusion reduced maternal blood pressure, platelet activation, and uterine artery resistance without further compromising fetal Doppler indices in a group of 10 women with severe preeclampsia at 21 to 33 weeks' gestation.

Several trials are now in progress to assess the efficacy of modulating the nitric oxide pathway, for instance by dietary supplementation of L-arginine, to prevent and treat preeclampsia. In addition, one randomized trial in a limited number of women considered at risk for preeclampsia (abnormal uterine Doppler study at 16 to 18 weeks' gestation) revealed a significant reduction in the rate of preeclampsia in the women receiving 1000 mg of vitamin C and 400 IU of vitamin E. The overall rates of hypertensive disorders, however, were similar, and there were no differences in perinatal outcome.[137]

References

1. Department of Health, Welsh Office, Scottish Home and Health Department, DHSS Northern Ireland. Report on Confidential Enquiries into Maternal Death in the United Kingdom 1985–1987. London: Her Majesty's Stationery Office, 1991.
2. Duley L. Maternal mortality associated with hypertensive disorders of pregnancy in Africa, Asia, Latin America, and the Caribbean. Br J Obstet Gynaecol 1992;99:547–553.
3. Naeye RL, Friedman CA: Causes of perinatal death associated with gestational hypertension and proteinuria. Am J Obstet Gynecol 1979;133:8–10.
4. Working Group on High Blood Pressure in Pregnancy. The National High Blood Pressure Education Program Working Group Report on High Blood Pressure in Pregnancy: Consensus Report. Am J Obstet Gynecol 2000;83:S1–S22.
5. Hauth JC, Ewell MG, Levine RJ, Sibai B, et al. Pregnancy outcome in healthy nulliparas who developed hypertension. Obstet Gynecol 2000;95:24–28.
6. Sibai BM. Preeclampsia-eclampsia. Curr Probl Obstet Gynecol Fertil 1990;13:3–45.
7. Hamlin RMJ. The prevention of eclampsia and preeclampsia. Lancet 1952;i:64–68.

8. Crowther C, Chalmers I. Bed rest and hospitalization during pregnancy. *In* Chalmers I, Enkin M, Keirse MJNC (eds). Effective Care in Pregnancy and Childbirth. Oxford: Oxford University Press, 1989, pp 624–632.

9. Roberts JM, Redman CWG. Pre-eclampsia: More than pregnancy-induced hypertension. Lancet 1993;341:1447–1451.

10. Dekker GA, van Geijn HP. Endothelial dysfunction in preeclampsia: Part I. Primary prevention: Therapeutic perspectives. J Perinat Med 1996;24:99–117.

11. Smarason AK, Sargent IL, Starkey PM, Redman CWG. The effect of placental syncytiotrophoblast microvillous membranes from normal and preeclamptic women on the growth of endothelial cells in vivo. Br J Obstet Gynaecol 1993;100:943–949.

12. Zeeman GG, Dekker GA. Pathogenesis of preeclampsia: A hypothesis. Clin Obstet Gynecol 1992;35:317–337.

13. Conrad KP, Benyo DF. Placental cytokines and the pathogenesis of preeclampsia. Am J Reprod Immunol 1997;37:240–249.

14. Cooper DW, Brennecke SP, Wilton AN. Genetics of preeclampsia. Hypertens Pregn 1993;12:1–23.

15. Robillard PY, Hulsey TC, Alexander GR, et al. Paternity patterns and risk of preeclampsia in the last pregnancy in multiparae. J Reprod Immunol 1993;24:1–12.

16. Trupin LS, Simon LP, Eskenazi B. Change in paternity: A risk factor for preeclampsia in multiparas. Epidemiology 1996;7:240–244.

17. Klonoff-Cohen HS, Savitz DA, Cefalo RC, McCann MF. An epidemiologic study of contraception and preeclampsia. JAMA 1989;262:3143–3147.

18. Robillard PY, Hulsey TC, Perianin J, et al. Association of pregnancy-induced hypertension with duration of sexual cohabitation before conception. Lancet 1994;344:973–975.

19. Clark DA. Does immunological intercourse prevent preeclampsia? Lancet 1994;344:969–970.

20. Dekker GA. Oral tolerization to paternal antigens and preeclampsia [Abstract SPO]. Am J Obstet Gynecol 1996;174:516.

21. Walsh SW. Lipid peroxidation in pregnancy. Hypertens Pregn 1994;13:1–31.

22. Halliwell B, Gutteridge JMC, Cross CE. Free radicals, antioxidants, and human disease: Where are we now? J Lab Clin Med 1992;119:598–620.

23. Lu B, Zhang SW, Huang B, Liu W, Li CF. Changes in selenium in patients with pregnancy-induced hypertension. Chin J Obstet Gynecol 1990;25:325–327.

24. Stark JM. Pre-eclampsia and cytokine induced oxidative stress. Br J Obstet Gynaecol 1993;100:105–109.

25. Shanklin DR, Sibai BM. Ultrastructural aspects of preeclampsia: I. Placental bed and uterine boundary vessels. Am J Obstet Gynecol 1989;161:735–741.

26. Shanklin DR, Sibai BM. Ultrastructural aspects of preeclampsia: II. Mitochondrial changes. Am J Obstet Gynecol 1990;163:943–953.

27. O'Brien WF. Predicting preeclampsia. Obstet Gynecol 1990;75:445–452.

28. Dekker GA, Sibai BM. Early detection of preeclampsia. Am J Obstet Gynecol 1991;165:160–172.

29. Magann EF, Martin JN Jr. The laboratory evaluation of hypertensive gravidas. Obstet Gynecol Surv 1995;50:138–145.

30. Villar MA, Sibai BM. Clinical significance of elevated mean arterial blood pressure in second trimester and threshold increase in systolic or diastolic blood pressure during the third trimester. Am J Obstet Gynecol 1989;160:419–423.

31. Conde-Agudelo A, Belizan JM, Lede R, Bergel EF. What does an elevated mean arterial pressure in the second half of pregnancy predict—gestational hypertension or preeclampsia? Am J Obstet Gynecol 1993;169:509–514.

32. Masse J, Forest J-C, Moutquin J-M, et al. A prospective study of several potential biologic markers for early prediction of preeclampsia. Am J Obstet Gynecol 1993;169:501–508.

33. Dekker GA, Makovitz JW, Wallenburg HCS. Comparison of prediction of pregnancy-induced hypertensive disease by angiotensin II sensitivity and supine pressor test. Br J Obstet Gynaecol 1990;97:817–821.

34. Dekker GA, Walker JJ. Maternal assessment in pregnancy-induced hypertensive disorders: Special investigations and their pathophysiological basis. *In* Walker JJ, Gant NF (eds). Hypertension in Pregnancy. London: Chapman & Hall, 1997, pp 107–161.

35. Sanchez-Ramos L, Sandroni S, Andres FJ, Kaunitz AM. Calcium excretion in preeclampsia. Obstet Gynecol 1991;77:510–513.

36. Rodriguez MH, Masaki DI, Mestman J, et al. Calcium/creatinine ratio and microalbuminuria in the prediction of preeclampsia. Am J Obstet Gynecol 1988;159:1452–1458.

37. Hutchesson ACJ, MacIntosh MC, Duncan SLB, et al. Hypocalciuria and hypertension in pregnancy: A prospective study. Clin Exp Hypertens Pregn 1990;B9:115–134.

38. Sorensen TK, Williams MA, Zingheim RW, et al. Elevated second-trimester human chorionic gonadotropin and subsequent pregnancy-induced hypertension. Am J Obstet Gynecol 1993;169:834–838.

39. Vaillant P, David E, Constant I, et al. Validity in nulliparas of increased beta-human chorionic gonadotrophin at mid-term for predicting pregnancy-induced hypertension complicated with proteinuria and intrauterine growth retardation. Nephron 1996;72:557–563.

40. Muller F, Savey L, Le Fiblec B, et al. Maternal serum human chorionic gonadotropin level at fifteen weeks is a predictor for preeclampsia. Am J Obstet Gynecol 1996;175:37–40.

41. Walker JJ, Dekker GA. Etiology and pathophysiology of hypertension in pregnancy. *In* Walker JJ, Gant NF (eds). Hypertension in Pregnancy. London: Chapman & Hall, 1997, pp 39–75.

42. Ballegeer V, Spitz B, Kieckens L, et al. Predictive value of increased plasma levels of fibronectin in gestational hypertension. Am J Obstet Gynecol 1989;161:432–436.

43. Halligan A, Bonnar J, Sheppard B, et al. Haemostatic, fibrinolytic and endothelial variables in normal pregnancies and pre-eclampsia. Br J Obstet Gynecol 1994;101:488–492.

44. Murphy JF, Newcombe RG, O'Riordan JO, et al. Relation of haemoglobin levels in first and second trimesters to outcome of pregnancy. Lancet 1986;i:992–994.

45. Pearce JM, MacParland P. Uteroplacental circulation. Contemp Rev Obstet Gynaecol 1991;3:6–12.

46. Campbell S, Pearce JMF, Hackett G, et al. Qualitative assessment of uteroplacental blood flow: Early screening test for high-risk pregnancies. Obstet Gynecol 1986;68:649–653.

47. Steel SA, Pearce JM, McParland P, et al. Early Doppler ultrasound screening in prediction of hypertensive disorders of pregnancy. Lancet 1990;335:1548–1551.

48. Harrington K, Cooper D, Lees C, et al. Doppler ultrasound of the uterine arteries: The importance of bilateral notching in the prediction of pre-eclampsia, placental abruption or delivery of a small-for-gestational-age baby. Ultrasound Obstet Gynecol 1996;7:182–188.

49. Harrington K, Goldfrad C, Carpenter RG, Campbell S. Transvaginal uterine and umbilical artery Doppler examination of 12–16 weeks and the subsequent development of pre-eclampsia and intrauterine growth retardation. Ultrasound Obstet Gynecol 1997;9:94–100.

50. Steegers EAP, Eskes TKAB, Jongsma HW, Hein PR. Dietary sodium restriction during pregnancy: A historical review. Eur J Obstet Gynecol Reprod Biol 1991;40:83–90.

51. Robinson M. Salt in pregnancy. Lancet 1958; i:178–181.

52. Van Buul BJA, Steegers EAP, Jongsma HW, et al. Dietary sodium restriction in the prophylaxis of hypertensive disorders of pregnancy: Effects on the intake of other nutrients. Am J Clin Nutrition 1995;62:49–57.

53. Baker PN. Possible dietary measures in the prevention of pre-eclampsia and eclampsia: Possible dietary measures in the prevention of pre-eclampsia and eclampsia. Baillieres Clin Obstet Gynaecol 1995;9:497–507.

54. Green J. Diet and the prevention of pre-eclampsia. *In* Chalmers I, Enkin M, Keirse MJNC (eds). Effective Care in Pregnancy and Childbirth. Oxford: Oxford University Press, 1989, pp 281–300.

55. Collins R, Yusuf S, Peto R. Overview of randomised trials of diuretics in pregnancy. Br Med J 1985;290:13–17.

56. Collins R, Wallenburg HCS. Pharmacological prevention and treatment of hypertensive disorders in pregnancy. *In* Chalmers I, Enkin M, Keirse MJNC (eds). Effective Care in Pregnancy and Childbirth. Oxford: Oxford University Press, 1989, pp 512–533.

57. Skajaa K, Dorup I, Sandstrom B-M. Magnesium intake and status and pregnancy outcome in a Danish population. Br J Obstet Gynaecol 1991; 98:919–928.

58. Sibai BM, Villar MA, Bray E. Magnesium supplementation during pregnancy: A double-blind randomized controlled clinical trial. Am J Obstet Gynecol 1989;161:115–119.

59. Repke JT. Prevention of preeclampsia. Clin Perinatol 1991;18:779–792.

60. Hunt IF, Murphy NJ, Cleaver AE, et al. Zinc supplementation during pregnancy: Effects on selected blood constituents and on progress and outcome of pregnancy in low-income women of Mexican descent. Am J Clin Nutr 1984;40:508–521.

61. Mahomed K, James DK, Golding J, McCabe R. Zinc supplementation during pregnancy: A double blind randomised controlled trial. BMJ 1989;199:826–830.

62. Thomson AM. Diet in pregnancy: 3. Diet in relation to the course and outcome of pregnancy. Br J Nutr 1959;13:509–525.

63. Belizan JM, Villar J, Gonzalez L, et al. Calcium supplementation to prevent hypertensive disorders of pregnancy. N Engl J Med 1991;325:1399–1405.

64. Bucher HC, Guyatt GH, Cook RJ, et al. Effect of calcium supplementation on pregnancy-induced hypertension and preeclampsia: A meta-analysis of randomized controlled trials. JAMA 1996; 275:1113–1117.

65. Marcoux S, Brisson J, Fabia J. Calcium intake from dairy products and supplements and the risks of preeclampsia and gestational hypertension. Am J Epidemiol 1991;133:1266–1272.

66. Levine RJ, Hauth JC, Curet LB. Trial of calcium to prevent preeclampsia. N Engl J Med 1997;337:69–76.

66a. Atallah AN, Hofmeyr GJ, Duley L. Calcium supplementation during pregnancy for preventing hypertensive disorders and related problems (Cochrane Review). *In* The Cochrane Library, Issue 1, 2000. Oxford: Update Software.

66b. DerSimonian R, Levine RJ. Resolving discrepancies between a meta-analysis and a subsequent large controlled trial. JAMA 1999;282:664–670.

66c. Crowther CA, Hiller JE, Pridmore B, et al. Calcium supplemetation in nulliparous women for the prevention of pregnancy-induced hypertension, preeclampsia and preterm birth: An Australian randomized trial. FRACOG and the ACT Study Group. Aust N Z J Obstet Gynecol 1999;39:12–18.

67. Wallenburg HCS. Changes in the coagulation system and platelets in pregnancy-induced hypertension and preeclampsia. *In* Sharp F, Symonds EM (eds). Hypertension in Pregnancy. Ithaca, NY: Perinatology Press, 1987, pp 227–248.

68. Redman CWG. Platelets and the beginning of preeclampsia. N Engl J Med 1991;323:478–480.

69. Middelkoop CM, Dekker GA, Kraayenbrink AA, Popp-Snijders C. Platelet-poor plasma serotonin in normal and preeclamptic pregnancy. Clin Chem 1993;39:1675–1678.

70. Gant NF, Daley GI, Chand S, et al. A study of angiotensin-II pressor response throughout primigravid pregnancy. J Clin Invest 1973;52:2682–2689.

71. Fitzgerald DJ, Entman SS, Mulloy K, Fitzgerald GA. Decreased prostacyclin biosynthesis preceding the clinical manifestation of pregnancy-induced hypertension. Circulation 1987;75:956–963.

72. Fitzgerald DJ, Rocki W, Murray R, et al. Thromboxane A_2 synthesis in pregnancy-induced hypertension. Lancet 1990;335:751–754.

73. Friedman SA. Preeclampsia: A review of the role of prostaglandins. Obstet Gynecol 1988;71:122–137.

74. Harker LA. Platelets and vascular thrombosis. N Engl J Med 1994;330:1006–1007.

75. Moran N, Fitzgerald GA. Mechanisms of action of antiplatelet drugs. *In* Colman RW, Hirsch J, Marder VJ, Salzman EW (eds). Hemostasis and Thrombosis: Basic Principles and Clinical Practice, 3rd ed. Philadelphia: JB Lippincott, 1994, pp 1623–1637.

76. Sibai BM, Mirro R, Chesney CM, Leffler C. Low-dose aspirin in pregnancy. Obstet Gynecol 1989;74:551–557.

77. Louden KA, Broughton Pipkin F, Symonds EM, et al. A randomized placebo-controlled study of the effect of low dose aspirin on platelet reactivity and serum thromboxane B_2 production in non-pregnant women, in normal pregnancy, and in gestational hypertension. Br J Obstet Gynaecol 1992;99:371–376.

78. Patrono C. Aspirin as an antiplatelet drug. N Engl J Med 1994;330:1287–1294.

79. Pedersen AK, FitzGerald GA. Dose-related kinetics of aspirin. N Engl J Med 1984;311:1206–1211.

80. Bjornsson TD, Schneider DE, Berger H Jr. Aspirin acetylates fibrinogen and enhances fibrinolysis: Fibrinolytic effect is independent of changes in plasminogen activator levels. J Pharmacol Experimental Therapy 1989;250:154–161.

81. Rinder CS, Student LA, Bonan JL, et al. Aspirin does not inhibit adenosine diphosphate-induced platelet alpha-granule release. Blood 1993;82:505–512.

82. Walsh SW, Wang Y, Kay HH, McCoy MC. Low-dose aspirin inhibits lipid peroxides and thromboxane but not prostacyclin in pregnant women. Am J Obstet Gynecol 1992;167:926–930.

83. Kaplanski G, Porat R, Aiura K, et al. Activated platelets induce endothelial secretion of interleukin-8 in vitro via an interleukin-1 mediated event. Blood 1993;81:2492–2495.

84. Crandon AJ, Isherwood DM. Effect of aspirin on incidence of pre-eclampsia. Lancet 1979;i:1356.

85. Sanchez-Ramos L, O'Sullivan MJ, Garrido Calderon J. Effect of low-dose aspirin on angiotensin II pressor response in human pregnancy. Am J Obstet Gynecol 1987;156:193–194.

86. Wallenburg HCS, Dekker GA, Makovitz JW, Rotmans N. Effect of low-dose aspirin on vascular refractoriness in angiotensin-sensitive primigravid women. Am J Obstet Gynecol 1991; 164:1169–1173.

87. Beaufils M, Donsimoni R, Uzan S, Colau JC. Prevention of pre-eclampsia by early antiplatelet therapy. Lancet 1985;i:840–842.

88. Dekker GA, Sibai BM. Low-dose aspirin in the prevention of preeclampsia and fetal growth retardation: Rationale, mechanisms, and clinical trials. Am J Obstet Gynecol 1993;168:214–227.

89. Parazzini F, Benedetto C, Frusca T, et al. Low-dose aspirin in prevention and treatment of intra-uterine growth retardation and pregnancy-induced hypertension. Lancet 1993;341:396–400.

90. Louden KA. Aspirin in pregnancy [letter]. Lancet 1993;341:753.

91. Hauth JC, Goldenberg RL, Parker R Jr, et al. Low-dose aspirin therapy to prevent preeclampsia. Am J Obstet Gynecol 1993;168:1083–1093.

92. Sibai BM, Caritis SN, Thom E, et al. Prevention of preeclampsia with low-dose aspirin in healthy nulliparous pregnant women. N Engl J Med 1993;329:1213–1218.

93. CLASP Collaborative Group. CLASP: A randomised trial of low-dose aspirin for the prevention and treatment of pre-eclampsia among 9364 pregnant women. Lancet 1994;343:619–629.

94. Lilford RJ. Report of a workshop. Where next for prophylaxis against pre-eclampsia? Br J Obstet Gynaecol 1996;103:603–607.

95. Wallenburg HCS, Dekker GA, Makowitz JW, Rotmans P. Low-dose aspirin prevents pregnancy-induced hypertension and pre-eclampsia in angiotensin-sensitive primigravidae. Lancet 1986; 1:1–3.

96. McParland P, Pearce JM, Chamberlain GVP. Doppler ultrasound and aspirin in recognition and prevention of pregnancy-induced hypertension. Lancet 1990;i:1552–1555.

97. Atallah AN. ECPPA: Randomised trial of low dose aspirin for the prevention of maternal and fetal complications in high risk pregnant women. Br J Obstet Gynecol 1996;103:39–47.

98. Caritis S, Sibai BM, Hauth J, et al. Low-dose aspirin for the prevention of preeclampsia in high-risk women. N Engl J Med 1998;338:701–705.

99. Rotchell YE, Cruickshank JK, Gay MP, et al. Barbados Low-dose Aspirin Study in Pregnancy (BLASP): A randomised trial for the prevention of pre-eclampsia and its complications. Br J Obstet Gynaecol 1998;105:286–292.

100. Golding J. A randomised trial of low dose aspirin for primiparae in pregnancy. Br J Obstet Gynaecol 1998;105:293–299.

101. Caspi E, Raziel A, Sherman D, et al. Prevention of pregnancy-induced hypertension in twins by early administration of low-dose aspirin: A preliminary report. Am J Reprod Immunol 1994; 31:19–24.

102. Ramaiya C, Mgaya HN. Low dose aspirin in prevention of pregnancy-induced hypertension in primigravidae at the Muhimbili Medical Centre, Dar Es Salaam. East Afr Med J 1995;72:690–693.

103. Wang Z, Li W. A prospective randomized placebo-controlled trial of low-dose aspirin for prevention of intra-uterine growth retardation. Chin Med J 1996;109:238–242.

104. Gilani A, Khan Z. Role of aspirin in management of pregnancy induced hypertension: A study in Pakistani population. Specialist 1994;10:323–325.

105. Grant JM. Multicentre trials in obstetrics and gynaecology: Smaller explanatory trials are required. Br J Obstet Gynaecol 1996;103:599–602.

106. Lindheimer MD. Pre-eclampsia-eclampsia 1996: Preventable? Have disputes on its treatment been resolved? Curr Opinion Nephrol Hypertens 1996;5:452–458.

107. Gallery EDM, Ross MR, Hawkins M, et al. Low-dose aspirin in high-risk pregnancy. Hypertens Pregn 1996;16:229–238.

108. Reynolds JEF (ed). Aspirin. *In* Martindale: The Extra Pharmacopoeia, 31st ed. London: The Pharmaceutical Press, 1996, p 17.

109. Meyer NL, Mercer BM, Friedman SA, et al. Urinary dipstick protein: A poor predictor of absent or severe proteinuria. Am J Obstet Gynecol 1994;170:137–141.

110. Knight M, Duley L, Henderson-Smart DJ, King JF. Antiplatelet agents and pre-eclampsia (Cochrane Review). *In* The Cochrane Library, Issue 1, 2000. Oxford: Update Software.

111. Harker LA, Maraganore JM, Hirsch J. Novel antithrombotic agents. *In* Colman RW, Hirsch J, Marder VJ, Salzman EW (eds). Hemostasis and Thrombosis: Basic Principles and Clinical Practice, 3rd ed. Philadelphia: JB Lippincott, 1994, pp 1638–1660.

112. Uzan S, Beaufils M, Breart G, et al. Prevention of fetal growth retardation with low-dose aspirin:

Findings of the EPREDA trial. Lancet 1991; 337:1427–1431.

113. Wilcox GR, Trudinger BJ. Fetal platelet consumption: A feature of placental insufficiency. Obstet Gynecol 1991;77:616–621.

114. Friedman SA, Schiff E, Emeis JJ, et al. Fetal plasma cellular fibronectin levels in preeclampsia [Abstract 486 SPO]. Am J Obstet Gynecol 1994;170:409.

115. Swiet de M, Fryers G. Review. The use of aspirin in pregnancy. J Obstet Gynaecol 1990;10:467–482.

116. Briggs GG, Freeman RK, Yaffe SJ. Drugs in Pregnancy and Lactation: A Reference Guide to Fetal and Neonatal Risk. Baltimore: Williams & Wilkins, 1994, pp 65–73.

117. Bremer HA, Wallenburg HCS. Aspirin in pregnancy. Fetal Matern Med Review 1992;4:37–57.

118. Sibai BM, Caritis SN, Thom E, et al. Low-dose aspirin in nulliparous women: Safety of continuous epidural block and correlation between bleeding time and maternal-neonatal bleeding complications. Am J Obstet Gynecol 1995; 172:1553–1557.

119. Dyerberg J, Bang BO, Hjorne N. Fatty acid composition of the plasma lipids in Greenland Eskimos. Am J Clin Nutr 1975;28:958–966.

120. Daviglus ML, Stamler J, Orencia AJ, et al. Fish consumption and the 30-year risk of fatal myocardial infarction. N Engl J Med 1997;336:1046–1053.

121. Leaf A, Weber PC. Cardiovascular effects of ω-3 fatty acids. N Engl J Med 1988;318:549–557.

122. Adair CD, Sanchez Ramos L, Briones DL, Ogburn P Jr. The effect of high dietary ω-3 fatty acid supplementation on angiotensin II pressor response in human pregnancy. Am J Obstet Gynecol 1996;175:688–691.

123. Olsen SF, Secher NJ. A possible preventive effect of low-dose fish oil on early delivery and preeclampsia: Indications from a 50-year-old controlled trial. Br J Nutr 1990;64:599–609.

124. Olsen SF, Olsen J, Frische G. Does fish consumption during pregnancy increase fetal growth? A study of the size of the newborn, placental weight and gestational age in relation to fish consumption during pregnancy. Int J Epidemiol 1990; 19:971–977.

125. Sorensen JD, Olsen SF, Pedersen AK, et al. Effects of fish oil supplementation in the third trimester of pregnancy on prostacyclin and thromboxane production. Am J Obstet Gynecol 1993;168:915–922.

126. Schiff E, Ben-Baruch G, Barkai G, et al. Reduction of thromboxane A_2 synthesis in pregnancy by polyunsaturated fatty acid supplements. Am J Obstet Gynecol 1993;168:122–124.

127. Olsen S, Secher W, Tabor A, et al. Randomized clinical trials of fish oil supplementation in high-risk pregnancies. Br J Obstet Gynaecol 2000; 107:382–395.

128. Dekker GA, Geijn van HP. Endothelial dysfunction in preeclampsia: Part II. Reducing the adverse consequences of endothelial cell dysfunction in preeclampsia: Therapeutic perspectives. J Perinat Med 1996;24:119–139.

129. Cotton DB, Longmire S, Jones MM, et al. Cardiovascular alterations in severe pregnancy-induced hypertension: Effects of intravenous nitroglycerin coupled with blood volume expansion. Am J Obstet Gynecol 1986;154:1053–1059.

130. Longmire S, Leduc L, Jones MM, et al. The hemodynamic effects of intubation during nitroglycerin infusion in severe preeclampsia. Am J Obstet Gynecol 1991;164:551–556.

131. Silver HM. Acute hypertensive crisis in pregnancy. Med Clin North Am 1989;73:623–638.

132. Grunewald C, Kublickas M, Carlstrom K, et al. Effects of nitroglycerin on the uterine and umbilical circulation in severe preeclampsia. Obstet Gynecol 1995;86:600–604.

133. Giles W, O'Callaghan S, Boura A, Walters W. Reduction in human fetal umbilical-placental vascular resistance by glyceryl trinitrate. Lancet 1992;340:856.

134. Ramsay B, de Belder A, Campbell S, et al. A nitric oxide donor improves uterine artery diastolic blood flow in normal early pregnancy and in women at high risk of pre-eclampsia. Eur J Clin Invest 1994;24:76–78.

135. de Belder A, Lees C, Moncada S, Campbell S. Treatment of HELLP syndrome with nitric oxide donor. Lancet 1995;345:124–125.

136. Lees C, Langford E, Brown AS, et al. The effects of S-nitrosoglutathione on platelet activation, and uterine and fetal Doppler in severe preeclampsia. Obstet Gynecol 1996;88:14–19.

137. Chappell LC, Seed PT, Briley AL, et al. Effects of antioxidants on the occurrence of preeclampsia in women at increased risk: A randomised trial. Lancet 1999;354:810–816.

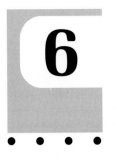

6 MEDICAL CONDITIONS ASSOCIATED with HYPERTENSIVE DISORDERS of PREGNANCY

Gustaaf A. Dekker and Nicholas H. Morris

The clinical syndrome of preeclampsia develops as a result of an impaired maternal vascular endothelial response to pregnancy or endothelial cell dysfunction and damage. The evidence for this vascular endothelial abnormality is supported not only by the established imbalance in endothelial vasodilator and vasoconstrictor prostanoid synthesis but also by other markers of endothelial cell damage, including (1) increased levels of factor VIII–related antigen (fVIIIrag), total fibronectin, cellular fibronectin, thrombomodulin, and growth factor activity and (2) an imbalance between tissue plasminogen activator and inhibitor.[1–12] Women with established insulin-dependent diabetes and chronic hypertension are at increased risk for development of preeclampsia. The increased incidence of (superimposed) preeclampsia in these disorders may be explained by the associated preexisting endothelial cell dysfunction.

This chapter reviews both the well-known association between preeclampsia and conditions, such as chronic hypertension and diabetes, and later findings on the association between preeclampsia and thrombophilic disorders, antiphospholipid antibodies, hyperhomocysteinemia, and the insulin resistance syndrome (syndrome X). Our focus is on presenting the pathophysiology of the interaction between these medical disorders and the clinical syndrome preeclampsia.

CHRONIC HYPERTENSION AND RENAL DISEASE

Chronic Hypertension

Chronic hypertension is a highly significant risk factor in the development of preeclampsia. This association is so frequent that it even "earned" a separate classification as *superimposed* preeclampsia. Women with chronic hypertension are at risk not only for superimposed preeclampsia but also for abruptio placentae (placental abruption) and renal failure, and the fetus is at risk for fetal growth restriction and second-trimester fetal compromise. Superimposed preeclampsia occurs in about 10% to 30% of pregnancies complicated by chronic hypertension. This may well be an overestimation and possibly reflects inclusion of cases in which a rise in the blood pressure in the third trimester represents a return to prepregnancy levels.[13] It is therefore important to measure blood pressure during the first trimester in order to identify women with chronic hypertension because many of these patients become normotensive in the second trimester. Women with long-standing severe hypertension and those with preexisting cardiovascular or renal disease are at particularly high risk for superimposed preeclampsia.

Several studies have now documented that in pregnancies complicated by severe early-onset preeclampsia, approximately 30% to 40% of the patients have chronic hypertension.[15–17] The incidence of chronic hypertension in pregnant women ranges from 1% to 5%.[13, 14] The rates are higher in women who are older, obese women, and black women.[16, 17] Most chronically hypertensive women have primary (essential) hypertension, which is sometimes related to obesity. (The relationship between obesity, insulin resistance, and hypertension is discussed later; see Obesity and Insulin Resistance.)

In babies born to pregnant women with chronic hypertension, perinatal outcome is determined primarily by the presence or absence of superimposed preeclampsia.[16, 17] The criteria used to diagnose superimposed preeclampsia vary but have included exacerbation of hypertension, edema, proteinuria, hyperuricemia, or a combination of these factors.[17] Neither the exacerbation of hypertension nor edema is a reliable indicator of superimposed preeclampsia. In the absence of renal disease, the onset of significant proteinuria is the best indicator of superimposed preeclampsia.[16]

Rey and Couturier,[18] in their assessment of pregnancy outcome in women with chronic hypertension, demonstrated that fetal outcome is worse in superimposed preeclampsia than in preeclampsia in previously normotensive women. They showed that there was a higher perinatal mortality rate (45/1000 versus 12/1000), an increased incidence in preeclampsia (21.2% versus 2.3%), premature delivery (34.4% versus 15.0%), and fetal growth restriction (15.5% versus 6.3%), a higher primary cesarean section rate (29.6% versus 14.2%), and an increase in gestational diabetes (33.1% versus 12.0%). Chronic hypertensive women who did not develop superimposed preeclampsia had also significantly higher frequencies of perinatal death (29/1000) and small-for-gestational-age (SGA) newborns (10.5%) than the normotensive control group (perinatal death rate 12/1000).

In summary, women with chronic hypertension have a 10-fold potential increased risk for development of preeclampsia. Perinatal deaths are substantially more frequent in pregnant women with chronic hypertension with superimposed preeclampsia (10%) compared with pregnant women who have chronic hypertension (0.3%) alone.[18] Chronically hypertensive women are at a significant risk for severe early-onset, recurrent preeclampsia, or both.[15–17] The women with hypertension who are more likely to develop superimposed preeclampsia are those with more severe underlying blood pressure elevations, as demonstrated by left ventricular hypertrophy, increased serum creatinine levels, or a diastolic blood pressure above 100 mmHg at less than 20 weeks' gestation.[19] The clinical features and management of chronic hypertension in pregnant women are detailed in Chapter 8.

Renal Disease

The incidence of superimposed preeclampsia is markedly increased in patients with chronic renal disease and coexisting hypertension. It is difficult, however, to establish the exact risks because the diagnosis can be questioned in many pregnant women with known renal disorders presenting with worsening hypertension and proteinuria.[20] In contrast, patients with intrinsic renal disease who are normotensive and who have minimal renal dysfunction tend to have uncomplicated pregnancies, but the risk of maternal and fetal complications in women with moderate or severe renal insufficiency remains uncertain.

Jones and Hayslett[21] have assessed the maternal and obstetric complications in 67 women with primary renal disease (82 pregnancies). The mean serum creatinine concentration increased from 168 ± 71 μmol/L in early pregnancy to 221 ± 115 μmol/L in the third trimester. The frequency of hypertension rose from 28% at initial examination to 48% in the third trimester, and the frequency of high-grade proteinuria (>3 g/L) rose from 23% to 41%. A pregnancy-related loss of renal function occurred in 43% of the women. There was a high rate of both preterm delivery (59%) and growth restriction (37%), but the infant survival rate was 93%.

Jungers and coworkers[22] reported on all pregnancies (43 pregnancies in 30 women) taking place over 20 years (1975–1994) in one specialized hospital, the Necker Hospital in Paris. Successful pregnancies were significantly more common in the second decade than in the preceding one (91% versus 65%; $P = .05$). The overall live birth rate was higher in pregnancies in which the initial serum creatinine levels were below 200 μmol/L than in pregnancies with creatinine levels above 200 μmol/L (80% versus 53%; $P = .02$). The upper preconceptional serum creatinine level associated with a successful fetal outcome was 270 μmol/L. The relative risk for adverse perinatal outcome was 10.6 times higher when hypertension was present at conception or early in pregnancy. Seven women (23%) underwent an accelerated course toward end-stage renal failure; all of these women had severe hypertension and heavy proteinuria at conception. Superimposed preeclampsia was a frequent complication (>50% of all pregnancies), again mainly in patients with preexisting hypertension.

In 1987, Ihle and colleagues,[23] reporting on a follow-up study of 84 patients with early-onset preeclampsia (<37 weeks' gestation), found a high prevalence of underlying renal disease. Renal abnormalities were found in 33 of the 49 primiparas (67%) and in 22 of the 35 multiparas (63%). Two thirds of the multiparous women with either underlying essential hypertension or renal disease developed recurrent preeclampsia. Idiopathic preeclampsia occurred in 10% of primiparas in the early-onset group, whereas it was the main condition in more than 75% of primiparas in the late-onset group. These authors also suggested that a presumptive diagnosis of idiopathic preeclampsia is likely to be correct only in primiparous women developing the disease after 37 weeks of pregnancy, and in all other cases further investigation would detect an underlying, predominantly renal abnormality. In contrast, Reiter and coworkers[24] showed that 10% of women with de novo hypertension in pregnancy were subsequently found to have essential hypertension, and underlying renal disease was rare.

The exact mechanism by which renal disease is associated with increased risk for (superimposed) preeclampsia is unclear. The association might be explained in part by the fact that not all patients demonstrating an increased blood pressure and/or proteinuria are correctly classified as having preeclampsia.[25] Other possible mechanisms are an increased renal production of thromboxane-A_2[26] and increased homocysteine levels (see Hyperhomocysteinemia).

OBESITY, INSULIN RESISTANCE, AND DIABETES

Obesity and Insulin Resistance

Obesity is a major contributor to morbidity and mortality in the developed world. Obesity, insulin resistance, and glucose intolerance are strongly associated with nonpregnant hypertension. Insulin resistance predisposes to occlusive vascular disorders in nonpregnant subjects. Essential hypertension is an insulin-resistant condition. Fasting and postglucose plasma insulin levels are increased in hypertensive patients, and this finding is independent of obesity, glucose intolerance, age, and antihypertensive medication.[27, 28]

Several mechanisms have been postulated by which insulin resistance or hyperinsulinemia may increase blood pressure. Insulin may raise blood pressure by:

- Increasing renal tubular sodium reabsorption
- Stimulating the sympathetic nervous system
- Causing hypertrophy of vascular smooth muscle

Because of the importance of the insulin–insulin resistance–vascular tone interaction, especially in understanding the relation with preeclampsia, we discuss these mechanisms in detail. Insulin resistance may also raise blood pressure by altering cellular cation transport in arterial smooth muscle, which results in an intracellular accumulation of sodium and calcium.

Paolisso and Barbagallo[29] have suggested that a reduced intracellular magnesium concentration may provide the missing link between non–insulin-dependent diabetes (NIDDM) and hypertension.[29] Intracellular magnesium accumulation is virtually dependent on the activation of the insulin receptor. Magnesium ions promote smooth muscle relaxation, and offset calcium-related excitation-contraction coupling. Magnesium ions decrease cellular responsiveness to depolarizing stimuli by stimulating Ca^{2+}-dependent K^+ channels, which serve to offset the potential depolarizing influence of cellular calcium.

Epidemiologic studies suggest that an inverse relationship exists between magnesium intake and hypertension.[29] Lower magnesium intake was associated with higher blood pressure, and hypomagnesemia is a common finding in diabetic patients. Hypomagnesemia is also a feature of NIDDM. A depletion of magnesium seems to be a cofactor for a further derangement of insulin resistance. The pathogenetic role of magnesium depletion in NIDDM, which is supported by the Nurses Health Study, shows an increased magnesium intake to be associated with a significant decline in the incidence of NIDDM.[30]

Insulin is a vasodilatory hormone, inducing frank hypotension in the absence of an adequate compensatory rise in sympathetic activity. Peripheral insulin resistance in hypertension may signal a lack of effective insulin action,[29] and it is the lack of insulin effect on the vasculature, rather than hyperinsulinemia, that results in the development of hypertension. This is a very important point, because most of the postulated mechanisms by which insulin resistance causes vascular dysfunction are based on the assumption that insulin resistance induces hyperinsulinemia.

Within this concept, this elevated level of insulin in turn causes abnormality of the vasculature, hypertension, and atherosclerosis. However, this postulate is feasible only if there is differential expression of resistance in vivo, with vascular tissue lacking the resistance to insulin. Otherwise, if there is a general resistance to insulin in all tissues, hyperinsulinemia should not have any more effect on the vasculature than it does on the classical insulin tissues, such as liver, fat, and muscle. Thus, within the alternative concept, it is the lack of insulin effect that causes the vascular dysfunctions and not the hyperinsulinemia.[31] The lack of insulin's metabolic actions will then allow other vasoconstrictors to mediate their effects unopposed.

Enhanced sympathetic drive may result in or at least contribute to the insulin resistance–dyslipidemia complex in patients with hypertension.[32] There are at least three mechanisms by which sympathetic overactivity may lead to insulin resistance[32]:

1. Stimulation of β-adrenergic receptors causes acute insulin resistance.

2. Chronic β-adrenergic stimulation increases the proportion of insulin-resistant fast-twitch fibers in rats. Because the skeletal muscle is the major site of insulin resistance in humans, a change in fiber composition can have a major impact on the total body insulin sensitivity.

3. Vasoconstriction may decrease nutritional (capillary) blood flow and decrease the delivery of glucose to skeletal muscle cells.

The mechanism of the insulin resistance syndrome or tendency is complex[33]: Resistance to the glucoregulatory actions of insulin results in compensatory hyperinsulinemia. Insulin stimulates sodium reabsorption and has a sympathomimetic effect, contributing to a rise in blood pressure. Insulin may stimulate hepatic triglyceride release, and insulin resistance is associated with increased nonesterified fatty acid flux owing to suppression of lipolysis. This augments triglyceride release, which drives high-density lipoprotein concentrations down via the mediation of cholesterol ester–transfer protein.

Resistance to insulin's stimulatory effects on lipoprotein lipase might also contribute. This complex of lipoprotein disturbances tends to increase concentrations of the more atherogenic small, low-density lipoprotein. Insulin stimulates hepatic and endothelial synthesis of the antifibrinolytic factor plasminogen activator inhibitor-1 (PAI-1). The recognition of manifold interactions between insulin and other cardiovascular risk factors led Reaven[34] to introduce the term *insulin resistance syndrome*, unfortunately dubbed "syndrome X," a term already used by Kemp in 1973 to describe patients with angina and angiographically normal coronary arteries.[34] Reaven[35] has characterized syndrome X with the following features:

- Insulin resistance
- Compensatory hyperinsulinemia
- Glucose intolerance to some degree
- Increased plasma triglycerides
- Decreased high-density lipoprotein cholesterol concentrations
- High blood pressure
- Hyperuricemia
- Smaller low-density lipoprotein particles
- Higher circulating levels of PAI-1

Studies in the 1990s also demonstrated other signs of endothelial cell activation, such as increased levels of fVIIIrag.[36]

About 25% of apparently healthy people may be considered to be insulin-resistant.[33, 35] Insulin resistance may represent a permissive factor in the development of serious vascular disease or reflect an underlying vascular dysfunction, which may progress to atherosclerosis. The vasodilatory actions of insulin are impaired in insulin-resistant states, as are those of other vasoactive agents, and transport of insulin across the capillary endothelium is one of the rate-limiting steps in insulin actions.[33] Insulin resistance may therefore be an early indicator of vascular endothelial dysfunction. A subsequent metabolic disturbance might then feed back on insulin action to augment, sustain, or even initiate a state of insulin resistance.[33]

Obesity is the most common cause of insulin resistance. Basal and total 24-hour rates of insulin secretion are three to four times higher in obese subjects than in lean subjects.[35, 37] Obesity can lead to a decrease in insulin-mediated glucose uptake, which is corrected by weight loss, resulting in enhanced in vivo insulin action.[35] Body weight and blood pressure are linked along an entire continuum of levels, not only along the upper limits of each parameter.[38] Obesity is the most common nutritional disorder of affluent societies.[39] Unger[40] has suggested that both insulin resistance and glucose incompetence of β cells in obesity-dependent NIDDM are both caused by a single abnormality extrinsic to β cells, this extrinsic factor being the delivery of free fatty acids to tissues. This concept is known as the *lipotoxic hypothesis* and is based on the following[40]:

1. Plasma levels of free fatty acids are elevated in obesity.
2. Chronic exposure of cultured islets to free fatty acids causes basal hypersecretion of insulin.
3. Free fatty acid levels are high in obesity because they are not fully suppressed by the hyperinsulinemia they induce; that is, there is attenuation of the feedback between β cells and adipocytes that normally would prevent the coexistence of high insulin and high free fatty acid levels.

Obesity, hyperinsulinemia, and insulin resistance have now been recognized as risk factors for preeclampsia.[14] Stone and associates[41] found that the only risk factors associated with the development of severe preeclampsia were severe obesity in all patients (odds ratio [OR] 3.5; 95% confidence interval [CI] 1.68–7.46) and a history of preeclampsia in multiparous patients (OR 7.2; 95% CI 2.74–18.74). Unlike the earlier study by Chesley,[42] this study excluded patients with chronic hypertension. Therefore, a high body mass index (BMI) is an independent risk factor for preeclampsia. Estimates of the relative risk range from 2.3 to 5.5, depending on the definition of overweight used.[19]

Solomon and associates[43] found significantly higher glucose levels on 50-g oral glucose loading test and a significantly higher frequency of abnormal glucose loading tests in pregnant women who subsequently developed hypertension than in women who remained normotensive. Relative glucose intolerance was particularly common in women who developed nonproteinuric hy-

pertension. Women with gestational hypertension had significantly higher BMIs and baseline systolic and diastolic blood pressures, although all subjects were normotensive at baseline measurement by study design. There was a nonsignificant trend toward higher insulin levels in women with gestational hypertension. The authors concluded that a high BMI and a relative glucose intolerance were associated with an increased risk of new-onset nonproteinuric hypertension of pregnancy.

Laivuori and coworkers[44] compared carbohydrate and lipid metabolism in 22 women who had preeclampsia in their first pregnancy and in 22 control women who had remained normotensive during their first pregnancy, about 17 years earlier. At follow-up, there was no difference in BMI. Women with prior preeclampsia were normoglycemic but showed a significant hyperinsulinemia in the fasting state and after a glucose load. The serum levels of total cholesterol, high-density lipoprotein (HDL) cholesterol (with its subfractions HDL-2 and HDL-3), low-density lipoprotein cholesterol, triglyceride, or uric acid did not differ significantly between the study groups. These authors concluded that a history of preeclampsia was associated with mild hyperinsulinemia in nonpregnant women.

In a longitudinal study, Sowers and associates[45] measured fasting levels of insulin and glucose at 18 to 25 weeks' gestation in 140 nulliparous African-American women observed prospectively to delivery. Women who subsequently developed preeclampsia had significantly higher fasting insulin levels of 51.0 ± 12.0 μU/mL at 20 weeks; control subjects had values of 29.0 ± 2.8 μU/mL. Only mean arterial pressure and insulin levels were related to the development of preeclampsia. The finding that elevated second-trimester insulin levels characterize the subsequent development of preeclampsia, when controlled for increased mean arterial pressure, supports the hypothesis that hyperinsulinemia and associated insulin resistance may contribute to the pathogenesis of preeclampsia.

According to Cioffi and colleagues,[46] Sowers' findings[45] were a result of the higher BMI in the affected African-American women. Cioffi's group found a significant correlation between blood pressure at 26 to 28 weeks' gestation and both fasting insulin levels and insulin-glucose ratios as well as systolic blood pressure at term and fasting insulin levels in a group of 292 women of mixed parity. However, when controlled for confounding variables including BMI, race, and age, there was no statistically significant relationship. According to the Cioffi study, insulin resistance and hyperinsulinemia are not major determinants of blood pressure during pregnancy. Ethnic origin and obesity, as defined by the BMI, were more important factors in the development of gestational hypertension. However, the number of patients who developed hypertension in their study was small, and the authors did not differentiate between nonproteinuric hypertension and preeclampsia.

Kraayenbrink and associates[47] studied the relationship between insulin sensitivity and the angiotensin II pressor dose at 24 and 32 weeks' gestation in 64 nulliparous women who had been preselected because of an abnormal uteroplacental Doppler flow pattern. They found that future preeclamptic women were insulin resistant (as judged by the "intravenous mini-model") and hyperinsulinemic, and that angiotensin II sensitivity is partially determined by insulin resistance and cannot be explained by prostacyclin deficiency.

Thus, most studies confirm the presence of a certain degree of insulin resistance and hyperinsulinemia in preeclamptic women during pregnancy and several months and even years after delivery.[48] To a large extent, the insulin resistance appears to be based on a higher mean BMI in women with preeclampsia. The exact mechanism by which obesity and insulin resistance are associated with an increased risk for preeclampsia is not completely understood. Several possible explanations are described next.

Characteristic Hemodynamics Associated With Obesity

Obesity is characterized by an expanded blood volume and an increase in cardiac output (increased stroke volume) in order to meet increased metabolic demands.[49] Hypertension results when the systemic vascular resistance fails to decrease as cardiac output increases. The larger size of the obese individual necessitates a higher cardiac output at any level of blood pressure; the systemic vascular resistance is low compared with those of lean individuals with the same blood pressure. Normotensive obese individuals have an elevated cardiac output similar to that of hypertensive obese patients.[49]

Easterling and coworkers,[50] using noninvasive Doppler technology, measured cardiac output serially in a blinded longitudinal study of nulliparous women with uncomplicated pregnancies. They found that the cardiac output was significantly elevated throughout pregnancy in the nine patients who became preeclamptic. Six weeks post partum, the hypertension of the preeclamptic subjects had resolved but cardiac output remained elevated and peripheral resistance remained lower than in the normotensive subjects. The authors concluded that preeclampsia was not a disease of systemic hypoperfusion and therefore challenged current vascular models of the disease. They hypothesized that, early in pregnancy, preeclamptic patients have an elevated cardiac output with compensatory vasodilatation and suggested that "the dilated systemic terminal arterioles and renal afferent arterioles may expose capillary beds to systemic pressures and increased flow," which would eventually lead to the endothelial cell damage.

Although their observation in itself is relevant, the hemodynamics observed by Easterling and coworkers[50] may not represent a specific preeclamptic hemodynamic pattern but merely reflect the relative obesity of the preeclamptic women. In the Easterling study,[50] the hypertensive patients were not only shorter but also much heavier (80.5 versus 68.8 kg) than the normotensive control group. This is supported by the significantly higher mean arterial blood pressure in the first trimester and the elevated cardiac output in the preeclamptic patients 6 weeks post partum. The preeclamptic patients (n = 9) delivered at the same gestational age (39.4 weeks) as the normotensive control patients; thus, the hemodynamic data show that, also in pregnancy, obesity is associated with a high cardiac output and a hyperdynamic circulation, which may result in an increased incidence of near-term preeclampsia, possibly by creating too much shear stress on the vessel wall.

Dyslipidemia

Obesity is associated not only with hypertension but also with increased lipid availability and delivery of free fatty acids to tissues, higher cholesterol and triglyceride levels, insulin resistance, and hyperinsulinemia. Serum in preeclamptic women is more cytotoxic to endothelial cells than that from healthy normotensive pregnant women, resulting in more triglyceride accumulation in cultured endothelial cells in an in vitro model. Circulating free fatty acids are increased in women who later develop preeclampsia, long before the clinical onset of the disease.

Sera from preeclamptic women have both a higher ratio of free fatty acids to albumin and increased lipolytic activity, resulting in enhanced endothelial cell uptake of free fatty acids, which are further esterified within the endothelial cells into triglycerides.[51, 52] Plasma albumin exists as several isoelectric species, which range from isoelectric point (pI) 4.8 to pI 5.6. The more nonesterified fatty acids are bound to albumin, the lower the pI. The proportions of these isoelectric species of plasma albumin change rapidly in response to the body's need to mobilize nonesterified fatty acids from adipose tissue and transport them to the liver for incorporation into very-low-density lipoprotein (VLDL). Plasma albumin exerts a toxicity-preventing activity (TxPA) if it is in the pI 5.6 form. Because higher ratios of nonesterified fatty acids to albumin cause a shift from the pI 5.6 to the pI 4.8 form of plasma albumin, preeclamptic patients have lower amounts of protective TxPA (pI 5.6) than normotensive pregnant women do. A low ratio of TxPA to VLDL results in in vitro triglyceride accumulation in endothelial cells and in cytotoxicity.

Arbogast and coworkers[53] suggested that it is the increased VLDL toxicity that results in endothelial cell dysfunction and damage in preeclampsia. They believe that in order to compensate for the increased energy demands of pregnancy, placental hormones increase the mobilization of nonesterified fatty acids from adipose tissue. In women with low albumin concentrations, the burden of transporting extra nonesterified fatty acids from the adipose tissue to the liver is likely to reduce the concentration of TxPA to a point where VLDL toxicity is expressed. VLDL will then damage the vascular endothelium. The effects of obesity and insulin resistance in the causation of an increased incidence of preeclampsia may thus be mediated by a further or earlier derangement of the VLDL/TxPA balance.[40, 53]

Adipocytes Produce Cytokines (Especially Tumor Necrosis Factor-α)

Adipose tissue has a characteristic and unique feature in its enormous potential for volume and mass change. The hypothalamic region controls the basal metabolic rate, appetite, and levels of energy expenditure.[54] One of the most exciting developments in the field of obesity is the discovery of specific genes responsible for excessive fatness in animal models. The Ob/Ob mouse has attracted particular attention because of the proven existence of a defective or even absent blood-borne factor responsible for the control of food intake. This circulating factor has been cloned. The gene was found to be expressed only in fat cells. The cause of obesity in Ob/Ob mice was predicted to be an absence of circulating Ob protein, called *leptin*. The mouse Ob gene also has a closely related human homologue.[55]

Total body fatness has been linked to deoxyribonucleic acid (DNA) polymorphisms in the gene encoding tumor necrosis factor-alpha (TNF-α), which appears to point to the existence of an intricate interaction between body fat, insulin, and cytokine levels. TNF-α is produced by human preadipocytes and adipocytes. Its production is higher in obesity, with up to threefold increases in TNF-α messenger ribonucleic acid (mRNA), protein, and circulating levels. With respect to adipocyte function, TNF-α induces insulin resistance by at least two mechanisms[54]:

1. Downregulation of insulin tyrosine kinase activity.
2. Induction of an abnormality in insulin receptor substrate I, which inhibits phosphorylation of components of the insulin signaling cascade.

TNF-α reduces adipose mass by a reduction in cell number and volume. It is for these reasons that TNF-α has been proposed to be the "link" between insulin resistance and obesity. It is also possible that the increase in adipocyte TNF-α production in obese individuals may be protective by limiting potential weight gain. However, this protective mechanism may result in long-term overnutrition, resulting in hyperlipidemia and an increased cardiovascular risk.[54]

Within this context, obesity, insulin resistance, and the associated hyperinsulinemia may be involved in aggravating cytokine-mediated oxidative stress and increased expression of endothelial adhesion molecules, which are intimately related to the endothelial cell dysfunction and thus the pathophysiology of the clinical syndrome preeclampsia.[56, 57]

Direct Hemodynamic Effects of Insulin Resistance and Hyperinsulinemia

As discussed earlier, insulin resistance itself and the subsequent hyperinsulinemia are associated with increased sympathetic activity, increased tubular sodium resorption, or both.[27, 28] The increased sympathetic activity may reflect a compensatory reaction to the vasodilatory effects of insulin or a leptin-related attempt to increase energy expenditure.[39]

Schobel and associates[58] used intraneural recordings of sympathetic nerve activity in muscle-nerve fascicles to show that preeclampsia is accompanied by increased sympathetic overactivity. Insulin resistance and hyperinsulinemia may be related to this state of increased sympathetic activity.[59]

Finally, an endogenous sodium pump inhibitor or digitalis-like factor has been postulated to mediate essential hypertension, and increased levels have been found in pregnant women with NIDDM and in preeclamptic patients.[60]

Hyperinsulinemia and Trophoblast Invasion

In addition to cytokines, fetal and placental growth are at least partially regulated by insulin growth factors (IGFs) and insulin-like growth factor binding proteins (IGFBPs).[61, 62] IGFBP-1 is produced by decidual stromal cells, and plasma IGFBP-1 concentrations have been found to be decreased in women who later develop preeclampsia. These lower IGFBP-1 levels may reflect impaired trophoblast invasion.[63] Insulin, at physiologic concentrations, causes a dose-dependent reduction of decidual IGFBP-1 secretion. Hyperinsulinemia in insulin-resistant states may interfere with the balance between the effects of IGF-I and IGFBP-1.[61–63]

The Barker Hypothesis

The Barker phenomenon[64–66] has shown that there is a startling relationship between fetal growth restriction and an increased chance of cardiovascular disease in adult life. Children not only inherit their X chromosome from their mother but also are affected by their prenatal environment. Long-term follow-up studies have demonstrated that babies who suffered intrauterine growth restriction are more likely to have hypertension, coronary artery disease, and diabetes in adult life.[64–66]

The increased incidence of raised blood pressure is not confined to offspring who sustained intrauterine growth restriction. Blood pressure falls progressively across the whole range of birth weights.[66] Hypertension and insulin resistance may be a part of syndrome X, the incidence of which is markedly increased in patients who were growth-restricted themselves at birth.[64–67] Men and women with low birth weights have a high prevalence of syndrome X, a syndrome associated with marked insulin resistance.[64] The prevalence of syndrome X is about 30% in adults who weighed 2.475 kg or less at birth and 6% in adults who weighed 4.275 kg or more.[64] Hence, the population distribution of blood pressure and insulin resistance appears to be at least partly programmed in intrauterine life.[66]

A potential explanation for the apparent "hereditary" characteristics of preeclampsia may be that the daughters born to a severely preeclamptic woman may have been in a poor intrauterine environment, with its adverse effects and long-term sequelae on the cardiovascular system. This results in an increased incidence of pregnancies complicated by intrauterine growth restriction and preeclampsia. In a group of 31 women with pregnancy-induced hypertension (eight with proteinuria), Kaaja and colleagues[68] determined the presence of the major features of syndrome X and found that the metabolic characteristics (hypertriglyceridemia, hyperinsulinemia, hyperuricemia, low HDL-2 cholesterol) in pregnancy-induced hypertension resemble the main features of the "insulin resistance syndrome."

Alternatively, insulin resistance may be the programmed response to fetal undernutrition.[69] The undernourished fetus makes metabolic adaptations, including becoming relatively insulin-resistant, from which it benefits in the short term by increasing fuel availability, after which these adaptations become permanently programmed and persist throughout life.[69]

Gestational Diabetes

The relation between gestational diabetes and preeclampsia is controversial.[70] In a study of 1249 nondiabetic women, Khan and Daya[71] found that even minor degrees of glucose intolerance are associated with a higher incidence of preeclampsia; the odds of having preeclampsia were increased by 20% (95% CI 0%–44%) per mmol/L rise in plasma glucose level in the glucose tolerance test.

Serner and coworkers,[72] in a study of 3637 patients without gestational diabetes carrying singleton fetuses, showed that increasing carbohydrate intolerance is an independent predictor for preeclampsia. In contrast, Suhonen and Teramo[73] found the frequency of pregnancy-induced hypertension and preeclampsia (19.8% versus 6.1%; $P < .001$) to be higher in the gestational diabetes group but not in the borderline group when compared with control pregnant women. In this study, the women with gestational diabetes and women in the borderline group were older and their prepregnancy weight and BMI were significantly higher than those in the control group. In addition, Schaffir and colleagues,[74] when comparing 197 gestational diabetic women with 197 control patients matched on the basis of age, race, parity, and prepregnancy weight, found no relation between gestational diabetes and pregnancy-induced hypertensive disorders.

Thus, the relation between gestational diabetes and pregnancy-induced hypertensive disorders remains controversial. We believe that obesity, which occurs in a significant percentage of gestational diabetic mothers, is probably the major factor contributing to the increased incidence of pregnancy-induced hypertensive disorders.

Diabetes Mellitus

Diabetes mellitus is associated with an increased incidence of preeclampsia, especially if there is established microvascular disease,[75] with incidences of 30% being reported among women with White classes D, F, and R. (The clinical features and management of pregnant diabetic women with hypertension are discussed in detail in Chapter 9.)

Van Assche and coworkers[76] suggested that the increased incidence of preeclampsia in women with type I diabetes was associated with an increased production of thromboxane-A_2. There is also an abnormal antioxidant status in women with impaired glucose tolerance and NIDDM.[77] Reactive oxygen species are formed in diabetes mellitus by the auto-oxidation of glucose and glycosylated proteins. There are increased lipid peroxidation and reduced levels of superoxide dismutase, catalase, glutathione, and ascorbic acid in NIDDM.[77]

Vijayalingam and associates[77] demonstrated that the altered antioxidant status is already present in individuals with impaired glucose tolerance before the onset of NIDDM, and the reactive oxygen species may even be involved in the progression from impaired glucose tolerance to NIDDM. In this way, hyperglycemia may lead to a higher incidence of preeclampsia by increasing overall oxidative stress.[56]

TNF may be relevant to the pathogenesis of both preeclampsia and type I diabetes.[78] Human TNF secretion to lipopolysaccharide is human leukocyte antigen (HLA) class II dependent. HLA-DR1, -DR3, and -DR4 individuals are high responders, whereas HLA-DR2 and -DR5 individuals are low responders, and it has been suggested that TNF plays a role in the pathogenesis of type I diabetes and is responsible for the HLA associations of the disease.[79]

Kilpatrick[78] tested the hypothesis that preeclampsia and diabetes may share a common immunogenetic susceptibility by comparing 92 preeclampsia patients with 264 general population controls. The relative frequencies of individual HLA-DR antigens in preeclamptic patients were found to correlate with reported relative TNF-α responses for those antigens. Moreover, putative high-responder HLA-DR1, -DR3 and -DR4 alleles were significantly ($P < .001$) more frequent in preeclampsia patients (79%) than in controls (59%). These findings confirm an association between preeclampsia and the group of HLA-DR specificities found in association with high TNF responders. This hypothesis may explain the weak association between preeclampsia and diabetes. In an earlier study, however, Liston and Kilpatrick[80] found no single DR4-bearing haplotype to be overrepresented in preeclampsia.

The Kilpatrick study[78] suggests that it is not necessary to invoke HLA-DR4 being linked to a susceptibility gene. Instead,

HLA-DR4 (and other DRβ alleles) may function as immune response genes, modulating the TNF-α response to (unspecified) stimulation. Such HLA associations, presumably, would be in addition to, and independent of, other disease susceptibility genes, and HLA would be part of a more complex genetic susceptibility, which would also include a fetal contribution.[79, 80]

OTHER ENDOCRINE DISORDERS

Disturbances of normal thyroid function—hypothyroidism and hyperthyroidism—are associated with an increased incidence of preeclampsia.[81, 82] The exact relationship is unclear. With autoimmune thyroid disorders, the increased incidence of preeclampsia may not reflect the abnormal thyroid function as such but may instead reflect the tendency for development of autoimmune antibodies.

THROMBOPHILIC DISORDERS, INCLUDING HYPERHOMOCYSTEINEMIA

In the 1990s, it was found that patients who had severe early-onset preeclampsia often had hemostatic or metabolic abnormalities known to be associated with vascular thrombosis.

Dekker and colleagues[15] evaluated a total of 101 patients with a history of severe early-onset preeclampsia. These patients were tested at least 10 weeks post partum for the presence of hyperhomocysteinemia, protein C, protein S, and antithrombin III deficiency as well as for activated protein C resistance (aPC-R), lupus anticoagulant, and immunoglobulin G or M anticardiolipin antibodies, or both. The authors found that chronic hypertension was the most common (39%) underlying disorder. However, the most exciting part of the study demonstrated the presence of a high incidence of thrombophilia. Eighty-five patients were tested for coagulation disturbances, and 21 (24.7%) had protein S deficiency. Fifty patients were tested for aPC-R, and eight (16.0%) showed positive findings. Seventy-nine patients were tested for hyperhomocysteinemia, and 14 (17.7%) had a positive methionine loading test result. Finally, 95 patients were tested for anticardiolipin antibodies; 27 (29.4%) had detectable immunoglobulin G or M anticardiolipin antibodies, or both.

A subsequent study of a larger group consisted of more than 300 patients with a history of severe preeclampsia, including patients with HELLP (*h*emolysis, *e*levated *l*iver enzymes, *l*ow *p*latelets) syndrome or eclampsia, or with both. The same authors were able to include a control group of 65 women with only uncomplicated pregnancies.[83] The main findings of this study are presented in Table 6–1.

After this first report, Preston and coworkers[84] reported on the relationship between heritable thrombophilic defects and fetal loss in a cohort of women with factor V Leiden mutation or deficiency of antithrombin, protein C, or protein S. The authors studied 1384 women enrolled in the European Prospective Cohort on Thrombophilia (EPCOT). They analyzed the frequencies of miscarriage (fetal loss at or before 28 weeks' gestation) and stillbirth (fetal loss after 28 weeks' gestation) jointly and separately.

The risk of fetal loss was increased in women with thrombophilia (168/571 versus 93/395; OR 1.35 [95% CI 1.01–1.82]). The

TABLE 6–1. PREVALENCE OF HEMOSTATIC ABNORMALITIES IN WOMEN WITH A HISTORY OF SEVERE PREECLAMPSIA

ABNORMALITY	CONTROLS	PREECLAMPSIA < 28 W*	PREECLAMPSIA > 28 W†
Protein S deficiency	6/65 (9.0%)	11/59 (19.0%)	26/251 (10.0%)
aPC-R	1/67 (1.5%)	9/50 (18.0%)	23/234 (9.8%)
fV Leiden	1/67 (1.5%)	4/50 (8.0%)	13/234 (5.6%)
HHC	3/67 (4.5%)	11/58 (19.0%)	35/289 (10.4%)
ACA	5/67 (7.5%)	17/62 (27.4%)	50/259 (19.3%)

*Preeclampsia and delivery before 28 weeks' gestation.
†Preeclampsia and delivery after 28 weeks' gestation.

ACA, detectable anticardiolipin IgG and/or IgM antibodies; aPC-R, activated protein C resistance; fV, factor V Leiden mutation; HIC, hyperhomocysteinemia.

OR was higher for stillbirth than for miscarriage (3.6 [CI 1.4–9.4] versus 1.27 [CI 0.94–1.71]). The highest OR for stillbirth was in women with combined defects (14.3 [CI 2.4–86.0]) compared with 5.2 (CI 1.5–18.1) in antithrombin deficiency, 2.3 (CI 0.6–8.3) in protein C deficiency, 3.3 (CI 1.0–11.3) in protein S deficiency, and 2.0 (CI 0.5–7.7) with factor V Leiden. The corresponding ORs for miscarriage in these subgroups were 0.8 (CI 0.2–3.6), 1.7 (CI 1.0–2.8), 1.4 (CI 0.9–2.2), 1.2 (CI 0.7–1.9), and 0.9 (CI 0.5–1.5).

The authors concluded that women with familial thrombophilia, especially those with combined defects or antithrombin deficiency, have an increased risk of fetal loss. Although the authors state that for all women with thrombophilia, the relative risk of stillbirth was greater than that for miscarriage, they do not provide data on the incidence of preeclampsia.

Another landmark study was published by Kupferminc and colleagues,[84a] who studied 110 women with obstetrical complications and 110 carefully matched controls. The fV Leiden mutation, homozygosity for MTHFR, and the prothrombin gene were found to be significantly more common in the women with obstetrical complications. Overall, 52% of women with an obstetrical complication had a thrombophilic mutation in contrast to 19% in women with normal pregnancies. In subgroup analyses, the prevalence of mutations in the three genes was 53% among the women with severe preeclampsia, 60% among those with abruptio placentae, 50% among women whose fetuses had growth restriction, and 42% among women whose infants were stillborn.

The following paragraphs review the relevant facts of these thrombophilic disorders.

Activated Protein C Resistance, Factor V Leiden

Protein C, protein S, and antithrombin III deficiencies are known to be associated with a marked increase in thrombotic disorders. The protein C pathway provides anticoagulant properties critical for limiting thrombosis. Thrombin activates the natural antithrombotic zymogen protein C, a vitamin K–dependent serine protease, by cleaving the amino-terminal dodecapeptide when bound to the endothelial cell surface factor thrombomodulin. In the presence of protein S, activated protein C (aPC) selectively degrades the coagulation factors Va and VIIIa. aPC also activates the fibrinolytic system by destroying fast-acting inhibitors of plasminogen activator.[85–88] In the 1990s, resistance to aPC was recognized as an important cause for familial thrombophilia.[85–88]

Protein S is another vitamin K–dependent protein and also serves as a cofactor for aPC.[89, 90] Both Protein S deficiency and aPC resistance result in an impaired aPC pathway. This impairment is apparently associated with a more aggressive course of the pathologic changes (thrombosis, acute atherosis) in the spiral arteries.

In 90% of cases of aPC resistance, the cause is a mutation of the coagulation factor V gene. Factor V is found in plasma and in platelet granules. Under the influence of thrombin, factor V is first activated and eventually inactivated after prolonged exposure to thrombin.

Factor V is the cofactor to factor Xa. Together with phospholipid and Ca^{2+}, it is responsible for factor II activation. The Leiden mutation of factor V leads to replacement of arginine 506 at position 1691 by a glutamine, resulting in preventing cleavage of activated factor V by aPC.[87, 88] The factor V Leiden molecules are resistant to degradation by aPC; however, they retain their procoagulant activity and predispose to thromboembolic disorders.

The factor V Leiden mutation is the most common genetic risk factor for deep vein thrombosis; it is present in about 5% of the white population. The highest prevalence, 15%, is found in Greece and Sweden. In contrast, the prevalence of the mutation in Asian and African countries seems much lower.[91]

Patients with this mutation have an estimated five to 10 times increased thrombotic risk in heterozygotes and a 50 to 100 times increased risk in homozygotes.[92] Hellgren and colleagues[93] found aPC resistance in about 60% of all patients with thromboembolic complications in connection with pregnancy. Because the factor V Leiden mutation responsible for aPC resistance is very common, it has been suggested that it would be reasonable to perform general screening for aPC resistance during early pregnancy or before prescribing any oral contraceptive pill.[93, 94]

Dizon-Townson and coworkers[94] found an allele frequency of 3% in a study in 407 women admitted to labor and delivery. Four of the 14 carriers had a deep vein thrombosis, one patient had a consumptive coagulopathy, and one patient had preeclampsia.

An increased incidence of aPC resistance and/or factor V Leiden mutation in women with a history of preeclampsia has since been noted by several groups.[94a–94c] In a relatively large case (n = 283)-control (n = 200) study, O'Shaughnessy et al[94d] found no evidence for the presence of an association between the fV Leiden mutation and preeclampsia. Although about 50% of these patients had severe preeclampsia and/or HELLP syndrome, information on the gestational age and birth weights are not mentioned. The absence of this association in the O'Shaughnessy study may well be related to the fact that most patients had preeclampsia in the near term period (>34 weeks' gestation).

In another prospective study, Murphy and coauthors[94e] found a similar frequency of the factor V Leiden mutation in preeclamptic (n = 12) and IUGR (n = 9) patients as in women with an uncomplicated pregnancy. Although this was a well-designed study, including nearly 600 nulliparous women, the incidence of severe early-onset preeclampsia (0.5%–1%) is so low that one needs an enormous sample size to evaluate the risk between any "high-risk" gene and severe early-onset preeclampsia. The patient cohorts studied in the two Amsterdam studies[15, 83] represent selected groups of very sick patients with early-onset preeclampsia referred to two large level III perinatal centers, from a densely populated area in The Netherlands with about 40,000 births per year.

The large series from the Amsterdam group (see Table 6–1) clearly demonstrates that the incidence of aPC resistance in patients with a history of severe preeclampsia is about six to seven times higher than in a control population; for patients with a history of early-onset preeclampsia, the incidence is about 10 to 12 times higher.[83] Interestingly, in the patients with aPC resistance, only half had a factor V mutation. Thus, aPC resistance not associated with a mutation in factor V appears to be prevalent in women with a history of severe preeclampsia, which is in concordance with observations in patients with cerebral ischemic disorders.[95] In the Amsterdam study, the investigators were able to show that their cases of aPC resistance were not due to the use of oral

contraceptives or recent pregnancies.[82, 83] An increased incidence of aPC resistance or factor V Leiden mutation, or both, in women with a history of preeclampsia has been verified by several other groups.[96–98] Of note, a certain degree of resistance to the effects of aPC is probably a physiologic feature of normal pregnancy, and a significant decrease in aPC sensitivity is present in about 50% of all pregnant women; this is maximal by week 28 of pregnancy.[99]

Protein S Deficiency

Even though hepatocytes are thought to be the major source of protein S production, vascular endothelial cells, megakaryocytes, osteoblasts, and neuroblast-derived tissue also synthesize significant amounts of protein S.[89, 90] Cytokines, such as TNF, and antiphospholipid antibodies are known to downregulate endothelial but not hepatic protein S secretion.[100] Protein S normally exists in plasma in two forms: (1) the functionally active free protein S and (2) protein S complexed with C4b-binding protein, which is functionally inactive. Thrombin degrades the protein S–C4b-binding protein complex and releases active free protein S.

Both free and bound protein S levels decrease early in pregnancy, with functional protein S remaining at levels of about 40% to 50% of normal through the first few days of the postpartum period. In contrast, no significant changes in the levels of protein C and antithrombin III occur during normal pregnancy.[101–103] Total protein S decreases in oral contraceptive users. The effect of oral contraceptives on free protein S is more controversial. According to Huisveld and associates,[104] oral contraceptives cause decreased total protein S, but because plasma levels of C4b-binding protein decrease as well, there is no net change in free protein S. In contrast, Malm and colleagues[105] found that oral contraceptives result in decreases of about 20% in both free and total protein S.

Compared with rates during normal pregnancy, preeclampsia is associated with increased thrombin/antithrombin III levels, reduced antithrombin III and protein C levels, but no further reduction of protein S.[101–103] Thrombophilia due to inherited deficiency of protein S was described in 1984.[106] The clinical manifestations of protein S deficiency are similar to those of deficiency of antithrombin III or protein C. In the normal population, the prevalence of protein S deficiency is not well known.

Tait and coworkers[107] measured total and free protein S antigen in 3971 blood donors. There was a marked interindividual variation in protein S results and mean values in males (total protein S 111%) were higher than in females (total protein S, 99%), whereas women taking oral contraceptives had even lower mean protein S antigen levels (total protein S, 91%). By applying arithmetically derived, gender-specific, 2 standard deviation "normal ranges" calculated from the whole cohort, the investigators identified 56 donors (1.4%) as having low total protein S antigen. Retesting 54 of these donors 6 months later established nine as having a persisting reduction in protein S antigen (0.2%).

According to Koster (personal communication, Leiden Thrombophilia Study, 1994) the incidence of protein S deficiency in the Netherlands is about 2%, which fits reasonably with the 1.4% reported by Tait and coworkers,[107] after a single protein S antigen measurement. In patients with deep venous thrombosis, the incidence of protein S deficiency seems only slightly higher, ranging between 1% and 8%.[107]

Very precise selection criteria were used in the Amsterdam study. All patients were tested at least 10 weeks post partum, and all were tested twice; only if the protein S antigen level was below 70% twice were patients considered to have protein S deficiency. Thus, the incidence of protein S deficiency in a population of patients with early-onset preeclampsia is about two to 10 times higher than in the control population, depending on which control population is used.[15, 83]

Several groups have demonstrated that antiphospholipids can interact with phospholipids and inhibit the protein S–dependent anticoagulant activity of aPC. A reduction in free protein S has also been reported in systemic lupus erythematosus (SLE) with or without antiphospholipids (aPLs). Interestingly, the most frequent combination of abnormal laboratory results reported by the Amsterdam group was protein S deficiency plus the presence of anticardiolipin antibodies.[15, 83]

All patients with a history of severe early-onset preeclampsia should be screened for protein S deficiency and aPC resistance (and factor V mutation) for the following reasons:

1. Results may be helpful in choosing appropriate pharmacologic management in future pregnancies.

2. Documentation of a thrombophilic disorder allows gynecologists to give safer and more balanced advice on contraception methods.

3. These disorders are hereditary; thus first-degree and second-degree relatives should be offered screening.

Antiphospholipids

Antiphospholipid (aPL) antibodies were first described by Wassermann in 1906 in patients with systemic lupus erythematosus (SLE).[108] Since then, it has been recognized that most cases of aPL syndrome neither meet international criteria for the classification of SLE nor have any recognizable features of the disease. The aPL syndrome is also seen in lupus variants such as discoid LE, subacute (Ro-positive) LE, and Sjögren syndrome, and it is rarely found in rheumatoid arthritis and primary inflammatory vasculitis.[109] The occurrence of a primary antiphospholipid syndrome (APS) was proposed by Harris[110, 111] with the following features:

- Recurrent venous or arterial thrombosis
- Recurrent fetal loss
- Thrombocytopenia
- Immunoglobulin G (IgG) anticardiolipin (aCL) above 20 IgG phospholipid units (GPLs)
- Lupus anticoagulant

Other features include[109–112]:

- Labile hypertension
- Migraine
- Epilepsy
- Transverse myelopathy
- Heart valve disease
- Ocular ischemia

APS is associated with both venous and arterial thrombosis, the latter distinguishing it from many other hypercoagulable disorders. Vessels of all sizes may be involved, including the aortic arch, carotid artery, pulmonary vessels, and smaller skin vessels. The antibodies persist for many years, and possibly for a lifetime.[109]

Antiphospholipid antibodies are a diverse family of autoantibodies that share in common a reactivity with negatively charged phospholipids. There are three clinically significant members[113]:

- The biologic false-positive test for syphilis
- Lupus anticoagulant
- Anticardiolipin antibodies

The standard tests for syphilis, such as the Venereal Diseases Research Laboratories (VDRL) and rapid plasma reagin (RPR), both use an antigen containing cardiolipin. The negatively charged cardiolipin reacts with antibodies produced in response to syphilitic infection. These antibodies have been called reagins. Moore and Mohr[114] in 1952 first used the term *biological false-positive test for syphilis* (BFP-STS) for patients who have positive reactions to reaginic tests but who have negative fluorescent treponemal antibody absorption (FTA-ABS) tests. These authors also demonstrated for the first time that two types of BFP-STS reactions might be encountered:

1. The "acute" reaction, a temporary positivity that appeared either during or following a nonsyphilitic infectious disease process and might disappear within days, weeks, or months (usually less than 6 months). These antibodies are not associated with thrombophilia.[113, 114]

2. The chronic reaction, seropositivity that might last for more than 6 months, years, or the lifetime of a patient. Moore and Lutz[115] showed that patients in the latter category have a high incidence of autoimmune disorders, especially SLE.

Lupus anticoagulant (LAC) derives its name from the fact that it originally was reported in patients with SLE. Although it is called anticoagulant, it is a misnomer since it is in fact associated with thrombosis instead of a bleeding tendency.[108] LAC comprises autoantibodies of either IgG or IgM class that prolong phospholipid-dependent coagulation assays by reacting with negatively charged phospholipids. A number of coagulation assays are currently used to screen for LAC. These include the activated partial thromboplastin time, kaolin clotting time, dilute Russell viper venom test, and the dilute tissue thromboplastin assay. There is no agreement in the literature as to which of these tests is most specific or

sensitive. There is common agreement that no single test can detect all LAC.[113, 116]

The third type of aPL, the *anticardiolipin antibody* (ACA), is detected by enzyme-linked immunosorbent assay or radioimmunoassay. Historically, the ACA assay may be considered to be a development from the RPR and VDRL for syphilis, which use a cardiolipin antigen. It was described that SLE patients with LAC often have a BFP-STS. The ACA assay has proved to be 200 to 400 times more sensitive than the VDRL test and detected 91% of the LAC in the original population studied.[113, 117] ACA enzyme-linked immunosorbent assays are subject to excessive interlaboratory variability. Although many factors may contribute to this variability, it has long been known that the sample diluent used in the assay is critical.[117–119] Only assays using bovine serum as the diluent are reliable. This is due to the requirement of the ACA cofactor, which is present in bovine serum. This cofactor has been identified as $\beta2$-glycoprotein-I (β_2-GP-I). A second hurdle to the usefulness of the ACA assay is the continued failure of the international community to agree on a standard from an international standardization workshop (Kingston Anti-Phospholipid Antibody Study) that utilizes the units GPL and MPL (IgG and IgM aCL units).[120–123]

Antiphospholipid antibodies have a well-established association with fetal loss,[113] half of which occurs in the second trimester. The aPL syndrome is associated with placental vascular thrombosis, decidual vasculopathy, intervillous fibrin deposition, and placental infarction. These pathologic changes in the placenta eventually result in abortion, fetal growth restriction, fetal demise, and severe preeclampsia. Although the clinical observations among patients with aPL antibodies unequivocally support a disturbance in coagulation as a central feature of this syndrome's pathophysiologic mechanism, it is still not completely understood by which pathway these antibodies promote thrombosis and why such a variable degree of expression exists among asymptomatic women and patients with overt autoimmune disease.[113, 124–126] A causal relationship between these antibodies and thrombosis or fetal loss has been proposed via interference with several natural phospholipid-dependent antithrombotic pathways, such as prostacyclin release, endothelial protein S production, thrombomodulin-dependent activation of protein C, endothelial cell surface expression of activated factor VII (in the presence of minimal levels of certain cytokines), contact-mediated fibrinolysis, and direct ACA-induced platelet adherence possibly mediated by platelet-activating factor.[113, 124, 126]

ACA, in the presence of β_2-GP-I, may induce thrombosis by inducing the expression of endothelial adhesion molecules. IgG purified from patients with aPL activates vascular endothelial cells, converting the steady-state, nonthrombotic endothelial surface into a prothrombotic state. The aPL-activated endothelial cells are characterized by the expression of leukocyte adhesion molecules, including intercellular adhesion molecule-1, vascular cell adhesion molecule, and E-selectin.[125]

Animal experiments in the 1990s have provided direct evidence for a pathogenic role of aPL antibodies. An experimental APS could be induced in naive mice upon active or passive immunization with ACA.[127, 128] Important progress has also been made by the recognition of the pathophysiologic importance of β_2-GP-I. ACAs are not directed against cardiolipin itself but against the complex that insolubilized cardiolipin forms with β_2-GP-I, a plasma protein with anticoagulant properties. That β_2-GP-I is important in its own right is demonstrated by the observation that immunization of normal mice with a mixture of cardiolipin and β_2-GP-I resulted in high titers of aPL, whereas cardiolipin alone was not immunogenic.[129] β_2-GP-I, a single-chain polypeptide consisting of 326 amino acids, inhibits the contact phase of the intrinsic coagulation pathway, platelet prothrombinase activity, and adenosine diphosphate–induced platelet aggregation, and is one of the naturally occurring anticoagulants. Many investigators now believe that β_2-GP-I as well as other phospholipid-associated proteins may be the actual epitopes for aPL binding. Moreover, β_2-GP-I–dependent ACA correlates better with clinical disorders associated with aPL antibodies; however, the clinical relevance of this is uncertain because assays currently used for ACA use β_2-GP-I–containing sera and thus ascertain β_2-GP-I–dependent antibodies.[130, 131] Antiphospholipid antibodies binding to other protein/phospholipid complexes such as protein C–phospholipid and protein S–phospholipid have meanwhile been found,[132] and a similar role has been reported also for annexin V, thrombomodulin, high- and low-molecular-weight kininogens.[132] Antiprothrombin antibodies are detected in approximately 50% of the aPL-positive patients, and these antibodies have been demonstrated to hamper the calcium-mediated prothrombin/lipid complex, thus causing the prolongation of the phospholipid-dependent coagulation reactions. The interaction between aPL antibodies and natural inhibitors of coagulation such as aPC, protein S, or thrombomodulin, might increase the risk for thromboembolic events. Similarly, the presence of antibodies to surface-bound annexin V has been hypothesized to play a role in recurrent abortions and fetal deaths.[132]

The prevalence of aPL antibodies in the general population is unclear. An Australian study has indicated that the prevalence of LAC is 3.6% and of ACA 4% to 6%.[133] According to a 1994 review,[113] the prevalence of aPL antibodies, both LAC and ACA, in the general obstetric population is approximately 2%. However, for ACA the range varied between 0.5% and 6.2% in different studies. This range of reported prevalences of aPL antibodies reflects disagreement in the cut-off levels for test positivity, population selection, and variation in assay methods and accuracy.[113] If a low cut-off level is chosen, the prevalence is high but association with fetal loss is less strong.

The association between aPL antibodies and pregnancy loss has been reported in case series and retrospective cohorts for several decades. The rate of pregnancy loss in untreated women with APS and prior fetal loss has been reported to be as high as 90%.[130] An unusually large proportion of pregnancy losses associated with aPL antibodies are second-trimester or third-trimester fetal deaths. Second-trimester fetal deaths account for only a small percentage of all pregnancy losses in the general population.[130] Recurrent abortion is also associated with APS.[134, 135]

The relationship between APS and preeclampsia is more controversial. In the series of more than 300 patients with severe preeclampsia reported by the Amsterdam group, an overall incidence was found of 20.9% of detectable (>10 GPL and/or MPL) ACAs, with a 27.4% incidence in the group with early-onset disease (delivery < 28 weeks' gestation), and a 19.3% incidence in the group with delivery later than 28 weeks' gestation (see Table 6–1).[15, 83] The incidence of detectable ACAs in their control group is 7.5%. With a cutoff above 15 GPL or MPL, the incidence of ACA-positive patients in a Dutch population of patients with a history of severe preeclampsia would be about 16%, which is consistent with other studies.

Branch and colleagues[136] found that 16% of women with severe preeclampsia that developed before 34 weeks' gestation had significant levels of aPL antibodies. Similar results were reported by Yamamoto and associates.[137] These investigators studied 43 cases of preeclampsia, including 26 cases of severe preeclampsia, and 47 normal pregnant women. Positive rates of ACAs in mild, severe, and total preeclampsia were 20.0%, 17.4%, and 18.4%, respectively. No ACA-positive cases were found in normal pregnancies.

Positive levels of aPL antibodies were also detected by Sletnes and coworkers[138] in seven (19%) of 37 preeclamptic women, compared with zero in a control group of 40 normotensive women at similar stage of pregnancy. Some studies found aPL antibodies related to preeclampsia and associated fetal growth restriction,[139] whereas other studies have found no relationship between aPL antibodies and fetal growth restriction.[140]

Several investigators found no correlation at all between ACA and preeclampsia. Rajah and colleagues[141] found no significant differences in ACA levels in 33 black women with severe preeclampsia as compared with 32 normotensive black women. Also Out and associates,[135] in a prospective, controlled, multicenter study, found no relationships between aPL antibodies and preeclampsia.

The clinical significance of low ACA titers remains controversial. Silver and associates[142] demonstrated that even low IgG ACA levels may be associated with increased maternal and perinatal risks, whereas the pathogenetic importance of low titers of IgM ACA is probably negligible.[124, 142, 143]

Though the results of animal studies suggested that aPL antibodies reactive with phosphatidylserine-dependent antigens are more relevant than those reactive with cardiolipin-dependent antigens,[144] Branch and colleagues[145] demonstrated that testing for aPL antibodies other than LACs and ACAs, such as antibodies against phosphatidic acid, phosphatidylserine, phosphatidylcholine, phosphatidylethanolamine, and phosphatidylinositol, is not clinically useful in patients with recurrent pregnancy loss.

Although the clinical significance of aPL antibodies in preeclamptic women is questionable, most studies found that 16% to 20% of patients with a history of early-onset preeclampsia have definitely positive ACAs. Laboratories involved in detecting the aPL syndrome should adhere to the most rigid qualifications and should always include an individual and adequate control group. Women whose positive aPL antibody status is diagnosed almost incidentally are not at high risk for aPL antibody–related obstetric complications, and Cowchock and Reece[146] advised that women should be considered at high risk for obstetric complications only if they have a clinical history and placental findings consistent with this diagnosis as well as persistently significant levels of antibodies cross-reactive with more than one negatively charged phospholipid.

In 1997 Rand and associates[147] described a mechanism by which aPL antibodies induce placental pathology. They found that aPL antibodies lower levels of annexin V, a surface anticoagulant present in vascular and trophoblast cells.[147] Annexin V has a powerful antithrombotic function at the apical surface of trophoblast and endothelial cells. The aPL antibody–induced reduction in the level of annexin V at these sites may account for the thrombosis that occurs in the APS.[147]

Although the interaction between SLE and pregnancy is not within the scope of this chapter, preeclampsia is more common in women with SLE (in 20%–30% of pregnancies). This high incidence is probably related to the combination of clinically apparent renal disease, underlying hypertension, and aPL antibodies in a high proportion of patients with SLE.[130]

Hyperhomocysteinemia

Hyperhomocysteinemia is now recognized as an independent risk factor for cardiovascular disease.[148–150] A meta-analysis of patients with hyperhomocysteinemia concluded that an increase in total homocysteine concentrations of 5 μmol/L gives an OR for coronary artery disease of 1.6 and for cerebrovascular disease of 1.5.[151] In classic homocysteinuria, 50% of the vascular complications occur in veins,[152] but in 1996 den

Heijer and coworkers[153] demonstrated that mild elevations of homocysteine levels are also a risk factor for deep vein thrombosis in the general population. It is intriguing that thrombosis develops in only about one third of patients with classic homocystein-uria; the reason for this variability, which is found even among siblings, remains unknown.

Mandel and coworkers[154] in 1997 demonstrated that the coexistence of additional genetic defects, such as factor V Leiden, increases the thrombosis risk in patients with homocystinuria. The reason for the variability in thrombosis risk can therefore be explained by the coexistence of other thrombophilic risk factors.

Homocysteine appears to affect both the coagulation system and endothelial cell resistance to thrombosis, and it may interfere with the vasodilator and antithrombotic functions of nitric oxide (NO). The reported vascular complications in patients with hyperhomocysteinemia are related to thrombosis rather than to atherosclerosis.[150] Homocysteine is thought to damage endothelial cells by several mechanisms, including the generation of hydrogen peroxide and depletion of nitric oxide–mediated detoxification of homocysteine.[155, 156] In addition, Rodgers and Kane[157] noted that cultured bovine aortic and human umbilical vein endothelial cells exhibit enhanced activity of factor V and increased prothrombin activation after treatment with homocysteine. Another study showed impaired thrombomodulin expression, also supporting the concept of an endothelial-based mechanism for the prothrombotic diathesis of hyperhomocysteinemia.[158] Homocysteine crystals in endothelial cells may act as pathologic surfaces for activation of the contact pathway for intrinsic coagulation.

Endothelial cells generate reduced bioactive nitric acid in response to shear stress when they are exposed to high concentrations of homocysteine. The adverse vascular effects of homocysteine are mitigated by the formation of S-nitroso-homocysteine. S-nitroso-homocysteine does not support hydrogen peroxide generation and does not undergo conversion to the corresponding thiolactone. In addition, similarly to other S-nitrosothiols, S-nitroso-homocysteine is a vasodilator and platelet inhibitor.

Stamler and colleagues[156] proposed that the damaging effects of homocysteine on the endothelium are a consequence of the inability of the endothelial cell to sustain adequate elaboration of nitric oxide in the presence of the elevations of homocysteine achieved in vivo in patients with hyperhomocysteinemia. Therefore, stimulation of endothelial cell nitric oxide synthesis provides a protective mechanism preventing homocysteine-induced endothelial cell injury; over time and with increasing homocysteine exposure, however, these protective effects become outstripped by the toxic effects of hydrogen peroxide and hydroxyl generation supported by homocysteine.[159] Other investigators postulated that homocysteine also induces increased superoxide generation.[160]

Methionine, an essential amino acid involved in cellular growth and cell division, is crucial in the donation of methyl groups to transfer RNA, DNA, and proteins. Methionine is the only source of the atherogenic amino acid homocysteine.[161] Homocysteine is an intermediate product, formed after transmethylation of methionine. The vascular endothelium expresses only two of the three crucial regulatory enzymes that control levels of homocysteine. These key enzymes are cystathionine-β synthase, a vitamin B_6–dependent enzyme, which catalyzes the transsulfuration of homocysteine to cystathionine; and 5,10-methylenetetrahydrafolate reductase, which catalyzes the remethylation of homocysteine to methionine. Folic acid and vitamin B_{12} are also required as cofactors for this remethylation pathway. However, betaine-homocysteine methyltransferase is inactive in endothelial cells, and it has been suggested that this inability to metabolize homocysteine completely causes endothelial cells to be more susceptible to the toxic effect of this amino acid.[161]

Defective transsulfuration as well as remethylation disorders result in increased blood and urine levels of homocysteine. Therefore, both *hyperhomocysteinemia* and *homocysteinuria* are used to describe elevated levels in blood and urine, respectively.

Classic homocysteinuria is the homozygous form of the autosomal recessively inherited cystathionine-β synthase deficiency. The main clinical cardiovascular characteristic is premature atherosclerosis. Heterozygous cystathionine-β synthetase deficiency and folate, vitamin B_{12}, and vitamin B_6 deficiency increase serum levels of homocysteine, which are usually not high enough to result in the excretion of homocysteine in urine.

Malinow and associates[162] have suggested use of the term *hyperhomocysteinemia* for transient or persistent elevation of serum homocysteine levels. The birth prevalence of heterozygosity for cystathionine-β synthase deficiency varies among several countries from 1:70 to 1:200.[163, 164] This enzyme is known to be vitamin B_6–dependent. Remethylation defects may be based on hereditary enzyme deficiencies, on deficiency of folic acid or vitamin B_{12}, or on both. Apart from cystathionine-β synthetase deficiency, a decreased activity of 5,10-methylenetetrahydrafolate reductase or other unknown enzyme deficiencies has been suggested.[148, 162, 165, 166] A common missense mutation in the methylenetetrahydrofolate reductase (MTHFR) gene, a C-to-T substitution at nucleotide 677, is responsible for reduced MTHFR activity and associated with modestly increased plasma homocysteine concentrations. Data from the 1990s have shown that, within the context of cardiovascular disorders, the MTHFR mutation is far more important than cystathionine synthetase deficiencies. Interestingly, the phenotype of this T677 variant, hyperhomocysteinemia, is only recognizable when there are suboptimal folate levels.[167]

Homocysteine levels in the fasting state and after standardized oral methionine loading in men and postmenopausal women are significantly higher when compared with premenopausal women, suggesting a unique efficiency of methionine handling in premenopausal women that is cardioprotective because it regulates homocysteine accumulation.[168]

Several case reports detailing pregnancies in women with homocysteinuria due to cystathionine-β synthase deficiency have been published. These have been reviewed by Mudd and colleagues,[163] and some women did have a poor obstetric history, especially in the untreated group. Until the 1990s, the outcome in mild to moderate hyperhomocysteinemia was unknown.

Burke and associates[169] examined the obstetric histories of eight women who were obligate heterozygotes for cystathionine-β synthase deficiency. These women had had a total of 34 pregnancies, with four ending in spontaneous abortion (12%). The mean birth weight for the remaining 30 infants was not significantly different from that of the control population. However, there were three perinatal deaths among these 30 infants. One infant, with a birth weight of 750 g, was stillborn. A second infant with a neural tube defect died 2 weeks after delivery. The third was an infant of 1220 g delivered at 31 weeks' gestation as a result of severe preeclampsia to a mother who had a previous uncomplicated pregnancy. These authors also studied fasting total homocysteine levels in mothers who delivered babies with growth restriction and found no significant differences in comparison with patients with an uncomplicated pregnancy.

Steegers-Theunissen and colleagues[170–171] found mild hyperhomocysteinemia to be associated with embryotoxicity (leading to neural tube defects or spontaneous abortion) or vascular toxicity (leading to placental infarcts or placental abruption), or with both.[172]

The relation between hyperhomocysteinemia and preeclampsia has now been assessed in a systematic way by Dekker and colleagues.[15] Using strict cut-off levels for defining hyperhomocysteinemia (fasting > 15 µmol/L and/or postloading > 51 µmol/L), they found that the incidence of hyperhomocysteinemia in patients with a history of severe early-onset preeclampsia is about sevenfold higher than the incidence in the normal population. In a subsequent study,[83] the authors again found a higher incidence of hyperhomocysteinemia in patients with a history of severe preeclampsia, but significant differences (19.0% versus 4.5%) were found only in patients with a history of early-onset preeclampsia (see Table 6–1).

In 1997, Sohda and coworkers[167] determined the MTHFR genotype in 67 preeclamptic patients and in 98 normal pregnant women. They found the T677 allele and the genotype homozygous for the T677 allele to be significantly increased in the preeclamptic group compared with the controls. The authors therefore concluded that the T677 variant of the MTHFR gene was one of the genetic risk factors for preeclampsia.

Currently, most[84a] but not all[94d, 173] investigators have found an association between the MTHFR polymorphism and preeclampsia. Patients with a history of severe preeclampsia may have a combination of hemostatic and metabolic problems.[174] Such a combination of underlying disorders is likely to increase the chance of adverse pregnancy outcome or thromboembolic problems.

Until recently, the only support for a pathogenetic impact of hyperhomocysteinemia was based on selected case-control studies. However, Sorensen and colleagues[175] have published data on a prospective case-control study from a base population of 3042 women who provided blood samples at an average gestational age of 16 weeks. Adjusted for maternal age, parity, and body mass index (BMI), a second-trimester elevated homocysteine level was associated with a 3.2 (95% CI 1.1–9.2)-fold increased risk of preeclampsia. There was evidence of an interaction between maternal adiposity and parity with second-trimester elevations in homocysteine levels. Nulliparous women with hyperhomocysteinemia experienced a 9.7-fold increased risk of preeclampsia as compared with multiparous women with normal homocysteine levels. Women with a prepregnancy BMI above the 50th percentile and hyperhomocysteinemia, as compared with leaner women without hyperhomocysteinemia, were 6.9 times more likely (95% CI 1.4–32.1) to later develop preeclampsia.

In the large (nearly 6000 women) retrospective Hordoland study,[176] in a comparison of the upper with lower quartile of plasma homocysteine, the adjusted risk for preeclampsia was 1.32 (95% CI 0.98–1.77), for prematurity 1.38 (95% CI 1.09–1.75), for very low birth weight 2.01 (95% CI 1.23–3.27), and for stillbirth 2.03 (95% CI 0.98–4.21). Abruptio placentae had no correlation with the homocysteine quartile, but the adjusted odds ratio, when homocysteine concentrations above 15 mol/L were compared with lower values, was 3.13 (95% CI 1.63–6.03).

In contrast, Murphy and coworkers[94e] found a similar frequency of the MTHFR polymorphism in preeclamptic (n = 12) and IUGR (n = 9) patients as in women with uncomplicated pregnancies (with nearly 600 nulliparous women).

The cases published by Dekker and colleagues[15] and by van Pampus and colleagues[83] represent a selected sample of early-onset preeclampsia referred to two large level III perinatal centers, essentially from a densely populated area in The Netherlands. The apparent controversial findings on hyperhomocysteinemia and MTHFR polymorphisms in their relationship with preeclampsia can be explained by considering the difference between phenotype and genotype and the selection of patients. The strongest association is found between the abnormal phenotype (hyperhomocysteinemia) and early-onset severe preeclampsia; no association is found between the abnormal gene and the large number of patients with near-term preeclampsia.

In a study of women with recurrent spontaneous miscarriages, Nelen et al[177] found that elevated homocysteine (fasting and after methionine loading) and decreased folate concentrations are more or less independent risk factors for recurrent pregnancy losses. In 1964, Hibbard[178] mentioned decreased folate as a risk factor for abruptio placentae, but prospective studies are needed to assess whether decreased folate per se is also a risk factor for preeclampsia. The systematic review by Ray and Laskin[179] shows the following data (Table 6–2). According to the results of this review, folate deficiency itself is not related to preeclampsia.

In summary, elevated homocysteine levels are now considered to be an established risk factor not only for occlusive arterial diseases, venous thrombosis, preeclampsia, IUGR, and abruptio placentae but also for recurrent spontaneous miscarriages, neural tube defects, and orofacial clefts. Hyperhomocysteinemia can easily be corrected from

TABLE 6–2. FOLATE DEFICIENCY, HYPERHOMOCYSTEINEMIA, AND THE MTHFR MUTATION AS RISK FACTORS FOR PLACENTAL VASCULOPATHY

	POOLED ODDS RATIO	95% CONFIDENCE INTERVAL
Placental Abruption		
Folate deficiency	25.9	0.9–736.3
Hyperhomocysteinemia	5.3	1.8–15.9
MTHFR mutation	2.3	1.1–4.9
Recurrent Pregnancy Loss		
Folate deficiency	3.4	1.2–9.9
Hyperhomocysteinemia	3.7	0.96–16.5
MTHFR mutation	3.3	1.2–9.2
Preeclampsia		
Folate deficiency	1.2	0.5–2.7
Hyperhomocysteinemia	20.9	3.6–121.6
MTHFR mutation	2.6	1.4–5.1

Data from Ray JG, Laskin CA. Folic acid and homocyst(e)ine metabolite defects and the risk of placental abruption, preeclampsia, and spontaneous pregnancy loss: A systematic review. Placenta 1999;20:519–529.

TABLE 6–3. RISK OF PREECLAMPSIA RANKED BY VARIOUS RISK FACTORS

RISK FACTOR	RISK	REFERENCE NO.
Chronic hypertension	10%–30%	13, 14, 182, 183
Renal disease	25%–50%	21, 22
Obesity	8%–15%	14, 19, 41
Gestational diabetes	5%–20%	71–74
Diabetes mellitus	20%–30%	75, 184
Activated protein C resistance	Elevated risk	15, 83, 94
Protein S deficiency	Elevated risk	15, 83
Antiphospholipid antibodies	Elevated risk?	15, 83, 135
Hyperhomocysteinemia	Elevated risk	15

the metabolic point of view, but it is unknown whether metabolic correction translates in improved perinatal outcome. More or less the same is true for the management of patients with previous adverse pregnancy outcome and documented aPC resistance or protein S deficiency with (low-molecular-weight) heparin. Several trials have been started to address these issues.

Patients with severe preeclampsia may have a combination of hemostatic and metabolic problems.[15, 83] This combination of underlying disorders is likely to increase the risk of an adverse pregnancy outcome or thromboembolic problems, or both. The coexistence of hyperhomocysteinemia and factor V Leiden has been demonstrated to be associated with an increased thrombosis risk.[154]

Lp(a) Lipoprotein

The levels of Lp(a) lipoprotein are genetically determined. High levels are associated with increased risk of cardiovascular disease. In a 1994 paper, Berg and coworkers[180] proposed that very high levels of Lp(a) lipoprotein might interfere with the placental circulation, resulting in fetal growth restriction. In 1997, Husby and associates[181] reported on a family with two cases of severe preeclampsia in which very high levels of Lp(a) were found. If confirmed, a very high level of Lp(a) lipoprotein may be another risk factor for preeclampsia that is genetically determined.

CONCLUSION

It is important to recognize the implications of the concept that preeclampsia is not just a hypertensive condition but a disease characterized by endothelial cell dysfunction. Hypertension is simply one symptom, just as is the case with pyrexia in many infectious disorders.

A history of severe early-onset preeclampsia may indicate the presence of underlying coagulation disturbances, hyperhomocysteinemia, or APS, or a combination of these conditions. On the other hand, the incidence of underlying disorders, associated with thrombophilia or early atherosclerosis, or with both, is probably very low in women with uncomplicated pregnancies only.

Table 6–3 summarizes the risk factors associated with preeclampsia. Although the risk of severe and early-onset preeclampsia appears to be increased in disorders associated with thrombophilia, the exact risk is unknown.

Pregnancy represents an in vivo, endothelial cell "stress" test. An uneventful pregnancy would indicate that the overall quality of the mother's cardiovascular and hemostatic system is likely to be good. Patients with a history of severe early-onset preeclampsia should be offered screening for chronic hypertension and renal disease as well as for protein S deficiency, aPC resistance, hyperhomocysteinemia, and APS. Abnormalities will be found in more than 50% of these patients. Recognizing the presence of these abnormalities has consequences in counseling about future pregnancies and in preconception care and may affect pharmacologic intervention in these women. Further studies are necessary to unravel the intricate relationships between insulin, insulin resistance, obesity, and preeclampsia.

References

1. Hsu CD, Iriye B, Johnson TRB, et al. Elevated circulating thrombomodulin in severe preeclampsia. Am J Obstet Gynecol 1993;169;148–149.

2. Dekker GA, Sibai BM. Early detection of pre-eclampsia. Am J Obstet Gynecol 1991;165:160–172.

3. Friedman SA, Schiff E, Emeis JJ, et al. Biochemical corroboration of endothelial involvement in severe preeclampsia. Am J Obstet Gynecol 1995;172:202–203.

4. Boer de K, Lecander I, ten Cate JW, et al. Placental-type plasminogen activator inhibitor in pre-eclampsia. Am J Obstet Gynecol 1988;158:518–522.

5. Lazarchick J, Stubbs TM, Romein L, et al. Predictive value of fibronectin levels in normotensive gravid women destined to become preeclamptic. Am J Obstet Gynecol 1986;154:1050–1052.

6. Lockwood CJ, Peters JH. Increased plasma levels of ED1+ cellular fibronectin precede the clinical signs of preeclampsia. Am J Obstet Gynecol 1990;162:358–362.

7. Rodgers GM, Taylor RN, Roberts JM. Preeclampsia is associated with a serum factor cytotoxic to human endothelial cells. Am J Obstet Gynecol 1988;159:908–914.

8. Ballegeer V, Spitz B, Kieckens L, et al. Predictive value of increased plasma levels of fibronectin in gestational hypertension. Am J Obstet Gynecol 1989;161:432–436.

9. Lazarchick J, Stubbs TM, Romein LA. Factor VIII procoagulant antigen levels in normal pregnancy and preeclampsia. Ann Clin Lab Sci 1986;16:395–398.

10. Stubbs TM, Lazarchick J, Horger EO III. Plasma fibronectin levels in pre-eclampsia: A possible marker for vascular endothelial damage. Am J Obstet Gynecol 1984;150:885–889.

11. Groot de CJM, Taylor RN. The role of endothelium in pregnancy and pregnancy-related diseases. Curr Obstet Med 1993;2:107–137.

12. Taylor RN, Heilbron DC, Roberts JM. Growth factor activity in the blood of women in whom pre-eclampsia develops is elevated from early pregnancy. Am J Obstet Gynecol 1990;163:1839–1844.

13. Working Group on High Blood Pressure in Pregnancy. The National high blood pressure education program working group report on high blood pressure in pregnancy: Consensus report. Am J Obstet Gynecol 2000;183(1):S1–S22.

14. Sibai BM, Lindheimer M, Hauth J, et al. Risk factors for preeclampsia, abruptio placentae, and adverse neonatal outcomes in women with chronic hypertension. N Engl J Med 1998;339:667–671.

15. Dekker GA, de Vries JIP, Doelitzsch PM, et al. Underlying disorders associated with severe early-onset preeclampsia. Am J Obstet Gynecol 1995;173:1042–1048.

16. Sibai BM. Treatment of hypertension in pregnant women. N Engl J Med 1996;335:257–265.

17. Sibai BM. Diagnosis and management of chronic hypertension in pregnancy. Obstet Gynecol 1991;78:451–461.

18. Rey E, Couturier A. The prognosis of pregnancy in women with chronic hypertension. Am J Obstet Gynecol 1994;171:410–416.

19. Ness RB, Roberts JM. Heterogeneous causes constituting the single syndrome of preeclampsia: A hypothesis and its implications. Am J Obstet Gynecol 1996;175:1365–1370.

20. Davison JD, Baylis C. Pregnancy in the patient with renal disease. In Walker JJ, Gant NF (eds). Hypertension in Pregnancy. London: Chapman & Hall, 1997, pp 213–251.

21. Jones DC, Hayslett JP. Outcome of pregnancy in women with moderate or severe renal insufficiency. N Engl J Med 1996;335:226–232.

22. Jungers P, Chauveau D, Choukroun G, et al. Pregnancy in women with impaired renal function. Clin Nephrol 1997;47:281–288.

23. Ihle BU, Long P, Oats J. Early onset pre-eclampsia recognition of underlying renal disease. Br Med J 1987;294:79–81.

24. Reiter L, Brown MA, Whitworth JA. Hypertension in pregnancy: The incidence of underlying renal disease and essential hypertension. Am J Kidney Dis 1994;24:883–887.

25. Lindheimer MD, Katz AI. Gestation in women with kidney disease: Prognosis and management. Ballieres Clin Obstet Gynaecol 1994;8:387–404.

26. Epstein FH. Pregnancy and renal disease. N Engl J Med 1996;335:277–278.

27. Modan M, Halkin H, Almog S, et al. Hyperinsulinemia: A link between hypertension, obesity and glucose intolerance. J Clin Invest 1985;75:809–817.

28. Ferrannini E, Buzzigoli G, Bonadonna R, et al. Insulin resistance in essential hypertension. N Engl J Med 1987;317:350–357.

29. Paolisso G, Barbagallo M: Hypertension, diabetes mellitus, and insulin resistance: The role of intracellular magnesium. Am J Hypertens 1997;10:346–355.

30. Colditz GA, Manson JAE, Stampfer MJ, et al. Diet and risk of clinical diabetes in women. Am J Clin Nutr 1993;55:1018–1023.

31. King GL. The role of hyperglycemia and hyperinsulinemia in causing vascular dysfunction in diabetes. Ann Med 1996;28:427–432.

32. Julius S, Jamerson K. Sympathetics, insulin resistance and coronary risk in hypertension: The "chicken-and-egg" question. J Hypertens 1994;12:495–502.

33. Godsland IF, Stevenson JC. Insulin resistance: Syndrome or tendency? Lancet 1995;346:100–103.

34. Reaven GM. Banting Lecture 1988: Role of insulin resistance in human disease. Diabetes 1988;37:1595–1607.

35. Reaven GM. Pathophysiology of insulin resistance in human disease. Physiol Rev 1995;75:473–485.

36. Heywood DM, Mansfield MW, Grant PJ. Levels of von Willebrand factor, insulin resistance syndrome, and a common vWF gene polymorphism in non–insulin-dependent (type 2) diabetes mellitus. Diabet Med 1996;13:720–725.

37. Polonsky KS, Sturis J, Bell GI. Non-insulin dependent diabetes mellitus: A genetically programmed failure of the beta cell to compensate for insulin resistance. N Engl J Med 1996;334:777–783.

38. Jones DW. Body weight and blood pressure: Effects of weight reduction on hypertension. Am J Hypertens 1996;9:50S–54S.

39. Roberts SR, Greenberg AS. The new obesity genes. Nutr Rev 1996;54:41–49.

40. Unger RH. Perspectives in diabetes: Lipotoxicity in the pathogenesis of obesity-dependent NIDDM: Genetic and clinical implications. Diabetes 1995;44:863–870.

41. Stone JL, Lockwood CJ, Berkowitz GS, et al. Risk

factors for severe preeclampsia. Obstet Gynecol 1994;83:357–361.

42. Chesley LC. History and epidemiology of preeclampsia-eclampsia. Clin Obstet Gynecol 1984;27:801–820.

43. Solomon CG, Graves SW, Greene MF, Seely EW. Glucose intolerance as a predictor of hypertension in pregnancy. Hypertension 1994;23:717–721.

44. Laivuori H, Tikkanen MJ, Ylikorkala O. Hyperinsulinemia 17 years after preeclamptic first pregnancy. J Clin Endocrinol Metab 1996;81:2908–2911.

45. Sowers JR, Saleh AA, Sokol RJ. Hyperinsulinemia and insulin resistance are associated with preeclampsia in African-Americans. Am J Hypertens 1995;8:1–4.

46. Cioffi FJ, Amorosa LF, Vintzileos AM, et al. Relationship of insulin resistance and hyperinsulinemia to blood pressure during pregnancy. J Maternal Fetal Med 1997;6:174–179.

47. Kraayenbrink AA, Gans ROB, van Geijn HP, Dekker GA. Insulin resistance, vasoactive mediators, and preeclampsia. Am J Obstet Gynecol 1997;176:S26.

48. Fuh MM, Chang-Sheng Y, Pei D, et al. Resistance to insulin-mediated glucose uptake and hyperinsulinemia in women who had preeclampsia during pregnancy. Am J Hypertens 1995;8:768–771.

49. Paulson DJ, Tahilani AG. Minireview: Cardiovascular abnormalities associated with human and rodent obesity. Life Sci 1991;51:1557–1569.

50. Easterling TR, Benedetti TJ, Schmucker BC, Millard SP. Maternal hemodynamics in normal and preeclamptic pregnancies: A longitudinal study. Obstet Gynecol 1990;76:1061–1069.

51. Lorentzen B, Endresen MJ, Clausen T, Henriksen T. Fasting serum free fatty acids and triglycerides are increased before 20 weeks of gestation in women who later develop preeclampsia. Hypertension in Pregnancy 1994;13:103–109.

52. Endresen MJ, Tosti E, Heimli H, et al. Effects of free fatty acids found increased in women who develop pre-eclampsia on the ability of endothelial cells to produce prostacyclin, cGMP and inhibit platelet aggregation. Scand J Clin Lab Invest 1994;54:549–557.

53. Arbogast BW, Leeper SC, Merrick RD, et al. Hypothesis: Which plasma factors bring about disturbance of endothelial function in pre-eclampsia? Lancet 1994;343:340–341.

54. Prins JB, O'Rahilly SO. Regulation of adipose cell number in man. Clin Sci 1997;92:3–11.

55. Zhang Y, Proenca R, Maffeik M, et al. Positional cloning of the mouse obese gene and its human homologue. Nature 1994;372:425–432.

56. Stark JM. Pre-eclampsia and cytokine induced oxidative stress. Br J Obstet Gynaecol 1993;100:105–109.

57. Greer IA, Lyall F, Perera T, et al. Increased concentrations of cytokines, interleukin-6 and interleukin-1 receptor antagonist in plasma of women with preeclampsia: A mechanism for endothelial dysfunction? Obstet Gynecol 1994;84:937–940.

58. Schobel HP, Fischer T, Heuszer K, et al. Preeclampsia—a state of sympathetic overactivity. N Engl J Med 1997;336:1326.

59. Gans ROB, Dekker GA. Preeclampsia—a state of sympathetic overactivity. N Engl J Med 1996;335:1480–1485.

60. Graves SW, Lincoln K, Cook SL, Seely EW. Digitalis-like factor and digoxin-like immunoreactive factor in diabetic women with preeclampsia, transient hypertension of pregnancy, and normotensive pregnancy. Am J Hypertens 1995;8:5–11.

61. Giudice LC. Growth factors and growth modulators in human uterine endometrium: Their potential relevance to reproductive medicine. Fertil Steril 1994;61:1–17.

62. Wang HS, Chard T. The role of insulin-like growth factor-I (IGF-I) and insulin-like growth factor binding protein-1 (IGFBP-1) in the control of human fetal growth. J Endocrinol 1992;132:11–19.

63. De Groot CJM, O'Brien TJ, Taylor RN. Biochemical evidence of impaired trophoblastic invasion of decidual stroma in women destined to have preeclampsia. Am J Obstet Gynecol 1996;175:24–29.

64. Barker DJP, Gluckman PD, Godfrey KM, et al. Fetal nutrition and cardiovascular disease in adult life. Lancet 1993;341:938–941.

65. Valdez R, Athens MA, Thompson GH, et al. Birth weight and adult health outcomes in a biethnic population in the USA. Diabetologia 1994;37:624–631.

66. Law CM, Barker DJP. Fetal influences on blood pressure. J Hypertens 1994;12:1329–1332.

67. Stern MP. Perspectives in diabetes. Diabetes and cardiovascular disease: The "common soil" hypothesis. Diabetes 1995;44:369–374.

68. Kaaja R, Tikkanen MJ, Viinikka L, Ylikorkala O. Serum lipoproteins, insulin, and urinary prostanoid metabolites in normal and hypertensive pregnant women. Obstet Gynecol 1995;85:353–356.

69. Philips DIW. Insulin resistance as a programmed response to fetal undernutrition. Diabetologica 1996;39:1119–1122.

70. Joffe GM, Esterliz JR, Levine RJ, et al. The relationship between abnormal glucose tolerance and hypertensive disorders of pregnancy in healthy nulliparous women. Am J Obstet Gynecol 1998;179:1032–1037.

71. Khan KS, Daya S. Plasma glucose and pre-eclampsia. Int J Gynecol Obstet 1996;53:111–116.

72. Serner M, Naylor CD, Gare DJ, et al. Impact of increasing carbohydrate intolerance on maternal-fetal outcomes in 3637 women without gestational diabetes. Am J Obstet Gynecol 1995;173:146–156.

73. Suhonen L, Teramo K. Hypertension and preeclampsia in women with gestational glucose intolerance. Acta Obstet Gynecol Scand 1993;72:269–272.

74. Schaffir JA, Lockwood CJ, Lapinski R, et al. Incidence of pregnancy-induced hypertension among gestational diabetics. Am J Perinat 1995;12:252–254.

75. Sibai BM. Risk factors, pregnancy complications, and prevention of hypertensive disorders in women with pregravid diabetes mellitus. J Matern Fetal Med 2000;9:62–65.

76. Van Assche FA, Spitz B, Hanssens M, et al. Increased thromboxane formation in diabetic pregnancy as a possible contributor to preeclampsia. Am J Obstet Gynecol 1993;168:84–87.

77. Vijayalingam S, Parthiban A, Shanmugasundaram KR, Mohan V. Abnormal antioxidant status in impaired glucose tolerance and non-insulin-dependent diabetes mellitus. Diabet Med 1996;13:715–719.

78. Kilpatrick DC. HLA-dependent TNF secretory re-

sponse may provide an immunogenetic link between pre-eclampsia and type 1 diabetes mellitus. Dis Markers 1996;13:43–47.

79. Pociot F, Briant L, Jongeneel CV, et al. Association of tumour necrosis factor (TNF) and class II major histocompatibility complex alleles with the secretion of TNF and TNF-β by human mononuclear cells: A possible link to insulin-dependent diabetes mellitus. Eur J Immunol 1993;23:224–231.

80. Liston WA, Kilpatrick DC. Is genetic susceptibility to pre-eclampsia conferred by homozygosity for the same single recessive gene in mother and fetus? Br J Obstet Gynaecol 1991;98:1079–1086.

81. Millar LK, Wing DA, Leung AS, et al. Low birth weight and preeclampsia in pregnancies complicated by hyperthyroidism. Obstet Gynecol 1994;84:946–949.

82. Leung AS, Millar LK, Koonings PP, et al. Perinatal outcome in hypothyroid pregnancies. Obstet Gynecol 1993;81:349–353.

83. van Pampus MG, Wolf H, Buller HR, et al. Underlying disorders associated with severe preeclampsia and HELLP syndrome. Am J Obstet Gynecol 1997;176:S26.

84. Preston FE, Rosendaal FR, Walker ID, et al. Increased fetal loss in women with heritable thrombophilia. Lancet 1996;348:913–916.

84a. Kupferminc MJ, Eldor A, Steinman N, et al. Increased frequency of genetic thrombophilia in women with complications of pregnancy. N Engl J Med 1999;340:9–13.

85. Dahlbäck H, Carlsson M, Svensson PJ. Familial thrombophilia due to a previously unrecognized mechanism characterized by poor anticoagulant response to activated protein C: Prediction of a cofactor to activated protein C. Proc Natl Acad Sci U S A 1993;90:1004–1008.

86. Koster T, Rosendaal FR, de Ronde H, et al. Venous thrombosis due to poor anticoagulant response to activated protein C: Leiden Thrombophilia Study. Lancet 1993;342:1503–1506.

87. Bertina RM, Koeleman BPC, Koster T, et al. Mutation in blood coagulation factor V associated with resistance to activated protein C. Nature 1994;369:64–67.

88. Majerus PW. Bad blood by mutation. Nature 1994;369:14–15.

89. Broze GJ, Miletich JP. Biochemistry and physiology of protein C, protein S, and thrombomodulin. In Colman RW, Hirsch J, Marder VJ, Salzman EW (eds). Hemostasis and Thrombosis. Basic Principles and Clinical Practice, 3rd ed. Philadelphia: Lippincott, 1994, pp 259–276.

90. Fair DS, Marlar RA, Levin EG. Human endothelial cells synthesize protein S. Blood 1986;67:1168–174.

91. Vandenbroucke JP, van der Meer FJM, Helmerhorst FM, Rosendaal FR. Factor V Leiden: Should we screen oral contraceptive users and pregnant women? BMJ 1996;313:127–130.

92. Svensson PJ, Dahlback B. Resistance to activated protein C as a basis for venous thrombosis. N Engl J Med 1994;300:517–522.

93. Hellgren M, Svensson PJ, Dahlback B. Resistance to activated protein C as a basis for venous thromboembolism associated with pregnancy and oral contraception. Am J Obstet Gynecol 1995;173:210–213.

94. Dizon-Townson DS, Nelson LM, Jang H, et al. The incidence of the factor V Leiden mutation in an obstetric population and its relationship to deep vein thrombosis. Am J Obstet Gynecol 1997;176:883–886.

94a. Dizon-Townson DS, Nelson LM, Easton K, Ward K. The factor V Leiden mutation may predispose women to severe preeclampsia. Am J Obstet Gynecol 1996;175:902–905.

94b. Lindoff C, Ingermarsson I, Martinsson G, et al. Preeclampsia is associated with a reduced response to activated protein C. Am J Obstet Gynecol 1996;176:457–460.

94c. Grisaru D, Fait G, Eldor A: Activated protein C resistance and pregnancy complications. Am J Obstet Gynecol 1996;174:801–802.

94d. O'Shaughnessy KM, Fu B, Ferraro F, Lewis I, et al. Factor V Leiden and Thermolabile Methylene Reductase Gene Variants in an East Anglian Preeclampsia Cohort. Hypertension 1999;33:1338–1341.

94e. Murphy RP, Donoghue C, Nallen RJ, et al. Prospective evaluation of the risk conferred by factor V Leiden and thermolabile methylenetetrahydrofolate reductase polymorphism in pregnancy. Arterioscler Thromb Vasc Biol 2000;20:266–270.

95. van der Bom JG, Bols ML, Haverkate F, et al. Reduced response to activated protein C is associated with increased risk for cerebrovascular disease. Ann Intern Med 1996;125:265–269.

96. Dizon-Townson DS, Nelson LM, Easton K, Ward K. The factor V Leiden mutation may predispose women to severe preeclampsia. Am J Obstet Gynecol 1996;175:902–905.

97. Lindoff C, Ingemarsson I, Martinsson G, et al. Preeclampsia is associated with a reduced response to activated protein C. Am J Obstet Gynecol 1996;176:457–460.

98. Grisaru D, Fait G, Eldor A. Activated protein C resistance and pregnancy complications. Am J Obstet Gynecol 1996;174:801–802.

99. Cumming AM, Tait RC, Fildes S, et al. Development of resistance to activated protein C during pregnancy. Br J Haematol 1995;90:725–727.

100. Hooper WC, Philips DJ, Ribeiro MJ, et al. Tumor necrosis factor-α downregulates protein S secretion in human microvascular and umbilical vein endothelial cells but not in the HepG- 2 hepatoma cell line. Blood 1994;84: 483–489.

101. Comp PC, Thurnau GR, Welsh J, Esmon CT. Functional and immunologic protein S levels are decreased during pregnancy. Blood 1986;8:881–885.

102. Gilabert J, Fernandez JA, Espana F, et al. Physiological coagulation inhibitors (protein S, protein C and antithrombin III) in severe preeclamptic states and in users of oral contraceptives. Thromb Res 1988;49:319–329.

103. de Boer K, Ten Cate JW, Sturk A, et al. Enhanced thrombin generation in normal and hypertensive pregnancy. Am J Obstet Gynecol 1989;160:95–100.

104. Huisveld IA, Hospers JE, Meijers JC, et al: Oral contraceptives reduce total protein S, but not free protein S. Thromb Res 1987;45:109–116.

105. Malm J, Laurell M, Dahlback B. Changes in the plasma levels of vitamin K-dependent protein C and S and of C4b-binding protein during pregnancy and oral contraception. Br J Haematol 1988;68:437–443.

106. Comp PC, Nixon RR, Cooper MR, Esmon CT: Fa-

milial protein S deficiency is associated with recurrent thrombosis. J Clin Invest 1984;74:2082–2087.

107. Tait RC, Walker ID, Islam SIAM, et al. Protein S deficiency in healthy blood donors. Br J Haematol 1994;86(Suppl 1):118.

108. Conley L, Hartmann R. A hemorrhagic disorder caused by circulating anticoagulant in patients with disseminated lupus erythematosus. J Clin Invest 1952;31:621–622.

109. Hughes GRV. The antiphospholipid syndrome: Ten years on. Lancet 1993;342:341–344.

110. Harris EN. The syndrome of the black swan. Br J Haematol 1987;26:324–326.

111. Harris EN, Asherson RA, Hughes GRV. Antiphospholipid antibodies: Autoantibodies with a difference. Annu Rev Med 1988;39:261–271.

112. Arnout J, Spitz B, van Assche A, Vermylen J. The antiphospholipid syndrome and pregnancy. Hypertens Pregn 1995;14:147–178.

113. Pattison NS, Birdsall MA, Chamley LW, Lubbe WF. Recurrent fetal loss and the antiphospholipid syndrome. Recent Adv Obstet Gynaecol 1994; 18:23–50.

114. Moore JE, Mohr CF. Biologically false positive serological test for syphilis: Type, incidence, and cause. JAMA 1952;150:467–473.

115. Moore JE, Lutz WB. Natural history of systemic lupus erythematosus: Approach to its study through chronic biologic false positive reactors. J Chron Dis 1955;1:297–316.

116. Triplett DA, Brandt JT. Laboratory identification of the lupus anticoagulant. Br J Haematol 1989;73:139–143.

117. Harris EN, Gharavi AE, Patel SP, Hughes GRV. Evaluation of the anticardiolipin antibody test: Report of an international workshop held 4 April 1986. Clin Exp Immunol 1987;68:215–222.

118. Harris EN, Gharavi AE, Boey ML, et al. Anticardiolipin antibodies detection by radioimmunoassay and association with thrombosis in systemic lupus erythematosus. Lancet 1983;ii:1211–1214.

119. Peaceman AM, Silver RK, MacGregor SN, Socol LM. Interlaboratory variation in antiphospholipid antibodies testing. Am J Obstet Gynecol 1992; 166:1780–1787.

120. Harris EN. A reassessment of the antiphospholipid antibody syndrome. J Rheumatol 1990; 17:733–735.

121. Harris EN. Annotation. Antiphospholipid antibodies. Br J Haematol 1990;74:1–9.

122. Harris EN. The second international anti-cardiolipin standardization workshop: The Kingston antiphospholipid antibody study (KAPS) group. Am J Clin Pathol 1990;94:476–484.

123. Rupin A, Gruel Y, Watier H, et al. ELISA for the detection of anticardiolipin antibodies. J Immunol Methods 1991;138:225–231.

124. Cowchock S. The role of antiphospholipid antibodies in obstetric medicine. Curr Obstet Med 1991;1:229–247.

125. Simantov R, Lo SK, Gharavi A, et al. Antiphospholipid antibodies activate vascular endothelial cells. Lupus 1996;5:440–441.

126. Silver RK, Mullen TA, Caplan MS, et al. Inducible platelet adherence to human umbilical vein endothelium by anticardiolipin antibody-positve sera. Am J Obstet Gynecol 1995;173:702–707.

127. Shoenfeld Y. Induction of experimental primary and secondary antiphospholipid syndromes in naive mice. Am J Reprod Immunol 1992;28:219–221.

128. Pierangeli SS, Liu XW, Barker JH, et al. Induction of thrombosis in a mouse model by IgG, IgM and IgA immunoglobulins from patients with the antiphospholipid syndrome. Thromb Haemost 1995;74:1361–1367.

129. Silver RM, Pierangeli SS, Gharavi AE, et al. Induction of high levels of anticardiolipin antibodies in mice by immunization with beta-2-glycoprotein I does not cause fetal death. Am J Obstet Gynecol 1995;173:1410–1415.

130. Silver RM, Ware Branch D: Autoimmune disease in pregnancy: Systemic lupus erythematosus and antiphospholipid syndrome. Clin Perinatol 1997;24:291–320.

131. Kandiah DA, Sheng YH, Krilis SA: Beta-2-glycoprotein I: Target antigen for autoantibodies in the (antiphospholipid syndrome). Lupus 1996;5:381–385.

132. Galli M: Non beta-2-glycoprotein I cofactors for antiphospholipid antibodies. Lupus 1996;5:388–392.

133. Shi W, Krilis SA, Chong BH, et al. Prevalence of lupus anticoagulant and anticardiolipin antibodies in a healthy population. Aust N Z J Med 1990;20:231–236.

134. Rai RS, Regan L, Clifford K, et al. Antiphospholipid antibodies and beta-2-glycoprotein-I in 500 women with recurrent miscarriage: Results of a comprehensive screening approach. Hum Reprod 1995;10:2001–2005.

135. Out HJ, Bruinse HW, Christiaens GCML, et al. A prospective, controlled multicenter study on the obstetric risks of pregnant women with antiphospholipid antibodies. Am J Obstet Gynecol 1992;167:26–32.

136. Branch DW, Andres R, Digre KB, et al. The association of antiphospholipid antibodies with severe preeclampsia. Obstet Gynecol 1989;73:541–545.

137. Yamamoto T, Yoshimura S, Geshi Y, et al. Measurement of antiphospholipid antibody by ELISA using purified beta-2-glycoprotein I in preeclampsia. Clin Exp Immunol 1993;94:196–200.

138. Sletnes KE, Wisloff F, Moe N, Dale PO. Antiphospholipid antibodies in pre-eclamptic women: Relation to growth retardation and neonatal outcome. Acta Obstet Gynecol Scand 1992; 71:112–117.

139. El-Roeiy A, Myers SA, Gleicher N. The relationship between autoantibodies and intrauterine growth retardation in hypertensive disorders of pregnancy. Am J Obstet Gynecol 1991;164:1253–1261.

140. Milliez J, Lelong F, Bayani N, et al. The prevalence of autoantibodies during third-trimester pregnancy complicated by hypertension or idiopathic fetal growth retardation. Am J Obstet Gynecol 1991;165:51–56.

141. Rajah SB, Moodley J, Pudifin D, Duursma J. Anticardiolipin antibodies in hypertensive emergencies. Clin Exper Hypertens Pregnancy 1990; B9:267–271.

142. Silver RM, Coulam C, Lyon JL, et al. Clinical consequences of low positive IgG anticardiolipin antibodies. Am J Obstet Gynecol 1994; 170(Suppl):336.

143. Pattison NS, Chamley LW, McKay EJ, et al. Anti-

phospholpid antibodies in pregnancy: Prevalence and clinical associations. Br J Obstet Gynaecol 1993;100:909–913.

144. Vogt EV, Ah-Kau Ng, Rote NS. A model for the antiphospholipid antibody syndrome: Monoclonal antiphosphatidylserine antibody induces intrauterine growth restriction in mice. Am J Obstet Gynecol 1996;174:700–707.

145. Branch DW, Silver R, Pierangeli S, et al. Antiphospholipid antibodies other than lupus anticoagulant and anticardiolipin antibodies in women with recurrent pregnancy loss, fertile controls, and antiphospholipid syndrome. Obstet Gynecol 1997;89:549–555.

146. Cowchock S, Reece EA. Do low-risk pregnant women with antiphospholipid antibodies need to be treated? Am J Obstet Gynecol 1997; 176:1099–1100.

147. Rand JH, Xiao-Xuan W, Andree HAM, et al. Pregnancy loss in the antiphospholid-antibody syndrome—a possible thrombogenic mechanism. N Engl J Med 1997;337:154–160.

148. Clarke R, Daly L, Robinson K, et al. Hyperhomocysteinemia: An independent risk factor for vascular disease. N Engl J Med 1991;324:1149–1155.

149. Malinow MR, Kang SS, Taylor LM, et al. Prevalence of hyperhomocyst(e)inemia in patients with peripheral arterial occlusive disease. Circulation 1989;79:1180–1188.

150. Nygard O, Nordrehaug JE, Refsum H, et al. Plasma homocysteine levels and mortality in patients with coronary artery disease. N Engl J Med 1997;337:230–236.

151. Boushey CJ, Beresford SAA, Omenn GS, Motulsky AG. A quantitative assessment of plasma homocysteine as a risk factor for cardiovascular disease. Probable benefits of increasing folate acid intake. JAMA 1995;274:1049–1057.

152. Mudd SH, Skovby F, Levy HL, et al. The natural history of homocysteinuria due to cystathionine β-synthase deficiency. Am J Hum Genet 1985; 37:1–31.

153. den Heijer M, Koster T, Blom HJ, et al. Hyperhomocysteinemia as a risk factor for deep-vein thrombosis. N Engl J Med 1996;334:759–762.

154. Mandel H, Brenner B, Berant M, et al. Coexistence of hereditary homocystinuria and factor V Leiden—effect on thrombosis. N Engl J Med 1997;334:763–768.

155. Starkebaum G, Harlan JM. Endothelial cell injury due to copper-catalyzed hydrogen peroxide generation from homocysteine. J Clin Invest 1986; 77:1370–1376.

156. Stamler JS, Osborne JA, Jaraki A, et al. Adverse vascular effects of homocysteine are modulated by endothelium-derived relaxing factor and related oxides of nitrogen. J Clin Invest 1993; 91:308–318.

157. Rodgers GM, Kane WH. Activation of endogenous factor V by a homocysteine-induced vascular endothelial cell activator J Clin Invest 1986;77:1909–1916.

158. Lentz SR, Sadler JE. Inhibition of thrombomodulin surface expression and protein C activation by the thrombogenic agent homocysteine. J Clin Invest 1991;83:1906–1909.

159. Upchurch GR, Welch GN, Loscalzo J. Homocysteine, EDRF, and endothelial function. J Nutr 1996;126:1290S–1294S.

160. Jia L, Furchgott RF. Inhibition by sulphydryl compounds of vascular relaxation induced by nitric oxide and endothelium-derived relaxing factor. J Pharmacol Exp Ther 1993;267:371–378.

161. Hennig B, Toborek M, Cader AA. Nutrition, endothelial cell metabolism, and atherosclerosis. Crit Rev Food Sci Nutr 1994;34:253–282.

162. Malinow MR, Kang SS, Taylor LM, et al. Prevalence of hyperhomocyst(e)inemia in patients with peripheral arterial occlusive disease. Circulation 1989;79:1180–1188.

163. Mudd SH, Skovby F, Levy HL, et al. The natural history of homocysteinuria due to cystathionine-β-synthase deficiency. Am J Hum Genet 1985; 37:1–31.

164. Boers GHJ, Smals AGH, Trijbels FJM, et al. Heterozygosity for homocysteinuria in premature peripheral and cerebral occlusive arterial disease. N Engl J Med 1985;313:709–715.

165. Dudman NPB, Wilcken DEL, Wang J, et al. Disordered methionine/homocysteine metabolism in premature vasular disease. Arterioscler Thromb 1993;13:1253–1260.

166. Engbersen AMT, Franken DG, Boers GHJ, et al. Thermolabile 5,10-methylenetetrahydrofolate reductase as a cause of mild hyperhomocysteinemia. Am J Hum Genet 1995;56:142–150.

167. Sohda S, Arinami T, Hamada H, et al. Methylenetetrahydrofolate reductase polymorphism and pre-eclampsia. J Med Genet 1997;34:525–526.

168. Boers GHJ, Smals AG, Trijbels FJ, et al. Unique efficiency of methionine metabolism in premenopausal women may protect against vascular disease in the reproductive years. J Clin Invest 1983;72:1971–1976.

169. Burke G, Robinson K, Refsum H, et al. Intrauterine growth retardation, perinatal death, and maternal homocysteine levels. N Engl J Med 1992;326:69–70.

170. Steegers-Theunissen RPM, Boers GHJ, Trijbels JMF, Eskes TKAB. Hyperhomocysteïnemia and recurrent abortion or abruptio placentae. Lancet 1992;339:1122–1123.

171. Steegers-Theunissen RPM, Boers GHJ, Trijbels JMF, Eskes TKAB. Neural-tube defects and derangement of homocysteine metabolism. N Engl J Med 1991;324:199.

172. Wouters MGAJ, Boers GHJ, Blom HJ, et al. Hyperhomocysteinemia: A risk factor in women with unexplained recurrent early pregnancy loss. Fertil Steril 1993;60:820–825.

173. Groot CJ de, Bloemenkamp KW, Duvekot EJ, et al. Preeclampsia and genetic risk factors for thrombosis: A case-control study. Am J Obstet Gynecol 1999;181:975–980.

174. van Pampus MG, Dekker GA, Wolf H, et al. High prevalence of hemostatic abnormalities in women with a history of severe preeclampsia. Am J Obstet Gynecol 1999;180:1146–1150.

175. Sorensen TK, Malinow MR, Williams MA, et al. Elevated second-trimester serum homocysteine levels and subsequent risk of preeclampsia. Gynecol Obstet Invest 1999;48:98–103.

176. Vollset SE, Refsum H, Irgens LM, et al. Plasma total homocysteine, pregnancy complications, and adverse pregnancy outcomes: The Hordoland Homocysteine Study. Am J Clin Nutrition 2000; 71:962–968.

177. Nelen WLDM, Blom HJ, Steegers EAP, et al. Ho-

mocysteine and folate levels as ridk factors for recurrent early pregnancy loss. Obstet Gynecol 2000;95:19–24.

178. Hibbard BM. The role of folic acid in pregnancy: With particular reference to anaemia, abruption and abortion. J Obstet Gynaecol Br Commonw 1964;71:529–542.

179. Ray JG, Laskin CA. Folic acid and homocyst(e)ine metabolite defects and the risk of placental abruption, pre-eclampsia, and spontaneous pregnancy loss: a systematic review. Placenta 1999;20:519–529.

180. Berg K, Roald B, Sande H. High Lp(a) lipoprotein level in maternal serum may interfere with placental circulation and cause fetal growth retardation. Clin Genet 1994;46:52–56.

181. Husby H, Roald B, Schjetlein R, et al. High levels of Lp(a) lipoprotein in a family with cases of severe pre-eclampsia. Clin Genet 1997;50:47–49.

182. Caritis S, Sibai BM, Hauth J, et al. Low-dose aspirin therapy for the prevention of preeclampsia in high-risk women. N Engl J Med (in press).

183. Samadi AR, Mayberry RM, Zaidi AA, et al. Maternal hypertension and associated pregnancy complications among African-American and other women in the United States. Obstet Gynecol 1996;87:557–563.

184. Rudge MVC, Calderon IMP, Ramos MD, et al. Hypertensive disorders in pregnant women with diabetes mellitus. Gynecol Obstet Invest 1997;44:11–15.

7 CONTRACEPTION for the WOMAN with HYPERTENSION

John T. Repke

Hypertension occurs in 15% to 20% of the adult population in the United States and is an important risk factor for the development of a number of health problems, including atherosclerosis, stroke, myocardial infarction, heart failure, and ultimately death. For the woman in her reproductive years, hypertension can also pose significant health risks. Every obstetrician and gynecologist is well aware of the high-risk nature of managing hypertension during pregnancy and the risks that such hypertension during pregnancy poses to both mother and fetus. Superimposed preeclampsia, hypertensive crisis, renal failure, HELLP (Hemolysis, Elevated Liver enzymes, Low Platelets) syndrome, and death are also severe complications of pregnancy.

Once a woman has successfully negotiated a pregnancy or once she is sexually active and desires to avoid pregnancy, issues of contraception become important. In the former setting, contraception may be important to avoid an inadvertent pregnancy, once again placing the woman's life at risk, depending on the severity of her disease. Although the Centers for Disease Control and Prevention (CDC) still lists barrier contraception with early pregnancy termination for contraceptive failure to be among the safest methods of contraception,[1] this approach is not always practical for a variety of reasons. The issue of contraception therefore must be addressed with the hypertensive women so that her needs can be safely met.

This chapter presents the different methods of contraception available for use in women of reproductive age, with specific attention given to hypertension in women.

OVERVIEW

If one includes vasectomy, permanent sterilization was the most common method of birth control used by American couples in 1996 (Fig. 7–1).[2] Oral contraceptives, however, remain the most widely used *reversible* method of contraception. Regardless of method, one of the most important factors in determining contraceptive efficacy is satisfaction with the contraceptive method by the patient and her partner. The woman with hypertension has specific medical needs that must be addressed, and different methods of contraception have variable effects.

BARRIER CONTRACEPTION

Barrier contraception is a safe and effective method of contraception for all women. The major risks of barrier contraception have centered around (1) user and method failure rates (relatively high), (2) concerns about spermicides and birth defects, and (3) inconvenience. The failure rate of barrier contraception methods is quite low. In addition to the contraceptive benefits of barrier contraception, particularly condoms with a nonoxynol-9–containing spermicide, is their ability to minimize the risk of infection with human immunodeficiency virus and other sexually transmitted diseases. A number of studies have been unable to demonstrate any increased risk of Down syndrome, hypospadias, limb reduction defects, neoplasms, or neural tube defects associated with conception and continued use of spermicides during early pregnancy (Fig. 7–2).[3]

As stated earlier, there are no contraindications to barrier contraception in the hypertensive patient. With all method selection, however, it is important to recognize the contribution of failure rates to overall morbidity if pregnancy were to be established in the setting of severe hypertensive

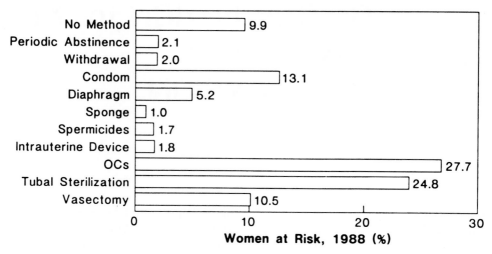

FIGURE 7–1. Birth control practices of American couples. OCs, oral contraceptives. (Adapted from Harlap et al. Preventing Pregnancy, Protecting Health. New York and Washington, DC: The Alan Guttmacher Institute, 1991.)

disease, especially when a termination of pregnancy was not an option.

INTRAUTERINE DEVICES

Intrauterine devices (IUDs) are an effective method of reversible contraception. IUDs became quite popular in the 1970s, but that popularity was short-lived due to emerging reports of pelvic inflammatory disease (PID) and septic abortion associated with IUD use, specifically with use of the Dalkon Shield. Nevertheless, the IUD remains an effective

reversible method for monogamous couples desiring or requiring long-term contraception.[4]

Multiple mechanisms of action have been reported for the IUD that in fact make it a morally acceptable alternative for virtually all patients.[5, 6] IUD myths have embodied such ideas as the IUD being essentially an abortifacient, resulting in failure of implantation of a fertilized embryo. This would create, or might potentially create, a moral dilemma for some individuals. In reality, the IUD exerts most of its action at the level of the cervical mucus, rendering it hostile to

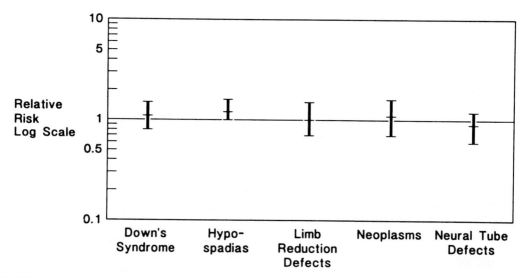

FIGURE 7–2. Spermicides: Risk of birth defects. (Adapted from data published by Louik C, Mitchell AA, Werler MPH, et al. Maternal exposure to spermicide in relation to certain birth defects. N Engl J Med 1987;317:474–478.)

TABLE 7-1. INTRAUTERINE DEVICES (IUDs): MECHANISMS OF ACTION

1. Studies show that IUD use decreases the number of sperm reaching the oviduct and their capacity to fertilize ova.
2. Depending on the type of IUD, the device acts by:
   a. Hindering sperm from penetrating the cervical mucus
   b. Precipitating head-tail separation in the presence of copper
   c. Causing cytotoxic effects in the IUD-altered uterine fluid
   d. Having deleterious effects on ova

Data from Alvarez F, Brache V, Fernandez E, et al. New insights on the mode of action of intrauterine contraceptive devices in women. Fertil Steril 1988;49:768–773; and Ortiz ME, Croxatto HB. The mode of action of IUDs. Contraception 1987;36:37–53.

sperm penetration; may interfere with cellule motility of the fallopian tube; and may interfere with fertilization through mechanisms yet undefined. Althought it is certainly possible that interfering with implantation of a fertilized egg might be a mechanism of action, it is clearly not the only mechanism of action (Table 7–1).

The risk of PID has also been a concern among women. It has been nicely demonstrated that if one eliminates all cases of PID attributable to the Dalkon Shield from analyses of PID incidents, the risk of PID from IUD use compares favorably with other methods of contraception or with no contraception at all (Fig. 7–3).[4]

Absolute contraindications to an IUD include:

- An established intrauterine pregnancy
- Suspected pregnancy
- Known or suspected genital malignancy
- Vaginal bleeding of unknown origin
- Acute pelvic or vaginal infection
- Allergy to copper (for IUDs containing copper)

Relative contraindications include:

- Chronic PID
- A history of ectopic pregnancy
- Congenital or acquired uterine anomalies
- Chronic anemia
- Leukemia
- Wilson's disease
- Valvular heart disease that would normally require streptococcal pyrogenic endotoxin prophylaxis for even minor surgical procedures

There are no contraindications to IUD use for hypertensive women; however, hypertensive women may have other medical complications and one should be cognizant of those co-morbid conditions before prescribing any method of contraception. An example would be a hypertensive woman who also has antiphospholipid syndrome requiring chronic anticoagulation therapy. She might not be an ideal candidate for an IUD because menorrhagia may result from such use.

In addition to the inert IUD, progesterone-

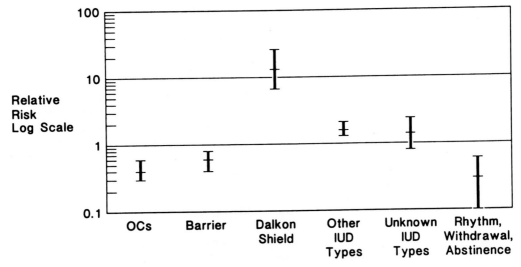

FIGURE 7–3. Intrauterine devices: Risk of pelvic inflammatory disease, Dalkon shield bias. OCs, oral contraceptives. (Adapted from Lee NC, Rubin GL, Borucki R. The intrauterine device and pelvic inflammatory disease revisited: New results from the Women's Health Study. Obstet Gynecol 1988;72:1–6.)

containing IUDs are also available. Because of the very low dose of progesterone, these devices are essentially metabolically neutral and the progesterone would be unlikely to exert any systemic metabolic effect. These devices are less popular because they require more frequent replacement.

From these data, one may see that an IUD may be a quite satisfactory method of contraception for nearly all women but particularly the hypertensive woman because of the following:

- The relative absence of systemic effects
- The relative absence of contraindications
- The fact that it is a method that allows for long-term reversible contraception, with current IUDs requiring replacement no more frequently than every 10 years

NATURAL FAMILY PLANNING

In this technical age, we as care providers not infrequently assume that all medical interventions must require a device or a pharmaceutical. For a variety of reasons, when it comes to contraception, these alternatives are not always viable. Natural family planning continues to be a popular and accepted method of contraception that, when used correctly, can be quite effective. There are several advantages to natural family planning:

1. It is culturally and morally widely acceptable.
2. It introduces an awareness of fertility to the couple that can be beneficial.
3. Little or no outlay of finances is needed.

At the family level, it does make procreation more of a shared responsibility, which can have positive effects on the relationship of the couple.

Of course, there are some disadvantages. Cycle regularity and close cooperation between both partners are requisites for a successful planning approach. A summary of 10 studies has estimated a failure rate associated with natural family planning ranging from 3.9% to 39.7%.[7] The advent of new technology, including "fertility" software, home use hormonal assays, and even bioelectric impedance measuring devices, however, has improved a woman's ability to identify when she is to become ovulatory; this knowledge can greatly assist in the successful implementation of a natural family planning program. Investigations of salivary assays of estradiol to predict impending ovulation are under way.

HORMONAL CONTRACEPTION

The major portion of the rest of this section covers hormonal contraception, specifically, combination oral contraceptive pills, which represent the most widely used method of reversible contraception in the United States today. Their contraceptive efficacy is well established, and there are proven noncontraceptive health benefits to their use.

One major advantage to hormonal contraception, particularly combined low-dose oral contraceptive pills, is their essential metabolic neutrality. With regard to oral contraception, several major disease states come to mind, and many of them are related to patients who have hypertension. Specifically, concerns over oral contraceptive ingestion can center around elevation of blood pressure, hyperlipidemia, thromboembolic disease and stroke, glucose intolerance, drug interactions, and neoplasia. With the exception of neoplasia, all of these categories relate directly to hypertension. Hypertensive patients are at higher risk for hyperlipidemia and for thromboembolic disease and stroke—or for concomitant illnesses that put them at risk for thromboembolic disease and stroke—such as certain collagen vascular disorders (e.g., lupus, antiphospholipid antibody syndrome). These patients are also at risk for glucose intolerance because hypertension is a well-known complication of diabetes.

Patients requiring antihypertensive therapy are also concerned about the potential for drug interaction. They are concerned not only about how oral contraceptives affect the efficacy of their antihypertensive medication but also about how the antihypertensive medication may affect the contraceptive efficacy of their oral contraceptive pill.

Hypertension

Blood pressure increases slightly among women who take combined oral contraceptive pills. It is thought that the oral contraceptive, via its effect on the renin-angiotensin-aldosterone system, can effectively elevate blood pressure by 7 to 8 mmHg.[8] Intravascular volume and cardiac output increases have also been reported in women taking higher-dose oral contraceptive pills (>50 μg ethinyl estradiol) but not in patients taking lower-dose pills. Although estrogen has generally been assumed to be the agent responsible for this modest blood pressure elevation, elevation of blood pressure has been observed in association with administration of depo-medroxyprogesterone acetate (Depo-Provera).[9]

Earlier studies, specifically the Walnut Creek Study,[10] suggested that about 4% of users of oral contraceptives who, presumably, had been normotensive before use) developed diastolic hypertension at a rate more than double the rate seen in nonusers. These results are similar to those reported by the Royal College of General Practitioners Study.[11] Because of these observations, it is recommended that blood pressure always be measured before treatment with all contraceptive pills and thereafter at every visit. Although clinically significant hypertension is rare, when it does occur, it should be detected early and oral contraceptive agents stopped because this hypertension is generally fully reversible.

The main risks of uncontrolled hypertension are stroke and, in some cases, myocardial infarction. Another confounder for risk of hypertension in those taking oral contraceptives is cigarette smoking. Oral contraceptives may be prescribed to smokers under age 30 years only with great caution and should not be prescribed to women over age 35 who are cigarette smokers.

In patients with established hypertension, other issues need to be considered. Specifically, the risk of pregnancy cannot be ignored in such patients, and the potentially morbid sequelae of hypertension in pregnancy have been mentioned. Established hypertension is not a contraindication to oral contraceptive use if this is the patient's only medical condition. Generally, with close medical follow-up, oral contraceptives may be prescribed in this setting and antihypertensive medication adjusted so as to maintain blood pressure in the normal range. With regard to interactions with medications, no current studies suggest that antihypertensive medications adversely affect the performance of oral contraceptive pills or vice versa.

The one class of drugs that has been fairly closely studied relative to its effects on oral contraceptive pills has been β-blockers. A number of studies comparing the effects of different β-blockers on contraceptive efficacy, and vice versa, have concluded that no clinically significant interactions occur that would require adjustment of the dose of either medication.[12]

In addition to the alterations in the renin-angiotensin-aldosterone system, other metabolic alterations have been proposed to account for the possible effects of oral contraceptives on blood pressure, such as alterations in prostacyclin formation among oral contraceptive users.[13] There does not seem to be a significant effect on prostacyclin production from the use of oral contraceptives alone. When smoking is included in the analyses, however, there is a significant reduction in prostacyclin formation among oral contraceptive users (Fig. 7–4). This may account for the increased incidence of hypertension and stroke among oral contraceptive users who smoke.

Many hypertensive women also have varying degrees of hyperlipidemia. Although oral contraceptives are thought to be predominantly metabolically neutral, at least at a clinical level, combined oral contraceptive pills do affect components of cholesterol and triglycerides. An early recognition of an increased risk of ischemic heart disease among oral contraceptive users, along with the association of hyperlipidemia, hypertension, and atherosclerotic coronary artery disease, has fueled the interest in lipid research pertaining to estrogen and progesterone-containing oral contraceptive pills. The association between hyperlipidemia and atherosclerotic coronary artery disease and the risk of myocardial infarction forces our consideration of oral contraceptive effects in these areas. A summary of these effects is presented in Table 7–2.

In the early 1980s, it was demonstrated that the incidence of coronary atherosclerosis in young women dying of myocardial infarction was higher among nonusers of oral contraceptives than among users. It has been suggested that this may be a selection bias because oral contraceptive users may have been screened as being healthier. Nonetheless, these data support the observations of Clarkson and coworkers,[14] suggesting that oral contraceptives not only may be metabolically neutral but also may

TABLE 7-2. EFFECTS OF ORAL CONTRACEPTIVES ON LIPID LEVELS

LIPID	ESTROGEN	PROGESTIN
Total cholesterol	No change; slightly increased	No change; slightly decreased
VLDL cholesterol	Increased	Decreased
LDL cholesterol	Decreased	Increased
HDL cholesterol	Increased	Decreased
Triglycerides	Increased	Decreased

HDL, high-density lipoprotein; LDL, low-density lipoprotein; VLDL, very-low-density lipoprotein.

have a protective role against the development of atherosclerotic coronary artery disease. It is now viewed that the more likely etiologic mechanism of myocardial infarction among oral contraceptive users is thrombogenic infarcts that are probably related to estrogen. A well-known principle, however, is that the epidemiology will tend to lag behind the science. Many of these observations of thrombogenic infarcts date back to a cohort of women who used primarily high estrogen containing oral contraceptive pills. A 1990 review by Stampfer and coworkers[15] (Fig. 7–5) suggests that among low-dose oral contraceptive users, there was no statistically significantly increased risk of myocardial infarction.

On the basis of current evidence, then, one might safely say that low-dose preparations of oral contraceptive pills today have a nearly neutral effect on lipid metabolism and that these low-dose pills should be first-line choices for patients contemplating the use of oral contraceptives, particularly patients with hypertension.

Thromboembolic Disease and Stroke

In 1967, the British Medical Research Council[16, 17] first described evidence of an association between oral contraceptive pills and thromboembolic disease. The relative risk was estimated to be from 2 to 11, with an absolute risk of 6 in 10,000. As stated earlier, however, these data reflected a population of women who were taking fairly high doses of estrogen in their oral contraceptive pills. Nevertheless, the concern over thromboembolic disease and stroke remains even with today's low-dose combined oral contraceptive pills. In the woman with hypertension, thromboembolic disease and stroke may represent particular risk factors because hypertension is associated with many illnesses

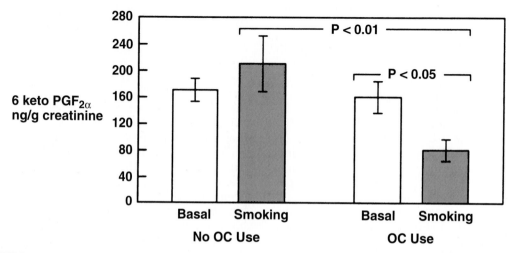

FIGURE 7–4. Alteration of prostacyclin formation in oral contraceptive (OC) users. (Adapted from Mileikowsky GN, Nadler JL, Huey F, et al. Evidence that smoking alters prostacyclin formation and platelet aggregation in women who use oral contraceptives. Am J Obstet Gynecol 1988;159:1547–1552.)

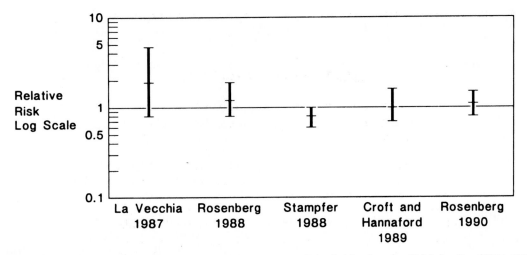

FIGURE 7-5. Published reports on past use of oral contraceptives and risk of myocardial infarction (1987–1990). (Adapted from Stampfer MJ, Willett WC, Colditz GA, et al. Past use of oral contraceptives and cardiovascular disease: A meta-analysis in the context of the Nurse's Health Study. Am J Obstet Gynecol 1990;163:285–291.)

that also predispose to these other conditions. Several issues therefore must be considered with regard to selecting women who might be candidates for oral contraceptives.

Thromboembolic Disease

Women with hypertension secondary to systemic illnesses such as antiphospholipid syndrome and lupus erythematosus may be at risk for hypercoagulability, thromboembolic disease, and stroke. There is significant controversy as to the appropriateness of oral contraceptives for this group of patients. In patients with no history of thromboembolic disease or stroke, after careful informed consent is reviewed with the patient, oral contraceptives may be an appropriate choice. It is recommended, however, that these women undergo screening for hypercoagulability although this measure remains controversial.

If screening for hypercoagulability is to be undertaken, the most cost-effective analyses as a first pass would include screening for the factor V Leiden mutation, a genetic mutation that causes resistance to activated protein C. Plasma homocysteine levels may also be measured; elevated levels constitute a treatable cause of hypercoagulability (with a cocktail of folic acid, pyridoxine, and cyanocobalamin).

In screening for lupus anticoagulant, the initial evaluation can detect 20% or more of patients with hypercoagulability. Lower yields can be achieved with screening for

protein C deficiency, protein S deficiency, and antithrombin III deficiency.

The relative risk of venous thromboembolism (VTE) among oral contraceptive users is significantly elevated in patients with the factor V Leiden mutation (Table 7–3). Data regarding third-generation oral contraceptives have suggested a possibly increased incidence of nonfatal VTE among third-generation progestin-containing oral contraceptives, specifically those containing desogestrel, and gestodene (which is not available in the United States (Table 7–4). It is currently recommended that first- or second-generation low-dose oral contraceptives be used for new users of oral contraceptive

TABLE 7-3. FACTOR V LEIDEN MUTATION INCREASES RISK OF VENOUS THROMBOEMBOLISM IN USERS OF ORAL CONTRACEPTIVES (OCs)

SCENARIO	NO.	PERSON-YEARS	INCIDENCE*
Leiden negative			
No OCs	36	437,870	0.8
Current OCs	84	275,858	3.0
Leiden positive			
No OCs	10	17,515	5.7
Current OCs	25	8,757	28.5

*Incidence per 10,000 person-years.
From Vandenbroucke JP, Koster T, Briet E, et al. Increased risk of venous thrombosis in oral-contraceptive users who are carriers of factor V Leiden mutation. Lancet 1994;344:1453–1457.

TABLE 7–4. RISK OF NONFATAL VENOUS THROMBOEMBOLISM WITH USE OF THIRD-GENERATION ORAL CONTRACEPTIVES: BOSTON COLLABORATIVE DRUG SURVEILLANCE

PROGESTAGENS	PERSON-YEARS	NO. PER 100,000	RR (95% CI)
Levonorgestrel*	143,255	16.1	1.0
Desogestrel	102,270	29.3	1.9 (1.1–3.2)
Gestodene	78,363	28.1	1.8 (1.0–3.2)

*Reference second-generation oral contraceptives.
CI, confidence interval; RR, relative risk.
From Jick H, Jick SS, Gurewich V, et al. Risk of idiopathic cardiovascular death and nonfatal venous thromboembolism in women using oral contraceptives with differing components. Lancet 1995;346:1589–1593.

pills until the data involving the risk of nonfatal VTE associated with third-generation oral contraceptives are further developed. Once again, as demonstrated in Figure 7–6, the risk of VTE is directly related to estrogen potency.

Stroke

The most common type of stroke among women of reproductive age is the hemorrhagic subarachnoid stroke. The Walnut Creek Study[18] suggested that oral contraceptive pills increased the relative risk (RR) of such strokes (RR=6.0). More than half of these cases, however, were more than 50 years old, and more recent data focusing primarily on users of low-dose oral contraceptives have not confirmed this association. Most hemorrhagic stroke would, however, be secondary to hypertension, which

once again underscores the need for very close surveillance of patients at risk for development of hypertension or for those overtly hypertensive patients in whom oral contraception is deemed to be a suitable method of contraception, provided there is the ability to carry out appropriate surveillance.

Again, smoking figures quite prominently into the risk of stroke among oral contraceptive users (Figs. 7–7 to 7–11). Whether the risk of cerebrovascular disease remains increased after discontinuation of oral contraceptive pills remains an unresolved issue, but the consensus suggests that it is not a significant risk.

Myocardial Infarction

In addition to hypertension, thromboembolic disease, and stroke, myocardial in-

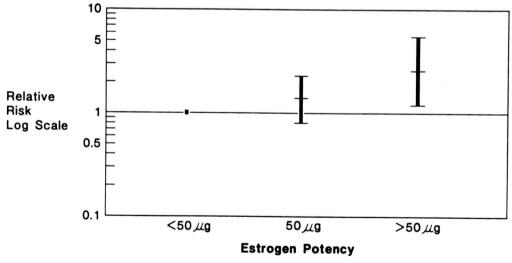

FIGURE 7–6. Relative risk of venous thromboembolism among oral contraceptive users, by estrogen potency. (Adapted from Gerstman BB, Piper JM, Freiman JP, et al. Oral contraceptive oestrogen and progestin potencies and the incidence of deep venous thromboembolism. Int J Epidemiol 1990;19:931–936. By permission of Oxford University Press.)

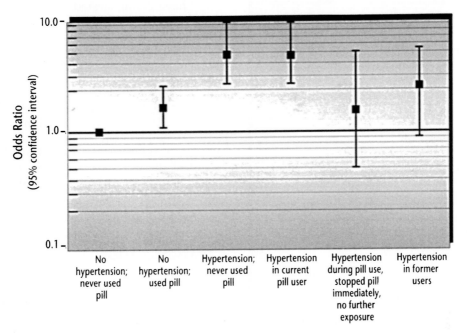

FIGURE 7–7. Adjusted odds ratios of first-ever stroke in oral contraceptive users and nonusers according to diagnosis of hypertension: Royal College of General Practitioners' oral contraception study. (From Hannaford PC, Croft PR, Kay CR. Oral contraception and stroke: Evidence from the Royal College of General Practitioners Oral Contraception Study. Stroke 1994;25:935–942.)

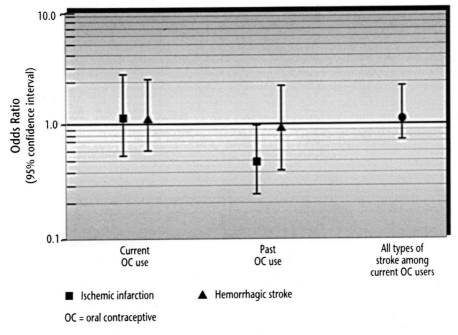

FIGURE 7–8. Adjusted odds ratios for ischemic, hemorrhagic, and all types of stroke according to oral contraceptive (OC) use in the Kaiser Permanente population. (Adapted from data published by Petitti DB, Sidney S, Bernstein A, et al. Stroke and users of low-dose oral contraceptives. N Engl J Med 1996;335:8–15.)

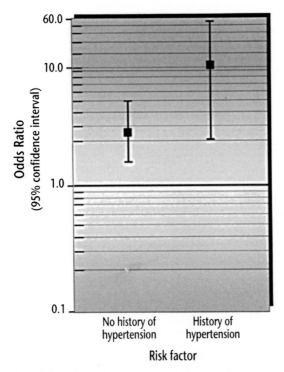

FIGURE 7–9. Odds ratios for ischemic stroke among European users of oral contraceptives according to history of hypertension. (From World Health Organization, Collaborative Study of Cardiovascular Diseases and Steroid Hormone Contraception. Ischemic stroke and combined oral contraceptives: Result of an international multi-center case-control study. Lancet 1996; 348:498–505.)

farction is also a perceived risk among oral contraceptive users. The best evidence suggests that oral contraceptive use is an unlikely independent risk factor for myocardial infarction but may compound the effects of other risk factors, such as hypercoagulability states, diabetes, hyperlipidemia, and cigarette smoking.

Carbohydrate Metabolism

Many women with hypertension have hypertension secondary to diabetes. Usually, contraindications to use of oral contraceptives by diabetic women pertain mostly to concomitant vascular disease. In the setting of insulin-dependent diabetes (see Chapter 9) not complicated by other vascular disease, oral contraceptives, as a result of their essential metabolic neutrality, may be offered as a method of birth control. Among otherwise healthy women, Hannaford and

Kay[19] have demonstrated no increase in the development of diabetes among users of low-dose oral contraceptive pills (Fig. 7–12). Although biochemical effects on glucose metabolism, glucagon secretion, and insulin secretion do occur in the presence of estrogen and progesterone, these effects appear to be clinically somewhat minor. Nevertheless, women with insulin-dependent diabetes who are being considered as candidates for oral contraceptive therapy should be advised of the possible need for increasing their insulin dosage in response to their oral contraceptive therapy.

PROGESTIN-ONLY HORMONAL CONTRACEPTION

Though less popular, primarily because of intermittent bleeding, amenorrhea, and weight gain, progesterone-only contraception is an option for hypertensive women. A variety of delivery systems for progesterone-only contraception exist, most notably the progestin-only pill (the mini-pill), Depo-

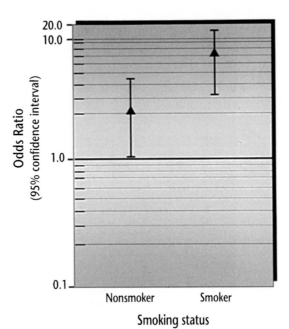

FIGURE 7–10. Odds ratios for ischemic stroke among European users of oral contraceptives according to smoking status. (From World Health Organization, Collaborative Study of Cardiovascular Diseases and Steroid Hormone Contraception. Hemorrhagic stroke, overall stroke risk, and combined oral contraceptives: Result of an international multi-center case-control study. Lancet 1996;348:505–510.)

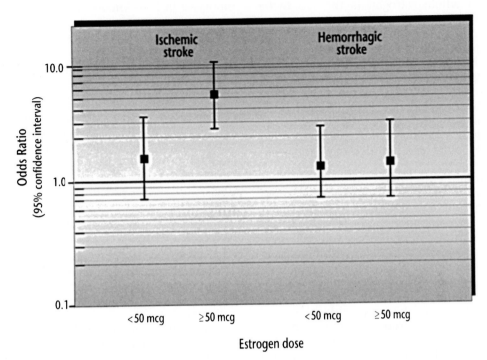

FIGURE 7–11. Adjusted odds ratios for ischemic and hemorrhagic stroke in European users of oral contraceptives by estrogen dose. (From World Health Organization, Collaborative Study of Cardiovascular Diseases and Steroid Hormone Contraception. Hemorrhagic stroke, overall stroke risk, and combined oral contraceptives: Result of an international multi-center case-control study. Lancet 1996;348:505–510.)

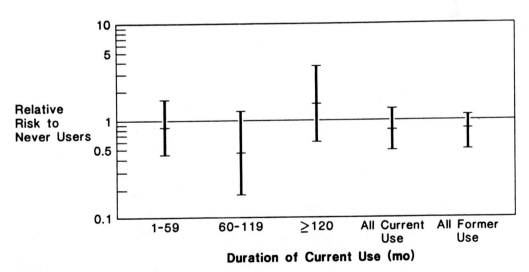

FIGURE 7–12. Relationship of oral contraceptive use and relative risk of diabetes. (Adapted from Hannaford PC, Kay CR. Oral contraceptives and diabetes mellitus. Br Med J 1989;299:1315–1316.)

Provera, and implanted levonorgestrel (Norplant). These are suitable alternatives for patients in whom estrogen is thought to be relatively contraindicated.

Specifically, patients with hypercoagulable states or those with nonfocal migraine headaches in whom combined oral contraceptives may be a relative contraindication may benefit from progesterone-only pills.[20] The side effects previously mentioned, however, including weight gain (most frequently attributed to Depo-Provera), result in these choices being less popular than those already reviewed.

Although combined oral contraceptive pills are thought to be relatively neutral from the metabolic perspective, progesterone-only preparations appear to have less effect on blood coagulation and carbohydrate metabolism compared with combined oral contraceptive pills; however, their effect on lipid metabolism is probably equivalent. Far fewer epidemiologic data are available on the risk of serious side effects of progesterone-only preparations (e.g., hypertension, thromboembolic disease and stroke, myocardial infarction, diabetes, and hyperlipidemia). Additionally, the overall contraceptive efficacy of progesterone-only preparations may be lower than that of combined oral contraceptives when only method failure rates, as opposed to user failure rates (actual failure rates), are analyzed.

CONCLUSIONS

In sum, a number of contraceptive choices are available to the hypertensive woman. Many of these choices present risks no different than those for her nonhypertensive counterpart. With respect to the most popular method of reversible contraception, specifically, combined oral contraceptives, the following metabolic effects have been observed:

1. Estrogen tends to result in an increase in β-globulin angiotensinogen, a variety of clotting factors, high-density lipoprotein cholesterol, total cholesterol, and triglycerides.

2. Low-density liproprotein cholesterol is generally diminished, and the effects on carbohydrate metabolism are negligible.

3. Progesterone effects include little effect on protein metabolism, decreases in high-density lipoprotein cholesterol and total cholesterol, minimal effect on triglycerides, increases in low-density lipoprotein cholesterol, and increases in insulin resistance. (An increase in insulin resistance may have implications for the hypertensive woman or the woman at risk for development of hypertension.)

In counseling women with regard to their contraceptive choices, the physician should explain all options. In women with hypertension, a thorough discussion is particularly important because of the risks that the hypertension may pose should a contraceptive failure occur. The physician should not ignore the noncontraceptive-related health benefits associated with oral contraceptive use. These include:

- Reduced risk for development of ovarian cancer or endometrial cancer
- Decreased incidence of fibroadenoma
- Reduced incidence of fibrocystic breast disease
- More regular menses with reduced menstrual blood loss, iron deficiency anemia, and dysmenorrhea
- Reduced incidence of acute pelvic inflammatory disease
- Decreased incidence of ectopic pregnancy
- Reduced incidence of functional ovarian cysts

With careful monitoring, regardless of method chosen, nearly all of the spectrum of contraceptive choices is available to hypertensive women provided that compliance and close follow-up can be guaranteed.

References

1. Hatcher RA, Trussell J, Stewart F, et al. Contraceptive Technology, 16th ed. New York: Irvington, 1994, pp 135, 268.
2. Riox JE. Female sterilization and its reversal. *In* Filshie M, Guillebaud J (eds). Contraception: Science and Practice. Boston: Butterworths, 1989.
3. Louik C, Mitchell AA, Werler MPH, et al. Maternal exposure to spermicides in relation to certain birth defects. N Eng J Med 1987;317:474–478.
4. The intrauterine device. ACOG Technical Bulletin, No. 164, February 1992.
5. Alvarez F, Brache V, Fernandez E, et al. New insights on the mode of action of intrauterine contraceptive devices in women. Fertil Steril 1988;49:768–773.
6. Ortiz ME, Croxatto HB. The mode of action of IUDs. Contraception 1987;36:37–53.
7. Flynn AM, Bonnar J. Natural family planning. *In*

Filshie M, Guillebaud J (eds). Contraception: Science and Practice. Boston: Butterworths, 1989.

8. Cardoso F, Polonia J, Santos A, et al. Low-dose oral contraceptives and 24-hour ambulatory blood pressure. Int J Gynaecol Obstet 1997;59:237–243.

9. Hall WD, Douglas MB, Blumestein BA, Hatcher RA. Blood pressure and oral progestational agents. Am J Obstet Gynecol 1980;136:344–350.

10. Rinehart W, Piotrow PT. OCs—update on usage and safety and side effects. Population Reports Series A 1979;5:A133–A186.

11. Dalen JE, Hickler RB. Oral contraceptives and cardiovascular disease. Am Heart J 1981;101:626–639.

12. Kendall MJ, Jack DB, Quarterman CP, et al. Beta adrenoceptor blocker pharmacokinetics and the oral contraceptive pill. Br J Clin Pharmacol 1984;17:87S–89S.

13. Mileikowsky GN, Nadler JL, Huey F, et al. Evidence that smoking alters prostacyclin formation and platelet aggregation in women who use oral contraceptives. Am J Obstet Gynecol 1988;159:1547–1552.

14. Clarkson TB, Shively CA, Morgan TM, et al. Oral contraceptives and coronary artery atherosclerosis of cynomolgus monkeys. Obstet Gynecol 1990;75:217–222.

15. Stampfer MJ, Willett WC, Colditz GA, et al. Past use of oral contraceptives and cardiovascular disease: A meta-analysis in the context of the Nurse's Health Study. Am J Obstet Gynecol 1990;163:285–291.

16. Vessey MP. Female hormones and vascular disease—an epidemiological overview. Br J Fam Plan 1980;6:1–12.

17. Inman WHW, Vessey MP, Westerholm B, Engleund A. Thromboembolic disease and the steroidal content of oral contraceptives: A report to the Committee on Safety on Drugs. Br J Med 1970;2:203–209.

18. Petitti DB, Wingerd J. Use of oral contraceptives, cigarette smoking, and risk of subarachnoid hemorrhage. Lancet 1978;2:235–236.

19. Hannaford PC, Kay CR. Oral contraceptives and diabetes mellitus. Br Med J 1989;299:1315–1316.

20. The use of hormonal contraception in women with coexisting medical conditions. Clinical Management Guidelines for Obstetrician-Gynecologists. ACOG Practice Bulletin, vol 18, 2000, pp 1–14.

8

CHRONIC HYPERTENSION in PREGNANCY

Bassam Haddad and Baha M. Sibai

Chronic hypertension is observed in 1% to 5% of pregnant women, depending on the population studied and the diagnostic criteria used.[1] In the 1990s, the incidence was 2.5% among African Americans and 1% among other racial groups.[2] In addition, the prevalence of chronic hypertension varies according to age. The reported rates range from 1.9% at 20 to 29 years to 5.7% at 30 to 39 years among African Americans and from 0.9% at 20 to 29 years to 5.2% at 40 to 49 years among other racial groups.[3] This is critical because the rate of birth in women between 40 and 44 years of age increased by 56% from 1980 to 1993, perhaps in relation to delayed pregnancy in order to achieve educational or career goals or to remarriage later in life.[4, 5]

DEFINITION AND DIAGNOSIS

Chronic hypertension is defined by elevated blood pressure occurring before pregnancy. In pregnant women whose prepregnancy blood pressure is unknown, the diagnosis of chronic hypertension is based on the presence of hypertension (either systolic blood pressure of at least 140 mmHg or diastolic blood pressure of at least 90 mmHg on at least two occasions at least at 4 hours apart), before 20 weeks' gestation.[1] However, the diagnosis in such women may be difficult to assess because hypertension before 20 weeks' gestation may be the first manifestation of preeclampsia.[6] Furthermore, the physiologic decrease in blood pressure observed in healthy pregnant women that occurs during the first and second trimester also occurs in many patients with chronic hypertension. Therefore, such patients are more likely to be erroneously diagnosed as having a transient hypertension or a pre-

eclampsia according to blood pressure criteria.[1, 7–9]

CLASSIFICATION AND ETIOLOGY

Chronic hypertension during pregnancy can be subclassified as either *mild* or *severe,* depending on systolic and diastolic values. A systolic and a diastolic (Korotkoff phase V) blood pressure of 160 mmHg or greater or 110 mmHg or greater, respectively, or both, constitutes severe chronic hypertension.[10]

The etiology of chronic hypertension is an important consideration in the management of pregnancy (Table 8–1). Chronic hypertension can be subdivided into *primary (idiopathic)* and *secondary.* Primary hypertension is by far the most common cause of

TABLE 8–1. CAUSES OF CHRONIC HYPERTENSION IN PREGNANCY

Idiopathic (90%)
Secondary (10%)
  Renal disease
    Glomerulonephritis
    Interstitial nephritis
    Nephropathy
    Polycystic kidneys
    Renal artery stenosis
    Renal transplant
  Collagen vascular disorders
    Lupus erythematosus
    Periarthritis nodosa
    Scleroderma
  Endocrine diseases
    Diabetes
    Hyperaldosteronism
    Pheochromocytoma
    Thyrotoxicosis
  Vascular disease
    Coarctation

From Sibai BM. Chronic hypertension in pregnancy. Clin Perinatol 1991;18:833–844.

chronic hypertension seen during pregnancy (90%). In 10% of the cases, chronic hypertension may be related to one or several underlying disorders such as renal disease, collagen vascular disorders, endocrine disease, or aortic coarctation.[11]

MATERNAL RISKS

Pregnancies complicated by chronic hypertension are at increased risk for development of superimposed preeclampsia and abruptio placentae (placental abruption).[12] The incidence of superimposed preeclampsia in women with chronic hypertension is under debate. The reported incidence ranges from 4.2% to 52%,[9, 13–23] with differences related to the population studied, severity of hypertension during pregnancy, and the diagnostic criteria used for superimposed preeclampsia. The incidence of superimposed preeclampsia in women with *severe* chronic hypertension ranges from 28.2% to 52%[13, 17, 18, 22]; it ranges from 4.8% to 15.6% in women with *mild* chronic hypertension.[7, 9, 16, 22]

In one study,[23] incidence of superimposed preeclampsia was studied in 763 women with documented chronic hypertension. This diagnosis of superimposed preeclampsia was based on strict clinical and laboratory criteria. The overall rate of superimposed preeclampsia was 25%. The rate was not affected by (1) maternal age (26% among women older than 35 years of age versus 25% among those younger than 35 years of age), (2) race (25% among black women versus 26% among white women), or (3) the presence of proteinuria at baseline measurement (27% among women with proteinuria versus 25% among those without it); however, the rate was significantly greater in women who had had hypertension for at least 4 years (31% versus 22%, $P < .001$), in those having preeclampsia during a previous pregnancy (32% versus 23%, $P = .02$), and in those whose diastolic blood pressure was 100 to 110 mmHg compared with those whose baseline diastolic blood pressure was below 100 mmHg (42% versus 24%, $P = .01$).[23]

In another study, the reported incidence of abruptio placentae in women with chronic hypertension ranged from 0.5 to 10%.[12] For those with mild chronic hypertension, the incidence was nearly 1.5% to 2% and was not influenced by antihypertensive treatment.[7, 9] The incidence of abruptio placentae in women with severe hypertension ranged from 2.3[13] to 9.5%.[7]

In a 1998 study that included 763 women with chronic hypertension,[23] the overall incidence of abruptio placentae was 1.5% and the frequency was significantly higher in women with superimposed preeclampsia than in those without this complication (3% versus 1%, $P = .04$). In addition, the incidence of abruptio placentae was similar in women older or younger than 35 years of age, and in those with a diastolic blood pressure of 90 to 100 mmHg versus those with a diastolic blood pressure of 100 to 110 mmHg at baseline. In addition, the incidence was not influenced by the duration of hypertension.

PERINATAL RISKS

Fetal and neonatal complications are closely related to maternal complications. The risk of fetal death and perinatal death is increased two to four times in women with complications compared with the general population.[24–26] In a follow-up study of 337 pregnancies among 298 women with chronic hypertension, the rate of perinatal mortality was 45/1000 compared with a rate of 12/1000 in the general population ($P < .001$).[24] Rates for premature deliveries and small-for-gestational-age (SGA) infants were increased in women with chronic hypertension.[22, 24–28] In addition, the rates of preterm delivery and SGA infants in women with severe chronic hypertension (62% and 31%, respectively) were significantly higher than the respective rates in women with mild chronic hypertension (16% and 11%, respectively).[22]

In 1998, Sibai and associates[23] reported risk factors for adverse perinatal outcome among 763 women with chronic hypertension who were evaluated prospectively at several university centers in the United States. The authors reported that the development of superimposed preeclampsia was associated with significantly higher rates of preterm delivery (56% versus 25%, $P < .001$), higher rates of neonatal intraventricular hemorrhage (3% versus 1%, $P < .01$), and higher rates of perinatal death (8% versus 4%, $P = .02$). In addition, in women with chronic hypertension, the presence of proteinuria early in pregnancy (13–26 weeks' gestation) was also an independent risk factor that was associated with higher rates of preterm delivery (53% versus 31%, $P < .001$), higher rates of SGA infants (23% versus 10%, $P < .001$), and higher rates of neonatal intraventricular hemorrhage (4% versus 1%, $P = .01$).[23]

GENERAL MANAGEMENT

The purpose of management of women with chronic hypertension is to reduce pregnancy-related complications (i.e., superimposed preeclampsia, abruptio placentae, etc.) and acute maternal cerebral hemorrhage, which may occur in cases of severe hypertension. Ideally, women should be evaluated before conception so that drugs that may have adverse side effects on the fetus, such as angiotensin-converting enzyme inhibitors, can be replaced by other drugs if necessary. Depending on the medical history and clinical and laboratory findings, pregnant women with chronic hypertension can be then divided into categories of low-risk or high-risk chronic hypertension.

LOW-RISK CHRONIC HYPERTENSION

Pregnant women with chronic hypertension are considered to be at low risk in cases of mild hypertension without any organ involvement. Because the maternal benefits of treating mild chronic hypertension are not clear, the question of whether antihypertensive treatment improves perinatal outcome becomes paramount. Few prospective randomized studies have been conducted to determine whether antihypertensive treatments in such women improve maternal or perinatal outcome (Table 8–2).[9, 14, 16, 19, 29–37]

Maternal Outcome

The effectiveness of antihypertensive treatment on prevention of adverse maternal outcome (superimposed preeclampsia, abruptio placentae) has been the subject of a limited number of randomized studies. In a prospective randomized trial, Sibai and colleagues[9] compared pregnancy outcome

among women receiving no medication (n = 90) versus methyldopa (n = 88) or labetalol (n = 86), and who were randomized between 6 and 13 weeks' gestation. The incidences of superimposed preeclampsia (15.6%, 18.4%, and 16.3%, respectively), abruptio placentae (2.2%, 1.1%, and 2.3%, respectively) were similar among the three groups.

Hirsch and coworkers[35] evaluated the effect of pindolol on pregnancy outcome in a prospective randomized placebo-controlled trial including 30 patients. The incidence of exacerbated hypertension was statistically similar (27% versus 50%) between the two groups.

A 1998 Italian study evaluated the effect of routine treatment with the calcium channel blocker nifedipine in pregnant women with mild to moderate hypertension.[32] A total of 145 women were assigned to take 10 mg slow-release nifedipine twice daily and 138 were assigned to no treatment. Of the women, 47% had mild chronic hypertension. The rate of preeclampsia was similar in both groups. It was concluded that in pregnant women with mild hypertension routine treatment with nifedipine had no benefit on pregnancy outcome. The authors did not, however, specifically provide the outcomes in women with chronic hypertension.

The usefulness of ketanserin and low-dose aspirin versus placebo and low-dose aspirin in the prevention of superimposed preeclampsia in chronic hypertensive patients has been evaluated in a prospective randomized placebo-controlled trial including 138 patients.[34] The treatment was started before 20 weeks' gestation. The rate of superimposed preeclampsia was significantly lower in women allocated to ketanserin as compared with those in the placebo group (3% versus 19%, $P = .006$). The rate of abruptio placentae was lower in the ketanserin group as compared with the placebo group (1% versus 8%); however, this finding was not statistically significant.

Overall, the usefulness of antihypertensive treatment in the prevention of superimposed preeclampsia in women with mild chronic hypertension remains controversial inasmuch as the two largest studies found contradictory results.[9, 34] Figure 8–1 shows the results of these randomized studies. Concerning abruptio placentae, the two studies (>100 patients) revealed a beneficial

TABLE 8–2. RANDOMIZED TRIALS OF ANTIHYPERTENSIVE DRUG THERAPY IN PREGNANCIES COMPLICATED WITH MILD CHRONIC HYPERTENSION

AUTHORS	NO. OF WOMEN	MEAN GESTATION AT ENTRY (WKS)	MEAN DBP AT ENTRY (mmHg)	TREATMENT	MAIN FINDINGS
Sibai et al[9]	263	<11	92, 91, and 91	Methyldopa vs. labetalol vs. no drug	No differences in outcomes
Arias and Zamora[14]	58	15 and 16	90 to 99	Methyldopa, diuretics, hydralazine vs. no drug	Compromised infants born to mother in whom severe hypertension developed despite treatment
Redman et al[16]	208	21 and 22	88 and 90	Methyldopa ± hydralazine vs. no drug	Fewer midpregnancy losses in treated women
Weitz et al[19]	25	<34	90	Double blind: methyldopa vs. placebo	No differences in outcomes
Leather et al[29]	47	<20	107	Methyldopa ± diuretics ± hydralazine vs. no drug	Longer gestation and fewer perinatal deaths
Sibai et al[30]	20	9 to 13	93	Diuretics vs. no drug	Lower plasma volume in treated women
Butters et al[31]	29	16	86	Double blind: atenolol vs. placebo	Poor fetal growth in treated women
Steyn and Odendaal[34]	138	12 to 19	—	Double blind: ketanserin + aspirin vs. placebo + aspirin	Decreased rate of superimposed preeclampsia in ketanserin group
Hirsch et al[35]	30	<35	91 and 90	Pindolol vs. placebo	No differences in outcomes
Welt et al[33]	16	19 to 22		Methyldopa, hydralazine, or hydrochlorothiazide vs. placebo	Limited number of patients included; unwarranted results
Hogstedt et al[36]*	161	29 and 31	91 and 91	Metoprolol + hydralazine vs. no drug	No differences in outcomes
Plouin et al[37]†	176	25 and 26	94 and 96	Labetalol vs. methyldopa	No differences in outcomes
Gruppo di Studio[32]‡	283	24	96 and 95	Nifedipine slow-release vs. no drug	No differences in outcomes

*19%, †33%, and ‡47% of the study population are patients with chronic hypertension; their specific outcomes are not outlined. DBP, diastolic blood pressure.

effect of treatment; however, this finding was not statistically significant (Fig. 8–2).[9, 34]

Perinatal Outcome

The prospective randomized trial of Sibai and colleagues[9] compared perinatal outcomes among women receiving no medication (n = 90) versus methyldopa (n = 88) or labetalol (n = 86). The incidences of preterm delivery (10%, 12.5%, and 11.6%, respectively), SGA (8.9%, 6.8%, and 8.1%, respectively), and perinatal death (1.1%, 1.1%, and 1.2%, respectively) were similar among the three groups.

Butters and associates[31] reported on a randomized trial comparing atenolol (n = 15) with a placebo (n = 14) in women with mild chronic hypertension enrolled at an average of 15.9 weeks' gestation. They found a significantly lower birth weight (2620 g versus 3530 g), a higher rate of SGA (67% versus 0%), and a lower mean placental

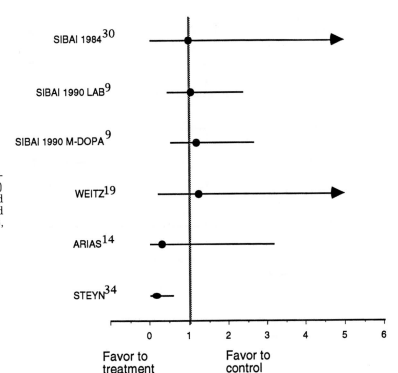

FIGURE 8–1. Summary odds ratios (95% confidence interval) comparing rates of superimposed preeclampsia between treated and control women in the trials. LAB, labetalol; M-DOPA, methyldopa.

weight in women treated by atenolol. In the late 1990s, two studies from the same team specifically found that atenolol was associated with low birth weight[38] and SGA.[39]

Lydakis and coworkers[39] found in a retrospective study that the rate of SGA infants was higher in patients treated with atenolol as compared with those without treatment (49% versus 21%, $P < .001$). The adverse effects of atenolol in these pregnancies may be due to the effects of atenolol on uteroplacental and fetal hemodynamics in such pregnancies.[40] Except for atenolol, the other antihypertensive treatments studied in the

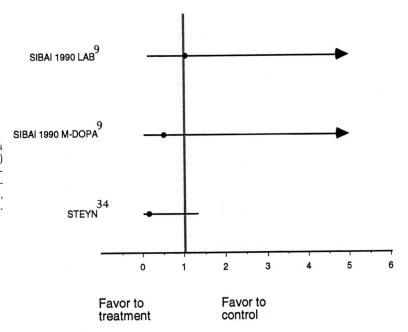

FIGURE 8–2. Summary odds ratios (95% confidence interval) comparing rates of abruptio placentae between treated and control women in the trials. LAB, labetalol; M-DOPA, methyldopa.

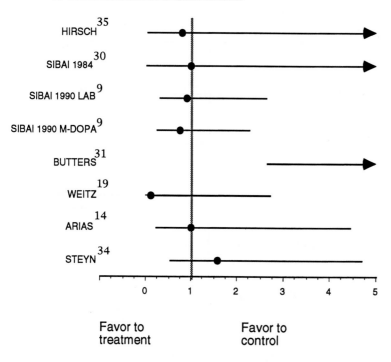

FIGURE 8–3. Summary odds ratios (95% confidence interval) comparing rates of small-for-gestational-age (SGA) infants between treated and control women in the trials. LAB, labetalol; M-DOPA, methyldopa.

prospective trials were not associated with any effect with respect to the rate of SGA infants (Fig. 8–3).

In sum, overall analysis of these trials showed that, regardless of the treatment used, perinatal mortality was not influenced by the use of antihypertensive medications (Fig. 8–4).[41]

Management

In general, most women with low-risk chronic hypertension without superimposed preeclampsia have a pregnancy outcome similar to that of the general population.[22] Our policy is to discontinue antihypertensive treatment at the first prenatal

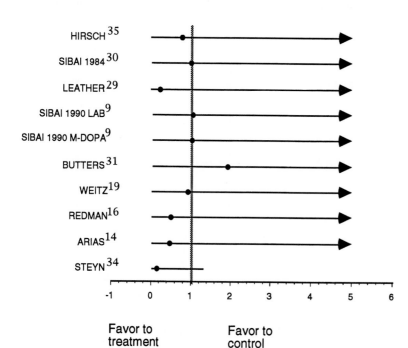

FIGURE 8–4. Summary odds ratios (95% confidence interval) comparing rates of perinatal mortality between treated and control women in the trials. LAB, labetalol; M-DOPA, methyldopa.

visit. Although these women do not require antihypertensive treatment, careful management is still essential because they may evolve into high-risk patients at any time during pregnancy.

Patients should be encouraged to avoid smoking. Frequency of outpatient assessment must be adjusted on the basis of clinical findings but it should be at least one visit per month. Maternal laboratory tests should include 24-hour urine collection for protein and creatinine clearance in the first trimester. Later during the pregnancy, further laboratory testing can be performed depending on clinical findings.

Fetal evaluation should include an ultrasound examination for estimation of fetal weight and amniotic fluid volume every 4 weeks during the third trimester, and weekly fetal heart rate testing, which can be started at 34 weeks' gestation.

Time of delivery must be individualized; however, low-risk patients may continue their pregnancy until the cervix becomes ripened or at 41 weeks' gestation. The development of severe hypertension, preeclampsia, or abnormal fetal growth dictates more frequent testing, or hospitalization or delivery, depending on the severity of complications and gestational age.

HIGH-RISK CHRONIC HYPERTENSION

Women with chronic hypertension should be considered at high risk when they have severe hypertension or mild hypertension associated with clinical or biologic signs of organ involvement or damage (Table 8–3). This group of patients is at high risk for pregnancy complications, including superimposed preeclampsia, abruptio placentae, SGA infants, and prematurity.[13, 22–24] Women with high-risk chronic hypertension must be evaluated before pregnancy, particularly when a target organ is involved. Women with renal insufficiency, diabetes (all classes), collagen vascular disease, and cardiomyopathy or coarctation of the aorta must have extensive counseling regarding maternal and fetal risks before starting a pregnancy.[12]

Interaction between target organs and pregnancy outcome is not reviewed here.

TABLE 8–3. CRITERIA FOR HIGH-RISK CHRONIC GESTATION HYPERTENSION

Severe hypertension (SBP $\geq$ 160 mmHg and/or DBP $\geq$ 110 mmHg) < 20 weeks' alone
Mild hypertension < 20 weeks' gestation associated with:
    Previous perinatal loss
    Previous preeclampsia
    Maternal age > 40 years
    Duration of hypertension $\geq$ 4 years
    Renal disease (all causes)
    Diabetes (class B to F)
    Cardiomyopathy
    Collagen vascular disease
    Presence of lupus anticoagulant
    Coarctation of the aorta
    Retinopathy

DBP, diastolic blood pressure; SBP, systolic blood pressure.

Management

It is generally agreed that pregnant women with severe hypertension must have pharmacologic treatment,[1, 42] although this principle has not been tested by large controlled trials.

At the first prenatal visit, the patient should be advised to avoid smoking and caffeine abuse. The patient should be given instructions on weight gain and nutritional requirements. During the first and second trimester, the patient should be seen every 2 to 3 weeks and preferably weekly in the third trimester. Frequency of outpatient assessment must be adjusted on the basis of clinical findings. Maternal laboratory tests should include 24-hour urine collection for protein and creatinine clearance in the first trimester. Later during the pregnancy, further laboratory testing can be performed, depending on clinical findings.

Fetal evaluation should include ultrasound examination for the estimation of fetal weight and amniotic fluid volume during the third trimester, every 4 weeks or more often, depending on clinical and ultrasound findings. Weekly fetal heart rate testing, or fetal biophysical profile when the non-stress test is nonreactive, may also be started at the beginning of the third trimester, depending on maternal or fetal complications (superimposed preeclampsia, fetal growth retardation).

All complications and uncontrolled severe hypertension must lead to hospitalization. Time of delivery must be individualized, but pregnancy should not be continued beyond 40 weeks' gestation.

For complications of high-risk chronic hypertension, it is advisable that these women be managed at a maternal-fetal referral center. If necessary, as a function of gestational age, delivery should take place at a tertiary care center.

PHARMACOLOGIC TREATMENT

The decision to initiate pharmacologic treatment in chronic hypertensive women must take into account both the severity of hypertension and the existence or the risk of target organ damage. In women with low-risk hypertension, we recommend antihypertensive therapy if systolic blood pressure is 160 mmHg or greater or if diastolic blood pressure is 105 mmHg or greater. For women with high-risk hypertension, we recommend treatment at diastolic blood pressure of 90 mmHg or greater.

Methyldopa

The published facts related to first-trimester use of methyldopa show no increase in congenital malformations.[43] Prospective trials that studied the effect of methyldopa in women with mild to moderate chronic hypertension revealed no adverse maternal or fetal outcome.[8, 14, 16, 19, 29, 33, 37] Moreover, methyldopa has the best safety record, which includes short-term[44] and long-term follow-up of children exposed in utero.[45, 46] It remains the agent of choice for oral nonemergent therapy.

Clonidine

Clonidine has not been evaluated by control trials in women with chronic hypertension. Only one case of a newborn with multiple birth defects exposed throughout gestation to clonidine has been reported in the literature.[47] Three birth defects (5.1%) have also been reported in 59 patients using clonidine in the first trimester. This malformation rate, however, was not significantly different from the one expected in the general population.[43]

Two prospective randomized trials have evaluated the effectiveness of clonidine in women with various hypertensive disorders during the third trimester.[48, 49] The use of clonidine was not associated with adverse fetal or neonatal outcomes.

β-Blocking Agents

β-Blocking agents have been extensively tested, mainly to treat hypertension in the third trimester, and are effective in the control of blood pressure.

First-trimester use of atenolol has been associated with an increase in birth defects (11.4%) in a series of 105 pregnant women registered in the Michigan Medicaid Surveillance Program.[43] Detailed study of these defects showed a possible relationship between the use of atenolol and hypospadias. The authors, however, assert caution in interpreting this relationship because several other drugs were used concomitantly. No evidence of teratogenicity was reported in three other studies with a limited number of patients treated (<10 patients) during the first trimester with atenolol.[50–52] No studies are available that address the use of acebutolol, oxprenolol, or pindolol during the first trimester.[43]

The use of atenolol begun during early pregnancy and continued for a long duration was associated with a lower birth weight[38] and fetal growth retardation.[31, 39] By 12 months of age, however, no difference in weight or any side effect was noted between the two groups.[53] Given late in pregnancy for the treatment of mild to moderate hypertension, atenolol,[40, 54, 55] metoprolol,[56] oxprenolol,[57–59] and pindolol[35, 40] were not associated with increased risk of adverse fetal outcome.

α-β Blocker: Labetalol

Of the 29 fetuses exposed in utero during the first trimester to labetalol and registered in the Michigan Medicaid Surveillance Program,[43] fetuses (13.8%) had nonspecified malformations but these were not in the categories of cardiovascular defects, oral clefts, spina bifida, polydactyly, limb reduction defects, or hypospadias. Moreover, the authors cautioned that the number of patients was small.

In a randomized controlled trial, 86 patients with mild chronic hypertension were enrolled between 6 and 13 weeks' gestation to be treated with labetalol.[9] None of the newborns had major congenital anomalies.

Rates for SGA infants related to the use of labetalol and reported in the literature are contradictory. Labetalol, when evaluated in women with mild pregnancy-induced hypertension in the second and third trimester, was found to be associated with an increased risk of SGA in some studies,[60–62] or with no increased rates in other studies.[9, 37] In a large and unique trial in which labetalol was started between 6 and 13 weeks' gestation in patients with chronic hypertension, labetalol was not associated with an increased rate of SGA infants.[9]

Calcium Channel Blockers

Calcium channel blockers, mainly nifedipine, have been tested as antihypertensive drugs (mainly in the second and third trimester) and tocolytic agents.

Knowledge regarding the risk of teratogenicity in humans is based on information regarding 211 pregnancy exposures during the first trimester.[43, 63–66] The Michigan Medicaid Surveillance Program[43] included 140 patients with first-trimester exposure to nifedipine (n = 37), diltiazem (n = 27), and verapamil (n = 76), which resulted in major birth defects in 5%, 14.8%, and 1.3% of the pregnancies, respectively. In a prospective multicenter cohort study in which 78 women were exposed to calcium channel blockers during the first trimester (mainly nifedipine and verapamil), Magee and associates[63] did not find any increase in rates of major birth defects.

The usefulness of nifedipine in pregnancy outcome was evaluated in a prospective randomized trial in which 47% of the participants had chronic hypertension. Women were enrolled between 12 and 34 weeks' gestation (mean, 24 weeks' gestation).[32] This study found no improvement in maternal or neonatal outcome. In the controlled trials involving women with pregnancy-induced hypertension, nifedipine,[32, 67] nicardipine,[68] nitrendipine,[69] and isradipine[70, 71] were not associated with adverse fetal outcomes. Cases of adverse maternal and fetal outcomes have been reported during the use of sublingual nifedipine such as myocardial infarction, or severe hypotension leading to fetal distress.[43, 72, 73]

Diuretics

Thiazide

From the diuretics of the thiazide group or those structurally related to this group, chlorothiazide, hydrochlorothiazide, and chlorthalidone are those for which data are available. These diuretics are rarely used during the first trimester. In the Collaborative Perinatal Project, where more than 50,000 mother-child pairs were monitored, 233 were exposed during the first trimester to thiazide or related diuretics.[74] Birth defects were increased in women exposed to chlorthalidone, but not with hydrochlorothiazide. These findings were not confirmed by the Michigan Medicaid Surveillance Program,[43] in which 635 first-trimester exposure to diuretics (20 chlorothiazide, 48 chlorthalidone, and 567 hydrochlorothiazide) was reported. Rates for major birth defects observed were 10%, 4.2%, and 4.2%, respectively; these rates, however, were not statistically higher than the expected rates. Although the number of exposures for two of the diuretics studied was small, these data do not support an increased risk of major congenital defects in women exposed to diuretics from this group during the first trimester.[43]

Later in the pregnancy, only one randomized trial evaluated the usefulness of diuretics on plasma volume expansion and perinatal outcome in women with chronic hypertension.[30] Unfortunately, the specific diuretics used are not provided and the number of patients included is small (20 patients in all). Nonetheless, diuretics induced a decrease of plasma volume expansion without influencing perinatal outcome.

Neonatal thrombocytopenia has been reported following the use of diuretics of this group,[75–78] and two of the babies died.[75, 76] In contrast, other studies did not find an increased risk of thrombocytopenia related to diuretics.[79, 80]

Furosemide

The Michigan Medicaid Surveillance Program[43] reported 350 cases of first-trimester exposure to furosemide. Major birth defects were observed in 5.1%. The detailed analysis of these anomalies revealed that only hypospadias might be associated with this drug. The authors caution, however, that other factors might be involved, such as the use of other medications. Later in pregnancy, use of furosemide seems safe.[43]

Regarding the potential side effects, diuretics should be used as a second-line or third-line treatment in combination with other drugs, particularly in women having a salt-sensitive hypertension.[1, 81]

Angiotensin-Converting Enzyme Inhibitors

The data regarding the use of ACE inhibitors are limited to captopril, enalapril, and lisinopril. The teratogenicity risk appears to be dependent on timing and dose. The Michigan Medicaid Surveillance Program[43] reported 141 newborns exposed in utero during the first trimester to ACE inhibitors. Birth defects were observed in 7%. A review of 85 case reports occuring before 1989 revealed the presence of anuria in 15%, and oligohydramnios in 14% of pregnancies exposed to ACE inhibitors after 16 weeks' gestation.[82] Exposure to ACE inhibitor during the second and third trimester appears to be responsible for altered kidney development.[83–86] The mechanism of the observed fetopathy may be related to persistent inhibition of the renin-angiotensin system, leading to tubular dysfunction.

ACE inhibitor agents have been associated with neonatal renal failure leading to death, renal dysgenesis, pulmonary hypoplasia, and fetal growth restriction.[43, 82, 87, 88] In other studies, the use of ACE inhibitors during the first trimester (before the start of tubular function) did not result in an increased teratogenic effect.[89–91] Clearly, ACE inhibitor agents are contraindicated in the second and third trimesters.

Vasodilating Agents: Hydralazine

Hydralazine is widely used to control blood pressure in women with severe preeclampsia. In contrast, first-trimester use of hydralazine is limited. The Michigan Medicaid Surveillance Program[43] reported 40 newborns exposed during the first trimester to hydralazine. Only one birth defect (2.5%) was observed.

Later in the pregnancy, no adverse maternal or fetal outcomes were observed in two controlled trials studying the usefulness of hydralazine in women with chronic hypertension[14, 33] or in the treatment of women with gestational hypertension.[36]

Low-Dose Aspirin for Prevention of Superimposed Preeclampsia
(see Chapter 5)

Initial reports studying the prophylactic use of low-dose aspirin ranging from 50 to 150 mg daily included a limited number of patients.[92, 93] Beaufils and colleagues[92] enrolled 102 patients in a prospective randomized trial. About one third had chronic hypertension. Fifty-two patients were treated with aspirin 150 mg/day and dipyridamole 300 mg/day, from 12 weeks' gestation until the delivery. The 50 control patients received no treatment. Preeclampsia occurred in six patients, all in the control group. Abruptio placentae complicated five pregnancies and led to three stillbirths, all in the control group. Major complications (fetal death or fetal growth retardation) occurred in nine patients in the control group, whereas no major complications were found in the treated group. However, the authors did not provide specific complications (if any) in the women with chronic hypertension.

Later, in 1993, Viinikka and associates[93] conducted a prospective, randomized, placebo-controlled trial to compare the effects on hypertensive diseases of 50 mg aspirin daily (n = 97) with a placebo (n = 100). Of the women, 89% had chronic hypertension. The use of 50 mg of aspirin did not reduce the rate of either severe hypertension only (12 versus 14) or preeclampsia (nine versus 11).

In 1998, Caritis and coworkers[94] studied the effect of low-dose aspirin (60 mg/day) for the prevention of preeclampsia. They conducted a prospective, randomized, double-blind, placebo-controlled trial that included 2539 pregnant women at high risk for preeclampsia. Of these patients, 774 had chronic hypertension. The women were enrolled between the 13th and the 26th gestational week and received either 60 mg of aspirin or placebo daily. The overall incidence of preeclampsia was similar in the 1254 women in the aspirin group and the 1249 women in the placebo group (18% versus 20%; $P = .23$). In addition, low-dose aspirin did not decrease the incidence of superimposed preeclampsia in women with chronic hypertension (26% in aspirin group versus 25% in placebo group; $P = 0.66$). The authors concluded that low-dose aspirin should not be given to prevent preeclampsia in women with chronic hypertension.

POSTPARTUM MANAGEMENT

Women with high-risk chronic hypertension are at risk for postpartum complications such as pulmonary edema, hypertensive encephalopathy, and renal failure.[12] These risks are particularly increased in women with a target organ involvement (Table 8–3), superimposed preeclampsia, or abruptio placentae. In these patients, blood pressure must be closely controlled for at least 48 hours after delivery. Intravenous labetalol or hydralazine can be used as needed[95] in addition to diuretics in women with circulatory congestion and pulmonary edema.[96]

Oral therapy may be needed to control blood pressure after delivery. Some patients may wish to breast-feed their infants. All antihypertensive drugs are found in the breast milk, although differences are found in the milk-plasma ratio of these drugs.[97] Additionally, the long-term effect of maternal antihypertensive drugs on breast-feeding infants has not been specifically studied. Milk concentrations of methyldopa appear to be low and are considered to be safe.[98] The β-blocking agents (atenolol and metoprolol) are concentrated in breast milk, whereas labetalol or propanolol have low concentrations.[99] Concentrations of diuretic agents in breast milk are low; however, they may induce a decrease in milk production.[97]

There is little information about the transfer of calcium channel blockers to breast milk, but there are no apparent side effects.[100] ACE inhibitors and angiotensin II receptor antagonists should be avoided because of their effects on neonatal renal function, even though their concentration appears to be low in breast milk.

Finally, in breast-feeding women, the use of methyldopa as a first-line oral therapy is a reasonable choice. If methyldopa is contraindicated, labetalol may be used.

CONCLUSION

Pregnant women with chronic hypertension are at risk for maternal and perinatal morbidity. Careful assessment and management of these patients during pregnancy are crucial for reducing maternal and fetal complications. Antihypertensive treatment is appropriate for women with high-risk chronic hypertension, but drug therapy does not improve pregnancy outcome in women at low risk. Prophylactic low-dose aspirin treatment started early in chronic hypertensive patients is not effective in reducing the frequency of superimposed preeclampsia.

References

1. National High Blood Pressure Education Program Working Group. National High Blood Pressure Education Program Working Group Report on High Blood Pressure in Pregnancy. Am J Obstet Gynecol 1990;163:1691–1712.
2. Samadi AR, Mayberry RM, Zaidi AA, et al. Maternal hypertension and associated pregnancy complications among African-American and other women in the United States. Obstet Gynecol 1996;87:557–563.
3. Burt VL, Whelton P, Roccella EJ, et al. Prevalence of hypertension in the U.S. adult population. Results from the Third National Health and Nutrition Examination Survey, 1988–1991. Hypertension 1995;24:305–313.
4. Ventura SJ, Martin JA, Taftel SM, et al. Advance report of final natality statistics, 1993. Monthly Vital Statistics Report 1995;44(Suppl 3):1–88.
5. Barton JR, Bergauer NK, Jacques DI, et al. Does advanced maternal age affect pregnancy outcome in women with mild hypertension remote from term? Am J Obstet Gynecol 1997;176:1236–1249, discussion, 1240–1243.
6. Sibai BM, Akl S, Fairlie F, Moretti M. A protocol for managing severe preeclampsia in the second trimester. Am J Obstet Gynecol 1990;163:733–738.
7. Sibai BM, Abdella TN, Anderson GD. Pregnancy outcome in 211 patients with mild chronic hypertension. Obstet Gynecol 1983;61:571–576.
8. Benedetto C, Zonca M, Marozio L, et al. Blood pressure patterns in normal pregnancy and in pregnancy-induced hypertension, preeclampsia, and chronic hypertension. Obstet Gynecol 1996;88:503–510.
9. Sibai BM, Mabie WC, Shamsa F, et al. A comparison of no medication versus methyldopa or labetalol in chronic hypertension during pregnancy. Am J Obstet Gynecol 1990;162:960–966.
10. Witlin AG, Sibai BM. Hypertensive diseases in pregnancy. In Reece EA, Hobbins JC (eds) Medicine of the Fetus and the Mother, 2nd ed. Philadelphia: Lippincott–Williams & Wikins, 1999, pp 997–1020.
11. Sibai BM. Chronic hypertension in pregnancy. Clin Perinatol 1991;18:833–844.
12. Sibai BM. Diagnosis and management of chronic hypertension in pregnancy. Obstet Gynecol 1991;78:451–461.
13. Sibai BM, Anderson GD. Pregnancy outcome of intensive therapy in severe hypertension in first trimester. Obstet Gynecol 1986;67:517–522.
14. Arias F, Zamora J. Antihypertensive treatment and pregnancy outcome in patients with mild chronic hypertension. Obstet Gynecol 1979;53:489–494.
15. Mabie WC, Pernoll ML, Biswas MK. Chronic

hypertension in pregnancy. Obstet Gynecol 1986;67:197–205.

16. Redman CWG, Beilin LJ, Bonnar J, Ounsted MK. Fetal outcome in trial of antihypertensive treatment in pregnancy. Lancet 1976;2:753–756.

17. Chesley LC, Annito JE. Pregnancy in the patient with hypertensive disease. Am J Obstet Gynecol 1947;53:372–381.

18. Landesman R, Holz W, Scherr L. Fetal mortality in essential hypertension. Obstet Gynecol 1955;6:354–365.

19. Weitz C, Khouzami V, Maxwell K, Johnson JWC. Treatment of hypertension in pregnancy with methyldopa, randomized double-blind study. Int J Gynaecol Obstet 1987;25:35–40.

20. CLASP (Collaborative Low-dose Aspirin Study in Pregnancy) Collaborative Group. CLASP: A randomized trial of low-dose aspirin for the prevention and treatment of pre-eclampsia among 9364 pregnant women. Lancet 1994;343:619–629.

21. Caritis S, Sibai B, Hauth J, et al. Predictors of pre-eclampsia in women at high risk. Am J Obstet Gynecol 1998;179:946–951.

22. McCowan LM, Buist RG, North RA, Gamble G. Perinatal morbidity in chronic hypertension. Br J Obstet Gynaecol 1996;103:123–129.

23. Sibai BM, Lindheimer M, Hauth J, et al. Risk factors for preeclampsia, abruptio placentae, and adverse neonatal outcomes among women with chronic hypertension. N Engl J Med 1998;339:667–671.

24. Rey E, Couturier A. The prognosis of pregnancy in women with chronic hypertension. Am J Obstet Gynecol 1994;171:410–416.

25. Ananth CV, Savitz DA, Bowes WA Jr. Hypertensive disorders of pregnancy and stillbirth in North Carolina, 1988 to 1991. Acta Obstet Gynecol Scand 1995;74:788–793.

26. Jain L. Effect of pregnancy-induced and chronic hypertension on pregnancy outcome. J Perinatol 1997;17:425–427.

27. Haelterman E, Breart G, Paris-Llado J, et al. Effect of uncomplicated chronic hypertension on the risk of small-for-gestational age birth. Am J Epidemiol 1997;145:689–695.

28. Meis PJ, Goldenberg RL, Mercer BM, et al. The preterm prediction study: Risk factors for indicated preterm births. Am J Obstet Gynecol 1998;178:562–567.

29. Leather HM, Humphreys DM, Baker P, Chadd MA. A controlled trial of hypotensive agents in hypertension in pregnancy. Lancet 1968;2:488–490.

30. Sibai BM, Grossman RA, Grossman HG. Effects of diuretics on plasma volume in pregnancies with long-term hypertension. Am J Obstet Gynecol 1984;150:831–835.

31. Butters L, Kennedy S, Rubin PC. Atenolol in essential hypertension during pregnancy. BMJ 1990;301:587–589.

32. Gruppo di Studio Ipertensione in Gravidanza. Nifedipine versus expectant management in mild to moderate hypertension in pregnancy. Br J Obstet Gynaecol 1998;105:718–722.

33. Welt SI, Dorminy JH III, Jelovsek FR, et al. The effects of prophylactic management and therapeutics on hypertensive disease in pregnancy: Preliminary studies. Obstet Gynecol 1981;57:557–565.

34. Steyn DW, Odendaal HJ. Randomised controlled trial of ketanserin and aspirin in prevention of pre-eclampsia. Lancet 1997;350:1267–1271.

35. Hirsch M, Bar J, Bott-Kanner G, et al. Effect of the beta-adrenergic blocker pindolol on platelet function in chronic hypertensive pregnancy. Hypertens Preg 1996;15:193–202.

36. Hogstedt S, Lindeberg S, Axelsson O, et al. A prospective controlled trial of metoprolol-hydralazine treatment in hypertension during pregnancy. Acta Obstet Gynecol Scand 1985;64:505–510.

37. Plouin PF, Breart G, Maillard F, et al. Comparison of antihypertensive efficacy and perinatal safety of labetalol and methyldopa in the treatment of hypertension in pregnancy: A randomized controlled trial. Br J Obstet Gynaecol 1988;95:868–876.

38. Lip GYH, Beevers M, Churchill D, et al. Effect of atenolol on birth weight. Am J Cardiol 1997;79:1436–1438.

39. Lydakis C, Lip GYH, Beevers M, Beevers G. Atenolol and fetal growth in pregnancies complicated by hypertension. Am J Hypertens 1999;12:541–547.

40. Montan S, Ingemarsson I, Marsal K, Sjoberg NO. Randomised controlled trial of atenolol and pindolol in human pregnancy: Effects on fetal haemodynamics. BMJ 1992;304:946–949.

41. Sibai BM. Treatment of hypertension in pregnant women. N Engl J Med 1996;335:257–265.

42. Redman CWG. Controlled trials of antihypertensive drugs in pregnancy. Am J Kidney Dis 1991;17:149–153.

43. Briggs GG, Freeman RK, Yaffee SJ. Drugs in Pregnancy and Lactation: A Reference Guide to Fetal and Neonatal Risk, 5th ed. Baltimore: Williams & Wilkins, 1998.

44. Montan S, Anandakumar C, Arulkumaran S, et al. Effects of methyldopa on uteroplacental and fetal hemodynamics in pregnancy-induced hypertension. Am J Obstet Gynecol 1993;168:152–156.

45. Mutch LM, Moar VA, Ounsted MK, Redman CW. Hypertension during pregnancy, with-and-without specific hypotensive treatment: II. The growth and development of the infant in the first year of life. Early Hum Dev 1977;191:59–67.

46. Cockburn J, Moar VA, Ounsted M, Redman CW. Final report of study on hypertension during pregnancy: The effects of specific treatment on the growth and development of the children. Lancet 1982;1:647–649.

47. Stoll C, Levy JM, Beshara D. Roberts' syndrome and clonidine. J Med Genet 1979;16:486–487.

48. Phippard AF, Fischer WE, Horvath JS, et al. Early blood pressure control improves pregnancy outcome in primigravid women with mild hypertension. Med J Aust 1991;154:378–382.

49. Horvath JS, Phippard A, Korda A, et al. Clonidine hydrochloride: A safe and effective antihypertensive agent in pregnancy. Obstet Gynecol 1985;66:634–638.

50. Rubin PC, Butters L, Low RA, Clark DC. Atenolol in the management of hypertension during pregnancy. Drugs 1983;25(Suppl 2):212–214.

51. Rubin PC, Butters L, Low RA, Reid JL. Atenolol in the treatment of essential hypertension during pregnancy. Br J Clin Pharmacol 1982;14:279–281.

52. Dubois D, Petitcolas J, Temperville B, Klepper A. Treatment of hypertension in pregnant women with beta-blockers: 60 cases [French, authors' translation]. Nouv Press Med 1980;9:2807–2810.

53. Reynolds B, Butters L, Evans J, et al. First year of life after the use of atenolol in pregnancy associated hypertension. Arch Dis Child 1984;59:1061–1063.

54. Rubin PC, Butters L, Clark D, et al. Obstetric aspects of the use in pregnancy-associated hypertension of the beta-adrenoreceptor antagonist atenolol. Am J Obstet Gynecol 1984;150:389–392.

55. Rubin PC, Butters L, Clark DM, et al. Placebo-controlled trial of atenolol in treatment of pregnancy-associated hypertension. Lancet 1983;1:431–434.

56. Williams ER, Morrissey JR. A comparison of acebutolol with methyldopa in hypertensive pregnancy. Pharmatherapeutica 1983;3:487–491.

57. Gallery ED, Saunders DM, Hunyor SN, Gyory AZ. Randomised comparison of methyldopa and oxprenolol for treatment of hypertension in pregnancy. Br Med J 1979;1:1591–1594.

58. Gallery ED, Ross MR, Gyory AZ. Antihypertensive treatment in pregnancy: Analysis of different responses to oxprenolol and methyldopa. Br Med J 1985;291:563–566.

59. Fidler J, Smith V, Fayers P, De Swiet M. Randomised controlled comparative study of methyldopa and oxprenolol in the treatment of hypertension in pregnancy. Br Med J 1983;286:1927–1930.

60. Cruikshank DJ, Robertson AA, Campbell DM, MacGillivray I. Does labetalol influence the development of proteinuria in pregnancy hypertension? A randomised controlled study. Eur J Obstet Gynecol Reprod Biol 1992;45:47–51.

61. Sibai BM, Gonzalez AR, Mabie WC, Moretti M. A comparison of labetalol plus hospitalization versus hospitalization alone in the management of preeclampsia remote from term. Obstet Gynecol 1987;70:323–327.

62. Pickles CJ, Symonds EM, Pipkin FB. The fetal outcome in a randomized double-blind controlled trial of labetalol versus placebo in pregnancy-induced hypertension. Br J Obstet Gynaecol 1989;96:38–43.

63. Magee LA, Schick B, Donnenfeld AE, et al. The safety of calcium channel blockers in human pregnancy: A prospective, multicenter cohort study. Am J Obstet Gynecol 1996;174:823–828.

64. Goodnick PJ. Verapamil prophylaxis in pregnant women with bipolar disorder [letter]. Am J Psychiatry 1993;150:1560.

65. Shen O, Entebi E, Yagel S. Congenital hypertrophic cardiomyopathy associated with in utero verapamil exposure [letter]. Prenat Diagn 1995;15:1088–1089.

66. Lubbe WF. Use of diltiazem during pregnancy [letter]. N Z J Med 1987;100:121.

67. Sibai BM, Barton JR, Akl S, et al. A randomized prospective comparison of nifedipine and bed rest versus bed rest alone in the management of preeclampsia remote from term. Am J Obstet Gynecol 1992;167:879–884.

68. Jannet D, Carbonne B, Sebban E, Milliez J. Nicardipine versus metoprolol in the treatment of hypertension during pregnancy: A randomized comparative trial. Obstet Gynecol 1994;84:354–359.

69. Lawrence MR, Broughton Pipkin F. Some observations on the effects of a calcium channel blocker, nitrendipine, in early human pregnancy. Br J Clin Pharmacol 1987;23:683–692.

70. Wide-Swensson DH, Ingemarsson I, Lunell NO, et al. Calcium channel blockade (isradipine) in the treatment of hypertension in pregnancy: A randomized placebo-controlled study. Am J Obstet Gynecol 1995;173:872–878.

71. Montan S, Anandakumnar C, Arulkumaran S, et al. Randomised controlled trial of methyldopa and isradipine in preeclampsia: Effects on uteroplacental and fetal hemodynamics. J Perinat Med 1996;24:177–184.

72. Impey L. Severe hypotension and fetal distress following sublingual administration of nifedipine to a patient with severe pregnancy-induced hypertension at 33 weeks. Br J Obstet Gynaecol 1993;100:959–961.

73. Oei SG, Oei SK, Brolmann HA. Myocardial infarction during nifedipine therapy for preterm labor [letter]. N Engl J Med 1999;340:154.

74. Heinonen OP, Slone D, Shapiro S. Birth Defects and Drugs in Pregnancy. Littleton, MA: Publishing Sciences Group, 1977, pp 371–373.

75. Rodriguez SU, Leikin SL, Hiller MC. Neonatal thrombocytopenia associated with antepartum administration of thiazide drugs. N Engl J Med 1964;270:881–884.

76. Menzies DN. Controlled trial of chlorothiazide in treatment of early pre-eclampsia. Br Med J 1964;1:739–742.

77. Leikin SL. Thiazide and neonatal thrombocytopenia [letter]. N Engl J Med 1964;271:161.

78. Prescott LF. Neonatal thrombocytopenia and thiazide drugs [letter]. Br Med J 1964;1:1438.

79. Finnerty FA Jr. Thiazide and neonatal thrombocytopenia [letter]. N Engl J Med 1964;271.

80. Jerkner K, Kutti J, Victorin L. Platelet counts in mothers and their newborn infants with respect to ante-partum administration of oral diuretics. Acta Med Scand 1973;194:473–475.

81. August P, Lindheimer MD. Chronic hypertension and pregnancy. In Lindheimer MD, Roberts JM, Cunningham FG (eds). Chesley's Hypertensive Disorders in Pregnancy, 2nd ed. Stamford, CT: Appleton & Lange, 1998, pp 605–633.

82. Hanssens M, Keirse MJ, Vankelecom F, Van Assche FA. Fetal and neonatal effects of treatment with angiotensin-converting enzyme inhibitors in pregnancy. Obstet Gynecol 1991;78:128–135.

83. Piper JM, Ray WA, Rosa FW. Pregnancy outcome following exposure to angiotensin-converting enzyme inhibitors. Obstet Gynecol 1992;80:429–432.

84. Cunniff C, Jones KL, Phillipson J, et al. Oligohydramnios sequence and renal tubular malformation associated with maternal enalapril use. Am J Obstet Gynecol 1990;162:187–189.

85. Lavoratti G, Seracini D, Fiorini P, et al. Neonatal anuria by ACE inhibitors during pregnancy [letter]. Nephron 1997;76:235–236.

86. Thorpe-Beeston JG, Armar NA, Dancy M, et al. Pregnancy and ACE inhibitors. Br J Obstet Gynaecol 1993;100:692–693.

87. Pryde PG, Sedman AB, Nugent CE, Barr M Jr. Angiotensin-converting enzyme inhibitor fetopathy. J Am Soc Nephrol 1993;3:1575–1582.

88. Buttar HS. An overview of the influence of ACE inhibitors on fetal-placental circulation and perinatal development. Mol Cell Biochem 1997;176:61–71.

89. Bar J, Hod M, Merlob P. Angiotensin-converting enzyme inhibitors use in the first trimester of pregnancy. Int J Risk Saf Med 1997;10:23–26.

90. Centers for Disease Control and Prevention. Postmarketing surveillance for angiotensin-converting enzyme inhibitor use during the first trimester of pregnancy—United States, Canada, and Israel, 1987–1995. JAMA 1997;277:1193–1194.

91. Postmarketing surveillance for angiotensin-converting enzyme inhibitor use during the first trimester of pregnancy—United States, Canada, and Israel, 1987–1995. MMWR Morb Mortal Wkly Rep 1997;46:240–242.

92. Beaufils M, Uzan S, Donsimoni R, Colau JC. Prevention of pre-eclampsia by early antiplatelet therapy. Lancet 1985;1:840–842.

93. Viinikka L, Hartikainen-Sorri AL, Lumme R, et al. Low-dose aspirin in hypertensive pregnant women: Effect on pregnancy outcome and prostacyclin-thromboxane balance in mother and newborn. Br J Obstet Gynaecol 1993;100:809–815.

94. Caritis S, Sibai B, Hauth J, et al. Low-dose aspirin to prevent preeclampsia in women at high risk. N Engl J Med 1998;338:701–705.

95. Mabie WC, Gonzalez AR, Sibai BM, Amon E. A comparative trial of labetalol and hydralazine in the acute management of severe hypertension complicating pregnancy. Obstet Gynecol 1987;70:328–333.

96. Mabie WC, Ratts TE, Ramanathan KB, Sibai BM. Circulatory congestion in obese hypertensive women: A subset of pulmonary edema in pregnancy. Obstet Gynecol 1988;72:553–558.

97. White WB. Management of hypertension during lactation. Hypertension 1984;6:297–300.

98. Umans JG, Lindheimer MD. Antihypertensive treatment. *In* Lindheimer MD, Roberts JM, Cunningham FG (eds). Chesley's Hypertensive Disorders in Pregnancy, 2nd ed. Stamford, CT: Appleton & Lange; 1998, pp 581–604.

99. Atkinson H, Begg EJ. Concentrations of beta-blocking drugs in human milk. J Pediatr 1990;116:156.

100. Ehrenkranz RA, Ackerman BA, Hulse JD. Nifedipine transfer into human milk. J Pediatr 1989;114:478–480.

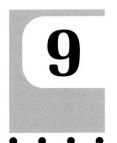

9

THE HYPERTENSIVE DIABETIC WOMAN

Lauren A. Plante and E. Albert Reece

Diabetes mellitus is among the most common of chronic diseases. Nearly 8 million Americans carried the diagnosis of diabetes mellitus as of 1993.[1] More than 90% of these have type 2, or non–insulin-dependent diabetes, and large population-based studies suggest that the ratio of diagnosed to undiagnosed type 2 cases is approximately 1:1, from which we may infer a total number of about 14 million diabetic Americans.[1]

Diabetes is more than simply a condition of hyperglycemia; it is a complex of metabolic abnormalities in which alterations in fuel handling have both immediate and distant repercussions. Co-morbidities associated with diabetes mellitus include renal failure, blindness, cardiac disease, cerebrovascular disease, and others. Diabetes is the cause of more than half of lower extremity amputations,[2] more than a third of all cases of end-stage renal disease,[3] and approximately 12% of new cases of blindness[4] in the United States each year. Mortality rates among diabetic patients are 2.5 times as high as for nondiabetic people.[5]

A heterogeneous group of disorders is subsumed under the single term *diabetes mellitus.* In 1979, the National Diabetes Data Group published the first widely used classification[6] in an attempt to standardize nomenclature and criteria for diagnosis. The three clinical classes described were those of diabetes mellitus (DM), impaired glucose tolerance (IGT), and gestational diabetes (GDM). Within the class of diabetes mellitus, four subtypes (Table 9–1) were identified:

- Type I, insulin-dependent diabetes mellitus (IDDM)
- Type II, non–insulin-dependent diabetes mellitus (NIDDM), including the so-called maturity-onset diabetes of the young, (MODY)
- Malnutrition-related diabetes mellitus

- Other types, including diabetes secondary to another medical condition (e.g., Cushing's disease, pheochromocytoma) or to the use of certain drugs

The diagnosis of either diabetes mellitus or impaired glucose tolerance was based on the results of an oral glucose tolerance test using a 75-g load ingested over 5 minutes, following a fast of at least 10 hours. Venous plasma glucose was measured in the fasting state and then at 30 minutes, 1 hour, 90 minutes, and 2 hours following the glucose load. The criteria for diagnosis appear in Table 9–2.

With some minor revisions, the World Health Organization accepted this classification in 1980[7] and 1985.[8] In 1997, however, the American Diabetes Association (ADA) convened an international Expert Committee to revise the diagnosis and classification of diabetes mellitus.[9] This revision bids to increase the number of diabetes diagnoses by several million in the United States alone.

The terminology of *IDDM* and *NIDDM* has been abandoned. The major classifications of type 1, type 2, GDM, and other types have been retained, whereas the category of malnutrition-related DM has been discarded. The stage of impaired glucose tolerance remains, referring to a metabolic stage intermediate between normal glucose homeostasis and frank diabetes. The new classification is shown in Table 9–3. The change from Roman to Arabic numerals is recommended. The most far-reaching change, however, is in the diagnosis of diabetes. The ADA now recommends that any one of the criteria given in Table 9–2 qualify the individual as diabetic.

The increased simplicity of measurement—only two samples are drawn for the oral glucose tolerance test, and only one

TABLE 9–1. CLASSIFICATION OF DIABETES MELLITUS

I. *Type 1 Diabetes (absolute insulin deficiency, β-cell destruction)*
  A. Immune-related
  B. Idiopathic

II. *Type 2 diabetes (insulin resistance)*

III. *Other specific types*
  A. Genetic defects of β-cell function
    1. Chromosome 12, HNF-1α (previously MODY3)
    2. Chromosome 7, glucokinase (previously MODY2)
    3. Chromosome 20, HNF-4α (formerly MODY1)
    4. Mitochondrial DNA
    5. Others
  B. Genetic defects in insulin action
    1. Type A insulin resistance
    2. Leprechaunism
    3. Rabson-Mendenhall syndrome
    4. Lipoatrophic diabetes
    5. Others
  C. Disease of the exocrine pancreas
    1. Pancreatitis
    2. Trauma, pancreatectomy
    3. Neoplasia
    4. Cystic fibrosis
    5. Hemochromatosis
    6. Fibrocalculous pancreatopathy
    7. Others
  D. Endocrinopathies
    1. Acromegaly
    2. Cushing's syndrome
    3. Glucagonoma
    4. Pheochromocytoma
    5. Hyperthyroidism
    6. Somatostatinoma
    7. Aldosteronoma
    8. Others
  E. Drug-induced or chemical-induced
    1. Vacor
    2. Pentamidine
    3. Nicotinic acid
    4. Glucocorticoids
    5. Thyroid hormone
    6. Diazoxide
    7. Beta-adrenergic agonists
    8. Thiazides
    9. Dilantin
    10. Alpha-interferon
    11. Others
  F. Infections
    1. Congenital rubella
    2. Cytomegalovirus
    3. Others
  G. Uncommon forms of immune-mediated diabetes
    1. Stiff-man syndrome
    2. Anti-insulin-receptor antibodies
    3. Others
  H. Other genetic syndromes associated with diabetes
    1. Down syndrome
    2. Klinefelter's syndrome
    3. Turner's syndrome
    4. Woffram syndrome
    5. Friedreich's ataxia
    6. Huntington's disease
    7. Laurence-Moon-Biedl syndrome
    8. Myotonic dystrophy
    9. Prader-Willi syndrome
    10. Porphyria
    11. Others

IV. *Gestational diabetes mellitus (GDM)*

MODY, maturity-onset diabetes of the young; DNA, deoxyribonucleic acid.
From American Diabetes Association. Report of the Expert Committee on the diagnosis and classification of diabetes mellitus. Diabetes Care 1997;20:1183–1197.

need be abnormal—as well as the lowered cut-off point of the fasting glucose ensures that diabetes will be diagnosed more frequently. The Expert Committee suggests a prevalence of 12.3% among adults aged 40 to 74 years using the new criteria, compared with a prevalence of 7.9% by history.[9] It is hoped that the reduction in the numbers of undiagnosed cases of diabetes will result in a decrease in vascular and other complications by providing earlier opportunities for intervention.

TYPE 1 DIABETES

Type 1 diabetes (formerly IDDM) is characterized by insulinopenia. It typically develops during childhood or adolescence, although up to 7% of cases of diabetes diagnosed after age 30 may in fact be type 1.[10] It is by far the most common chronic disease of childhood, with approximately 13,000 new cases diagnosed each year in the United States alone. Tremendous geographic, racial, and ethnic differences have been observed in type 1 DM; rates range from the Finnish (nearly 35/100,000 population/year) to the Chinese and Korean (<1/100,000 population/year).[10] Within the United States population, whites have the highest rates and blacks the lowest, with children of Hispanic background intermediate. There is no significant gender differential.

TABLE 9-2. CRITERIA FOR THE DIAGNOSIS OF DIABETES

1. Symptoms of diabetes (e.g., weight loss, polydipsia, polyuria) plus causal plasma glucose concentration ≥ 200 mg/dL (11.1 mmol/L), with "causal" defined as any time of day irrespective of timing of last meal

    or

2. Fasting plasma glucose level ≥ 126 mg/dL (7 mmol/L), where "fasting" implies a period of at least 8 h since last calorie intake

    or

3. A 2-hr plasma glucose level ≥ 200 during a 75-g oral glucose tolerance test; plasma glucose levels at 30, 60, and 90 min no longer need to be measured.

From American Diabetes Association. Report of the Expert Committee on the diagnosis and classification of diabetes mellitus. Diabetes Care 1997;20:1183–1197.

Presentation is usually acute in type 1 DM, and the diagnosis is apparent from the clinical picture, easily confirmed by measurement of urinary and serum glucose. The classic signs of polydipsia, polyuria, and polyphagia are associated with weight loss, fatigue, and irritability. Ketoacidosis is common; it may, in fact, be the initial presentation in up to 25% of type 1 diabetes.[11] Insulin is the only treatment for type 1 diabetes. These patients are dependent on insulin for life.

The exact etiologic mechanism of type 1 DM is unclear. There appears to be a genetic predisposition, but frank disease expression requires a specific trigger, such as a viral infection. Genetic susceptibility to type 1 DM is located in the human leukocyte antigen (HLA) region of chromosome 6; individuals with DR3 and DR4 haplotypes appear to be more prone to diabetes.[12] More sophisticated molecular mapping has demonstrated that variants in the DQB1 and DQA1 genes are highly associated with susceptibility to type 1 diabetes.[12] The genetic background is not sufficient for development of the disease, as demonstrated by a concordance of only 36% among monozygotic twin pairs.[13]

Several viruses have been associated with development of diabetes, specifically Coxsackie B, mumps, cytomegalovirus, and congenital rubella infection.[12] In addition, several nutritional risk factors have been implicated, among them high intake of nitrosamines[14] and infant feeding with cow's milk–based formula.[15, 16]

The unified theory for development of type 1 diabetes mellitus is summarized as follows. An individual with a genetic vulnerability to diabetes has normal pancreatic function until some insult is sustained, such as infection with a β-cell–tropic virus. The individual then elaborates antibodies that are capable of destroying β cells, or that, by an autoimmune mechanism, cross-react with β-cells. It is unclear whether the islet cell cytoplasmic antibodies and anti-insulin antibodies that are so prevalent in type 1 diabetes actually cause or merely reflect tissue damage. In either case, destruction of islet cells ends production of insulin.

TABLE 9-3. CLASSIFICATION AND DIAGNOSIS OF DIABETES MELLITUS

1. If a fasting plasma glucose level is > 140 mg/dL on more than one occasion, formal glucose tolerance testing is unnecessary.

2. Pretest preparation: Subjects consume a diet containing at least 150 to 200 g of carbonydrate for at least 3 days. The test is performed after an overnight fast of at least 10 h.

3. Subjects consume 75 g of glucose dissolved in 300 mL water. During test, no eating, drinking, or smoking is permitted.

4. Venous plasma glucose is measured fasting and at ½ h, 1 h, 1½ h, and 2 h after ingestion of a glucose beverage.

SAMPLE TIME	NORMAL	IMPAIRED GLUCOSE TOLERANCE (IGT)	DIABETES
Fasting	< 115 mg/dL *and*	< 140 mg/dL *plus*	≥ 140 mg/dL (sufficient for diagnosis), *or*
½ h, 1 h, and 1½ h	All three < 200, *and*	Any of these ≥ 200, *plus*	Any of these ≥ 200, *plus*
2 h	< 140	≥ 140 but < 200	≥ 200

From American Diabetes Association. Report of the Expert Committee on the diagnosis and classification of diabetes mellitus. Diabetes Care 1979;28:1039–1057.

TYPE 2 DIABETES

Type 2 diabetes (formerly NIDDM, or non–insulin-dependent diabetes) resembles type 1 only in that the end point is also hyperglycemia. The individual continues to produce insulin, usually in large quantities. Target tissues are, however, resistant to the effects of insulin.[17, 18]

The epidemiology, pathophysiology, genetics, presentation, and treatment of type 2 diabetes differ from type 1 in many ways. This is typically a disease of middle-aged and older adults. On the basis of the older criteria for diagnosis,[6] the prevalence of diagnosed diabetes among American women is less than 1% for the group under 45 years of age, rising to about 6% in the 45 to 64-year-old group and 10% in the group aged 65 years and older.[19] Prevalence varies widely among subpopulations.

In every age group, type 2 diabetes is more common in blacks than whites, usually approximately double, whereas Hispanic Americans fall in an intermediate range.[19] Black women are disproportionately likely to have this type of diabetes, compared with either black men or white women. Including all types of carbohydrate intolerance (diagnosed and undiagnosed diabetes in addition to glucose tolerance), Harris and associates estimated that 25% of black women aged 55 or older have some degree of diabetes.[20]

For populations worldwide, great variation is seen in prevalence, ranging from a rate of 0% in Melanesians to nearly 50% in the Pima Indians of the American Southwest.[21] Gender diffences are inconsistent within populations, and are easily confounded by other factors.

A strong genetic component is present in type 2 diabetes. Concordance rates between monozygotic twin pairs range from 60% to 100%.[21] A parental history of type 2 diabetes is an established risk factor for the disease, with a relative risk of 2.4 to 3.4 compared with those without the family history.[22] A discussion of the candidate genes that may be involved is beyond the scope of this chapter.

Persons with type 2 diabetes are much less likely than their type 1 counterparts to present acutely. They are also, therefore, less likely to be diagnosed; with the pre-1997 criteria, only 50% of cases of type 2 diabetics in America have been diagnosed.[1] The disease may exist for many years before any symptoms develop. In fact, the diagnosis may be made only after the development of a vascular complication, such as myocardial infarction. It is in this group, therefore, that screening programs would be expected to have the most impact.

Type 2 diabetes is also strongly associated with other metabolic and lifestyle factors.[21, 22] Obesity has a pronounced impact. Among American women in general, 3% of those with a body mass index (BMI) below 25 kg/m^2 are diabetic, a figure that rises to 8% with BMI greater than 25, and to 25% with a BMI above 35.[22] Not only the degree but the duration of obesity appears to be important. Central fat deposition, expressed as waist-to-hip ratio, is predictive of increased risk. Diets that are high in fat seem to be associated with greater risk; high fiber intake may be protective.[21] Increased levels of physical activity predict a decreased risk of diabetes.[21] Lower socioeconomic status, urban residence, and rapid Westernization of autochthonous populations are all associated with a higher rate of diabetes.[21] Advancing age is associated with increased risk.

The metabolic profile of type 2 diabetes is characterized by more than hyperglycemia.[23] Abnormal islet cell function leads to a downregulation of insulin receptors, so that the β-cell secretory response to glucose is impaired. (This has sometimes been designated *glucose resistance*.) Basal hepatic glucose production is increased. In addition, the response of target tissues to insulin is diminished; a given concentration of insulin stimulates less glucose uptake than in normal individuals. If the pancreas can compensate, this insulin resistance drives circulating insulin levels higher, which may allow for either normal or mildly impaired glucose tolerance. When compensation fails, overt hyperglycemia develops, until at some point insulin secretion declines, typically when fasting glucose levels exceed 140 mg/dL. The exact mechanism accounting for this decline in insulin secretion is unknown, but it is believed to be a manifestation of glucose toxicity.[18] A precursor state, the condition of impaired glucose tolerance, can be identified.

In a Pima Indian population (having the highest rate of type 2 diabetes in the world), the condition of subjects with impaired glucose tolerance frequently deteriorates to frank diabetes, 25% progress to diabetes within 5 years, and nearly two thirds within 10 years.[24] The higher the plasma insulin level at time of entry into the study, the higher the diabetes risk. A similar relation has been shown in other populations.[25] In a longitudinal study of offspring of two diabetic parents, all of whom had normal glucose tolerance testing at the start, diabetes was most likely to develop in those with the lowest insulin sensitivity. When insulin resistance was seen concomitantly with glucose resistance, diabetes developed in nearly 80% of subjects within 25 years.[26]

The hyperinsulinemic and insulin-resistant state is associated with many metabolic and vascular changes. Insulin reduces sodium excretion and sodium clearance by a direct effect at the renal tubule, decreases tubular sensitivity to atrial natriuretic peptide, and promotes plasma volume expansion.[27] Insulin also stimulates the sympathetic nervous system and provokes increases in plasma catecholamine concentrations, because of mitogenic activity, it may contribute to vascular remodeling.[28] Furthermore, insulin affects vascular smooth muscle reactivity by altering intracellular cation metabolism.[29, 30] Hyperinsulinemia also appears to stimulate the secretion of very-low-density lipoproteins (VLDLs),[17] raise triglyceride levels, and diminish production of high-density lipoprotein (HDL).[30]

Reaven described the infelicitously named *Syndrome X,* a cluster of variables related to insulin resistance that were predictive of the development of coronary artery disease.[17] These variables included glucose intolerance, hyperinsulinemia, resistance to insulin-stimulated glucose uptake, hypertriglyceridemia, decreased HDL cholesterol, increased VLDL, and hypertension. He suggested that the tendency to insulin resistance may be genetically determined, but because obesity and inactivity further exacerbate insulin resistance, the individual at risk might forestall development of coronary artery disease by maintaining a physically active lifestyle and a normal weight.

HYPERTENSION AND DIABETES

Hypertension frequently coexists with diabetes. Overall, the prevalence of hypertension among diabetic patients is nearly twice as high as among people with normal glucose tolerance.[31] The natural history of hypertension as well as the reasons for its development differ, however, for type 1 and type 2.

In type 1 diabetes, blood pressure is typically normal at the time of diagnosis and remains normal unless and until albuminuria develops. The first stage in the development of diabetic nephropathy is an increase in urinary albumin excretion in the range of 30 to 300 mg/day, referred to as *microalbuminuria* (Fig. 9–1).[32] This is rarely observed within the first 5 years after diagnosis.[33] Albuminuria tends to increase gradually, 10% to 30% per year, correlating with poor glycemic control.[33] Structural changes can be observed in the diabetic kidney even at this early stage. First there is an increase in kidney size and in protein content, accompanied by glomerular hyperfiltration.[34] A tendency to increased blood pressure is seen in diabetic persons with microalbuminuria,[35] although diagnostic criteria for hypertension (i.e., 140/90 mmHg) may not be met. When ambulatory 24-hour recordings of blood pressure are used, type 1 diabetics with microalbuminuria have more frequent elevations of blood pressure than either control subjects or diabetics without microalbuminuria.[35] They also lack the normal nocturnal drop in blood pressure, suggesting that the total daily pressure load on the kidneys is higher.[35]

Persistence of microalbuminurua predicts a decline in glomerular filtration rate (GFR) and the development of diabetic nephropathy within 10 years.[36] As the degree of microalbuminuria increases, blood pressure tends to increase at an equal pace. Once overt proteinuria develops (>300 mg of albumin/day, a range that is detectable by conventional dipstick assessment), the blood pressure begins to rise further, with systolic pressure increasing by an average of 1 mmHg per month.[37] During this time, GFR declines an average of 1 ml/min per month.[38] Within 15 years after diagnosis, 30% to 40% of type 1 diabetic patients will have developed nephropathy and will be hypertensive. The lifetime risk of hypertension is 40% to 50% among patients with type 1 diabetes. Hypertension in the absence of diabetic nephropathy is rare among this population.[31]

Type 2 diabetic patients tend to be older, heavier, and, at least in the United States

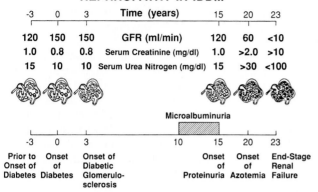

NATURAL HISTORY OF DIABETIC NEPHROPATHY IN IDDM

FIGURE 9–1. Natural history of diabetic nephropathy in type 1 diabetes. Note the appearance of microalbuminuria years before overt proteinuria. GFR, glomerular filtration rate. (Adapted from DeFronzo RA. Diabetes and the kidney: An update. *In* Olefsky JM, Sherwin RS (eds). Diabetes Mellitus: Management and Complications. New York, Churchill Livingstone, 1985, pp 1159–1222; reprinted from Porte Jr D, Sherwin RS. Ellenberg and Rifkin's Diabetes Mellitus, 5th ed. Stamford, CT: Appleton & Lange, 1997, p. 974.)

more frequently black, all factors independently associated with hypertension. Although these individuals make up more than 90% of those carrying both diagnoses—diabetes and hypertension—the age-adjusted prevalence of hypertension in type 2 diabetes is actually somewhat lower than in type 1.[39, 40] Without adjusting for age, almost 75% of type 2 diabetic patients are hypertensive as defined by a blood pressure of 140/90 mmHg, with approximately two thirds of cases uncontrolled.[39] Women with type 2 diabetes are, as a rule, more likely to be hypertensive than men, although the magnitude of this difference varies with ethnic background. Among American black women older than age 45 years with diabetes, an astonishing 90% also have hypertension.[39]

In the San Antonio Heart Study, a population-based study of diabetes and cardiovascular disease among Mexican-American and non-Hispanic whites, abnormal glucose tolerance was a stronger predictor of the development of hypertension in women than in men.[41] Compared with women with normal glucose tolerance, those with impaired glucose tolerance had a relative risk of 1.94 of development of hypertension, whereas those with NIDDM (type 2) had a relative risk of 2.65. The corresponding relative risks among men were 0.91 for impaired glucose tolerance and 1.61 for type 2 diabetes, compared with normal men. This differential impact of gender persisted even after controlling for age, obesity, and other confounding factors.

Impaired glucose tolerance may precede the development of hypertension, or hypertension may be seen first. At the time of diagnosis of diabetes, 28% of individuals are already known to be hypertensive.[31] Conversely, the prevalence of diabetes or impaired glucose tolerance among hypertensive patients is as high as 50% if formal glucose tolerance testing is performed.[42, 43] Underlying subtle defects in fuel metabolism appear to be even more common among hypertensive persons. In a study of 2475 Israelis, plasma insulin levels were elevated in hypertensive subjects compared with normotensive controls, even in the group with normal glucose tolerance testing.[44] Although this effect was seen in both the obese and normal-weight groups, its magnitude was greater among the lean hypertensive population.

In the San Antonio Heart Study, both fasting and postprandial insulin levels were 35% higher in hypertensive subjects than in their normotensive counterparts, adjusted for age, sex, ethnicity and BMI.[45] The implication to be drawn is, of course, that essential hypertension is an insulin-resistant state, and that these individuals are at risk for development of diabetes. Thus, it is not surprising that patients with type 2 diabetes are commonly hypertensive.

Nephropathy develops in 10% to 20% of type 2 diabetic patients.[40] The progression of renal disease is the same as in type 1, with microalbuminuria presaging overt proteinuria and with the same changes in GFR and blood pressure. Increased blood pressure appears to be both a cause and a result of nephropathy in type 2 diabetes. Once overt proteinuria develops, no methods are available to prevent or retard the progression of diabetic nephropathy; there is, however, room to intervene at the stage of microalbuminuria. Factors predicting progression of renal disease include poor glycemic control, hypertension, smoking, and dyslipidemia.[46, 47]

Leading causes of death in patients with diabetes include renal failure and cardiovascular disease. Diabetes is the only condition in which women manifest heart disease rates similar to those of men.[5] Among diabetic men in the Framingham Study, the risk ratio for the development of coronary disease among diabetic men was 2.3 and 2.9 for diabetic women.[48] The Nurses' Health Study, which observed 115,000 women aged 30 to 55 over 8 years, demonstrated an age-adjusted risk ratio for coronary disease of 6.7 among diabetics patients who did not require insulin and 12.2 among diabetic patients requiring insulin.[49] Thus, diabetes has a greater effect on women than on men in terms of cardiac disease. Furthermore, case-fatality rates after myocardial infarction are disproportionately higher for women than for men, and for diabetic women compared with women having normal glucose tolerance.[48, 50]

Hypertension is approximately twice as common among diabetic patients, and as many as 3 million Americans may have both.[51] Patients who have both diabetes and hypertension are at increased risk for diabetic complications, including coronary artery disease, cerebrovascular disease, renal failure, peripheral vascular disease, and diabetic retinopathy. The risk is more than additive. In a group of 3000 men monitored for 4 years, in whom the background rate of coronary artery disease was 6/1000, the presence of either diabetes or hypertension more than doubled that risk (14/1000 and 15/1000, respectively), whereas the presence of both increased the risk eightfold.[52] Hence, the presence of either diabetes or hypertension should prompt surveillance for the other and control of both.

Treatment of Hypertension in Diabetic Patients

Recommendations for the detection, evaluation, and treatment of hypertension have been published, in which preferred initial drug therapy is either a diuretic or a β blocker.[53] In diabetic people, however, some antihypertensive drugs have been found to worsen hyperglycemia or to have an adverse effect on the lipid profile.[54] Conversely, certain other drugs improve renal function in the diabetic: the angiotensin-converting enzyme inhibitors (ACE-Is) have specific renoprotective effects in decreasing albuminuria and in slowing the rate of decline of GFR.[55, 56] In fact, even normotensive type 2 diabetic patients in the earliest stages of nephropathy appear to profit from the use of ACE-Is in terms of stabilization of serum creatinine levels and progression of albuminuria.[57]

Guidelines for the management of hypertension in diabetes have been published by the National High Blood Pressure Education Program Working Group,[51] the Canadian Hypertension Society,[58] and the ADA.[59] These guidelines are summarized in Table 9–4.

Weight loss in obese patients can alleviate both hypertension and diabetes and improves insulin sensitivity. Weight loss is also associated with a more favorable lipid profile because HDL is increased and both low-density liproprotein (LDL) and triglycerides are reduced.[51] Both diet and exercise play a role (Table 9–5).[60, 61]

When nonpharmacologic approaches prove inadequate, drug therapy should be employed. In the evaluation and management of the diabetic patient with hypertension, the possibility of impaired autonomic

---

TABLE 9–4. GUIDELINES FOR MANAGEMENT OF HYPERTENSION IN DIABETES

1. Goals are to prevent mortality and morbidity associated with hypertension while disturbing quality of life as little as possible.

2. The optimal blood pressure in diabetic patients is unknown. In the absence of evidence to the contrary, a target level of below 130 mmHg systolic and below 85 mmHg diastolic is suggested.

3. Target organ damage should be assessed because modifications of treatment may be required.

4. Lifestyle modification should be made first, such as weight loss, dietary modification, increased physical activity, cessation of smoking, and curtailment of alcohol use.

Adapted from The National High Blood Pressure Working Group. National High Blood Pressure Education Program Working Group report on hypertension in diabetes. Hypertension 1994;23:145–158; Dawson KG, McKenzie JK, Ross SA, et al. Report of the Canadian Hypertension Society Consensus Conference: 5. Hypertension and diabetes. Can Med Assoc J 1993;149:821–826; and American Diabetes Association. Clinical Practice Guidelines 1996. Treatment of hypertension in diabetes. Diabetes Care 1996;19(suppl 1):S107–S113.

TABLE 9–5. GUIDELINES FOR MEAL PLANNING AND EXERCISE IN DIABETES

MEAL PLANNING

1. Obtain 50–60% of total calories from carbohydrates, especially complex carbohydrates.
2. Increase dietary fiber to 20–35 g per day.
3. Keep dietary fat content under 30% of total calories.
4. Maintain saturated fat at less than 10% of calories.
5. Consider moderate restriction of salt intake (< 2.3 g/day).
6. Consult a dietitian for help in devising meal plans.

EXERCISE PROGRAM

1. Consider general physical condition and clear program with your physician before embarking on an exercise regimen.
2. If unfit, build up exercise tolerance gradually.
3. Aim for aerobic exercise lasting 20–45 min, at least 3 days/wk, at a level of 50–75% of your maximum oxygen uptake.

responses to posture change must be kept in mind, so that it is desirable to assess blood pressure in standing, seated, and supine positions.[51] Home or ambulatory blood pressure monitoring should also be considered in these patients.

A number of classes of antihypertensive agents may be effective. In a meta-analysis of antihypertensive therapy in diabetics,[62] no single drug stood out as more effective than others in achieving blood pressure control. ACE-Is were unique among antihypertensive agents, however, in decreasing proteinuria and increasing GFR independent of any improvement associated with the lowering of blood pressure alone. The effects of ACE-Is on proteinuria were seen for microalbuminuria, for clinically apparent proteinuria, and for both types of diabetes; these effects have been seen even in diabetic patients with normal blood pressure and have not been associated with any adverse metabolic effects in diabetic patients.[51] Thus these drugs are an attractive option for the treatment of hypertension in diabetes, and may well be the first-line therapy for diabetics with any degree of renal disease. Both hyperkalemia and acute renal failure can develop, the former in patients with renal insufficiency, the latter in persons with renal artery stenosis, so that serum potassium and creatinine levels must be carefully moni-

tored after initiation of ACE-I therapy.[53] These drugs must be administered with caution to patients already receiving diuretics, because of the potential for profound hypotension.[53]

An alternative first-line drug in the hypertensive diabetic may be a calcium blocker.[54, 58] Both diltiazem and verapamil reduce albuminuria, although results with nifedipine and other dihydropyridines have been mixed.[58] Calcium antagonists do not appear to have ill effects on either glycemic control or serum lipids.[59] In a small Dutch study, nifedipine actually increased insulin absorption at the injection site.[63] Calcium blockers do have, however, some potential to induce orthostatic hypotension, which may be accentuated in patients with diabetics when autonomic reflexes are impaired.[51] α_1-Blockers (e.g., doxazosin, prazosin) are another good choice, because they may provide some mild benefit in lipid profile and do not alter glycemic control.[64] Like the calcium channel blockers, they retain potential to provoke or exacerbate postural hypotension.

Thiazide diuretics have long been a mainstay in the treatment of hypertension in diabetes. In small doses (i.e, 12.5–25 mg hydrochlorothiazide or equivalent daily), they are often effective in controlling blood pressure, but they have also been implicated in the development of insulin resistance and dyslipidemia,[59] especially as doses are increased. Unless the diuretics are in low doses, their use in the diabetic population has been discouraged.[54]

β-Blockers raise several other concerns. They can reduce hypoglycemia awareness among diabetics by blunting catecholamine release, can reduce peripheral blood flow (a potential problem for diabetic patients whose peripheral circulation may already be impaired), and are associated with worsening of glucose and lipid metabolism.[51, 53] Their ability to cause peripheral vasoconstriction also reduces insulin absorption at the injection site.[63] Their use has also been discouraged in hypertensive diabetic patients.

In all cases, an inadequate response to the first-line drug should prompt either an increase in dose or the substitution of another agent. Two algorithms suggested by Christlieb are reproduced in Figure 9–2.[54] Surveillance of the associated side effects

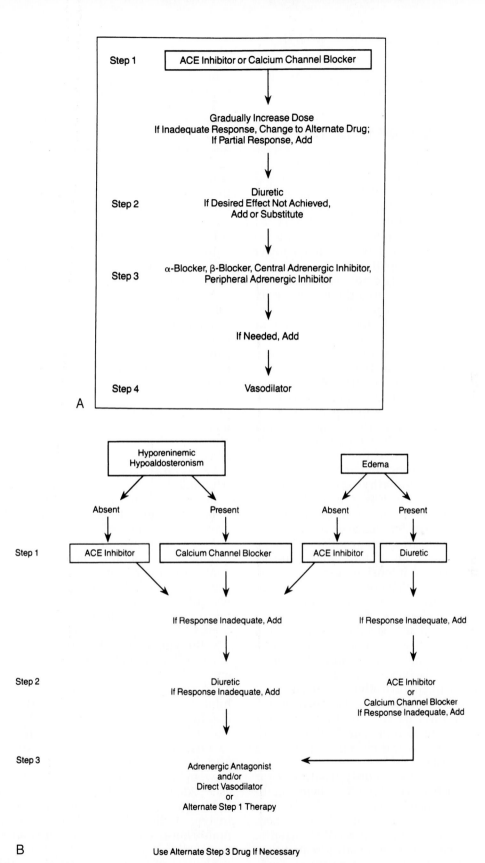

FIGURE 9–2. *A*, An approach to the treatment of hypertension in patients with diabetic nephropathy. *B*, An approach to the treatment of hypertension in patients with diabetic neuropathy. ACE, angiotensin-converting enzyme. (*A* and *B*, From Christlieb AR. Treatment selection considerations for the hypertensive diabetic. Arch Intern Med 1990;150:1171–1172; Copyright 1990, American Medical Association.)

(autonomic hypotension, dyslipidemias, hyperkalemia) is important.

MANAGEMENT OF DIABETES

Equally important as the management of hypertension is the maintenance of good glucose control. In the Diabetes Control and Complications Trial (DCCT), in which 1441 patients with type 1 diabete were monitored over a period of up to 9 years, tight glucose control was associated with a much lower likelihood of retinopathy, nephropathy, or neuropathy.[65] Patients randomly assigned to intensive therapy required three or more injections daily or an insulin pump, and monitored capillary blood glucose at least four times a day, with the goal of maintaining preprandial values 70 to 120 mg/dL, postprandial values below 180 mg/dL, and glycosylated hemoglobin below 6.05%. The conventional therapy group, in comparison, monitored urine or blood glucose once daily, took one or two insulin injections per day, and did not adjust dosage on a daily basis. In the intensive therapy group, the risk of development of microalbuminuria, proteinuria, retinopathy, and neuropathy was markedly reduced (Fig. 9–3). These results were, however, achieved at the cost of a threefold higher incidence of severe hypoglycemia. There was also a tendency toward transient worsening of retinopathy during the first year of intensive therapy among patients who had diabetic retinopathy at enrollment, which was usually corrected within 18 months. The DCCT research group recommended that type 1 diabetes be treated with intensive therapy so as to maintain glycemic status as close to the normal range as feasible. No similar study has been completed with type 2 diabetic patients, although hyperglycemia has also been associated with a higher risk of complications among this population. The National Institutes of Health (NIH) is currently sponsoring such a project.

Insulin remains the only treatment for type 1 diabetes. With type 2 diabetes mellitus, although insulin may be used, a number of other agents are available. Because there are many more type 2 diabetic patients, however, the number of insulin-treated type 2 diabetic patients is two or three times higher than the number with type 1 diabetes, a fact that has in the past led to some confusion about the designations *insulin-dependent* and *non–insulin-dependent*.[66]

The majority of patients with type 2 diabetes are obese. Weight loss has been advocated as the initial treatment in these cases, and even small achievements in this area, in the 10-pound range, may improve glucose control.[60] Unfortunately, weight loss is often difficult to achieve. Available pharmacologic treatments other than insulin include the sulfonylureas, biguanides, α_1-glucosidase inhibitors, and thiazolidinediones (Table 9–6).

The sulfonylureas have been the primary choice among the oral hypoglycemic agents for many years. They include tolbutamide, tolazamide, and chlorpropamide in the first generation and glipizide and glyburide in the second. All of these drugs stimulate insulin secretion by the pancreas: in some patients, they may improve sensitivity of target tissues to insulin.[67] They are often associated, as is insulin, with weight gain. Sulfonylurea therapy is unsuccessful in approximately 20% of type 2 patients.[67] For many others, euglycemia cannot be restored; but glycemic control can be improved.

Metformin is the first of the biguanides. Although it has been available in Europe for decades, it has been available in the United States only since 1995. Unlike the sulfonylureas, it does not stimulate insulin output but does improve insulin sensitivity.[67] Its mechanism of action remains unknown. In contrast to the sulfonylureas and insulin, it promotes weight loss or at least maintains weight without further gain, which may make it the better choice for obese patients. It can also be given in combination with a sulfonylurea, which provides more of a glucose-lowering effect than when either is given alone.[67]

Acarbose is the only alpha-glucosidase inhibitor available in the United States. It is an oligosaccharide that inhibits the conversion of complex carbohydrates into monosaccharides, thus decreasing postprandial glucose excursions, although overall improvement in blood glucose control is modest.[67] Alone among the oral agents, then, it holds some promise as an ancillary agent in type 1 diabetes, and is useful as either monotherapy or as combined therapy for type 2 diabetes.

The last group of oral agents is the thiazolidinediones. The first of these, troglitazone, was approved in 1997 in the United States

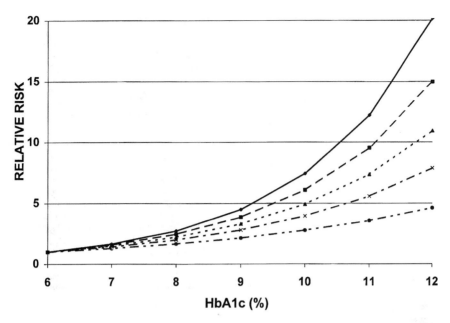

FIGURE 9–3. Relative risks for development of microvascular complications as a function of mean HbA1c (glycosylated hemoglobin), based on the Diabetes Control and Complications Trial (DCCT). The lines depict a stylized relationship for the risk of retinopathy (—♦), progression to clinical nephropathy (urinary albumin excretion ≥300 mg/24 h) (----■), progression to severe nonproliferative or proliferative retinopathy (...▲), progression to clinical neuropathy (----×), and progression to microalbuminuria (urinary albumin excretion ≥40 mg/24 hr) (----●). (Modified from Skyler JS. Diabetic complications: The importance of glucose control. Endocrinol Metab Clin North Am 1996;25:243–254; reprinted from Porte Jr D, Sherwin RS. Ellenberg and Rifkin's Diabetes Mellitus, 5th ed. Stamford, CT: Appleton & Lange, 1997.)

but taken off the market in 2000 because of hepatotoxicity. These agents, whose exact mode of action remains unknown, increase insulin sensitivity.[68–70] In a study of 284 type 2 patients for whom diet therapy was unsuccessful, although only 45% responded to troglitazone, those who did respond manifested an average drop in fasting plasma glucose of 24 mg/dL and a drop in fasting insulin level of about 12% while also showing decreasing plasma triglycerides.[71] Patients with a greater BMI were more likely to respond to the drug.

Troglitazone was also evaluated in individuals with impaired glucose tolerance; in 80% of these subjects, glucose tolerance became normal after 6 weeks of treatment along with normalization of fasting and postchallenge insulin levels and reduction of fasting triglycerides.[70] In obese subjects with either normal or impaired glucose tolerance (patients with overt diabetes were excluded from this study), a small decrease in fasting plasma glucose and a 44% drop in fasting insulin were seen, again confirming an improvement in insulin sensitivity.[68] A small decrement in both systolic and dia-

stolic blood pressure was observed in this group as well.

Finally, in a group of women considered to be at high risk for development of type 2 diabetes (obese, largely Mexican-American, and with a history of gestational diabetes), 3 months of thiazolidinedione treatment not only improved insulin sensitivity by 88% above baseline levels but also lowered total and LDL cholesterol levels.[69]

These studies suggest that the thiazolidinediones are likely to be helpful in improving the metabolic profile of type 2 diabetics and may also help slow progression to diabetes in individuals with recognized risk factors. Currently available agents in the United States include rosiglitazone and pioglitazone.

In type 2 diabetic patients who do not achieve satisfactory glucose control by taking oral agents, insulin is either added or substituted. One author estimates that 30% to 50% of these patients diabetics require treatment with insulin.[66] Insulin is well known to promote weight gain, which may worsen the metabolic profile in such patients. Combination therapy (with insulin

TABLE 9-6. ORALLY ACTIVE AGENTS IN THE CONTROL OF DIABETES

AGENT	DOSAGE
Sulfonylureas (stimulate pancreatic secretion of insulin)	
Tolbutamide	250–1000 mg bid–tid (maximum dose 2000 mg/day)
Tolazamide	100–500 mg qd–bid (maximum dose 1000 mg/day)
Chlorpropamide	100–250 mg qd–bid
Glipizide	2.5–20 mg qd–bid
Glyburide	1.25–10 mg qd–bid
Biguanides (improve insulin sensitivity)	
Metformin	500 bid or 850 mg qd, to maximum dose 1000 mg bid or 850 mg tid
α-Glucosidase Inhibitors (block breakdown of complex carbohydrates)	
Acarbose	25–75 mg tid (take with beginning of each meal)
Thiazolidinediones (increase insulin sensitivity)	
Rosiglitazone	4 mg, administered either once a day or in divided doses twice daily (may increase to 8 mg/day)
Pioglitazone	15–45 mg taken once daily

bid, twice a day; tid, three times a day; qd, once a day.

and sulfonylureas,[72] metformin and insulin,[73] or acarbose and insulin[74] has proved superior to insulin monotherapy in type 2 diabetes.

SPECIFIC HEALTH ISSUES FOR WOMEN WITH DIABETES

In caring for diabetic women, the practitioner must also keep in mind those aspects of health care not shared by men. The diabetic woman, hypertensive or not, may be dealing with puberty, infertility or menstrual irregularity, contraception, pregnancy, lactation, cancer of the breast and reproductive organs, or menopause. These issues are discussed briefly.

Menstruation and Infertility

Poretsky and Kalin have speculated that insulin and the insulin-like growth factors have some gonadotropic effect on the ovary.[75] The average age of menarche lags by about 1 year among girls with type 1 diabetes.[76] In the preinsulin era, in fact, primary amenorrhea was the rule among young diabetic patients.[77] Syndromes of insulin resistance and acanthosis nigricans are associated with hyperandrogenism, anovulation, and sometimes ovarian hyperstimulation.[75] Although a number of these are rare entities, polycystic ovary syndrome (PCOS) remains the most common endocrine disorder in women of reproductive age, with 5% to 10% of premenopausal women manifesting this syndrome of chronic anovulation, hyperandrogenism, and polycystic ovaries.[78] Women with PCOS not only are at a fourfold risk for development of type 2 diabetes but also tend to do so at an earlier age than the general population.[79,80] In a retrospective study of postmenopausal Swedish women who had undergone wedge resection for PCOS 20 to 30 years earlier, the women were 3.5 times more likely to have hypertension and 6.5 times more likely to have diabetes than age-matched controls[81] despite similarities in BMI between the groups.

Women with PCOS, whether obese or not, have higher circulating insulin levels, higher fasting and 2-hour plasma glucose levels, and decreased insulin sensitivity compared with weight-matched controls.[79] Despite their higher insulin levels, hepatic glucose production is more difficult to suppress, a characteristic of insulin resistance. The major metabolic malfunction in PCOS is believed to be a specific postreceptor defect in the adipocyte.[78] PCOS is, of course, a leading cause of oligomenorrhea and infertility. It may be a marker for the presence or eventual development of both hypertension and diabetes.

Contraception

Contraception is important in women's life choices. When a woman is diabetic or hypertensive or both, her choice of contraceptive method may influence her disease process. In addition, her disease should be optimally controlled before she attempts conception, so that the contraceptive method will be reliable. There should be no unplanned pregnancies in patients with diabetes because preconceptional glycemic control has important implications for pregnancy.

Barrier methods—condom and diaphragm—are safe, have no side effects, and provide protection against sexually transmitted diseases as well as pregnancy. Unfortunately, they are among the least effective methods.[82]

The intrauterine contraceptive device. (IUD) provides excellent contraceptive protection for up to 10 years if it (1) contains copper, (2) calls for no user motivation once it is inserted, and (3) does not alter the metabolic profile.[82] Historical concerns about the risk of pelvic inflammatory disease (PID) in IUD users have often kept providers from recommending its use in diabetics. Studies performed after the Dalkon Shield debacle have shown, however, that when that one particular device is excluded, the risk for development of PID is small and confined to a brief period following insertion of the device.[83–85] Excluding the first 4 months following insertion, the relative risk of PID in women using an IUD other than the Dalkon Shield is approximately 1.1 compared with controls using no method.[84] Even this slight increase in risk is limited to women with multiple coital partners, a history of PID, or those who were nulliparae under 25 years of age. Current recommendations for IUD use commonly restrict its use to women considered at low risk for exposure to sexually transmitted disease (e.g., monogamous, parous women without a recent history of sexually transmitted disease).[86] (Risk group assignment may, of course, be difficult.) Aside from these general risk factors, there is no evidence to support any increased risk of pelvic infection among IUD users who have diabetes.[86–88]

The IUD remains an important contraceptive option for diabetic women who are otherwise at low risk for PID (see earlier), and it is especially useful in diabetic patients with evidence of vascular disease, hypertension, or retinopathy because the copper-based devices are metabolically neutral. The use of antibiotic prophylaxis at time of insertion is recommended; regimens include doxycycline 200 mg, followed by 100 mg 12 hours after insertion; erythromycin 500 mg at insertion and 6 hours later; or azithromycin as a single 500-mg dose.[86] Obviously, any sign of pelvic infection would mandate appropriate examination, and any documented sexually transmitted disease or pelvic infection should be treated with IUD removal and aggressive antibiotic therapy.

Clinicians have also been hesitant in the past to prescribe hormonal methods of contraception for diabetic women. Two basic types of hormonal contraceptives are available: (1) those containing an estrogen plus a progestin and (2) those containing only a progestin, which may be delivered orally, intramuscularly, or by sustained release from implants beneath the skin.

The combination of estrogen and progestin is available only in oral form but with multiple choices as to type and dosage of both components. Currently available formulations contain much less of each of these than the first generation of oral contraceptives and are considered low-dose forms because they contain 50 μg or less of ethinyl estradiol or its derivative, mestranol. Formulations containing higher estrogen doses had been associated with an increase in thromboembolic complications, including myocardial infarction, stroke, pulmonary embolism, and deep venous thrombosis.[89, 90] The increased risk of myocardial infarction was related to arterial thrombosis rather than to acceleration of atherosclerosis. Diabetic patients, already at risk for several of these macrovascular vascular disorders, were previously advised to avoid oral contraceptives. The current low-dose preparations generally have not been associated with an increased risk of vascular complications.[91–93]

Ethinyl estradiol has been shown to increase levels of angiotensinogen, associated with a modest rise in blood pressure.[94] This effect appears to be dose-dependent, so that in women who are hypertensive or who are at risk for hypertension, including those with diabetes, the lowest effective dose of ethinyl estradiol should be prescribed—20 to 35 μg. The progestin-only oral contraceptive may be a good alternative if blood pressure control is an issue.

The progestin component of the combination oral contraceptive must also be considered during selection. In order of increasing androgenicity, the available progestins in the United States are gestodene, desogestrel, norgestimate, ethynodiol diacetate, norethindrone, and levonorgestrel. The more androgenic the progestin, or the higher the dose, the greater the adverse metabolic effect. In a sophisticated metabolic study of nearly 1500 oral contraceptive users, a number of different combination pills were evaluated.[95] With all three of the progestins studied, whether in monophasic or triphasic preparations and regardless of dose, both fasting plasma insulin and the response of insulin to glucose tolerance testing were increased. Although fasting plasma glucose changed little, overall glucose levels during glucose tolerance testing were increased. Thus, progestin in combination oral contraceptives appears to induce insulin resistance. The effect of ethinyl estradiol on insulin resistance is not clear, in as much as some researchers believe that it improves[96] and others believe that it worsens[95, 97] insulin sensitivity.

Overall, combined oral contraceptives have a slight effect on blood pressure,[98, 99] and have effects on insulin resistance and lipid profile that vary according to the specific agent and dose employed. The effects on serum lipids are summarized in Table 9–7. The newer, less androgenic progestins—gestodene, desogestrel, and norgestimate—seem to be preferable from the point of view of lipid effects, and there may be a slight beneficial effect if desogestrel is used. These issues are likely to be important in selecting a formulation for the type 2 patients, in whom insulin resistance and lipid abnormalities are the rule. Studies that have specifically evaluated oral contraceptive use in type 1 patients have found little effect on glycemic control.[100–102]

Little information is available relating oral contraceptive use among diabetics to long-term diabetes complications. When obesity, duration of diabetes, and presence of proteinuria were controlled for, a cross-sectional study of 384 insulin-dependent diabetics patients was unable to demonstrate any effect of current or prior use of oral contraceptives on hypertension, severity of retinopathy, or glycosylated hemoglobin.[102] In contract, a retrospective case-control study of nearly 2000 Danish women,[103] evaluating cerebral thromboembolism as an end point, demonstrated an odds ratio of 5.5 among diabetic patients, with no difference between users and nonusers of combination oral contraceptives. The use of oral contraceptives, regardless of diabetes state, doubled the odds of cerebrovascular thrombosis, which prompted the authors to conclude that a diabetic woman who uses combination oral contraceptives increases her risk of cerebrovascular accident tenfold compared with a woman who is neither diabetic nor an oral contraceptive user. The presence of hypertension increased the odds of cerebral embolism threefold, with no further analysis made of oral contraceptive use or of the concomitant presence of diabetes.[103] Still, if risk factors are multiplicative, one might extrapolate that a woman with both diabetes and hypertension who is an oral contraceptive user might have 30 times the risk of stroke of a woman with none of these factors.

In her review of the subject, Kjos[86] concludes that women with diabetes of either type who have no significant vascular disease may be candidates for oral contraceptives with either a progestin-only pill or the lowest-dose combination pill that is effective. Formulations containing 20 to 35 µg ethinyl estradiol are recommended from the latter category, and these should contain a low dose of a progestin with low androgenicity (Table 9–8). Kjos recommends baseline evaluation of weight, blood pressure, glucose control, and fasting lipids, repeated after the first cycle of pills and every 3 to 6 months thereafter. In this scheme, deterioration in glucose or lipid values would be managed by adjustment of diet, weight loss, exercise, or drug therapy before a change to another contraceptive method. We believe, however, that combination oral contracep-

TABLE 9–7. CONTRACEPTIVE PROGESTINS AND EFFECT ON SERUM LIPIDS

PROGESTIN	LOW-DENSITY LIPOPROTEIN	HIGH-DENSITY LIPOPROTEIN	TRIGLYCERIDES
Levonorgestrel	Slight increase	Large decrease	Increase
Norethindrone	Slight decrease	Slight decrease	Minimal effect
Desogestrel	Decrease	Increase	No effect
Norgestimate	Decrease	Increase	No effect

TABLE 9–8. COMPOSITION OF COMMONLY PRESCRIBED COMBINATION ORAL CONTRACEPTIVES

	ESTROGEN	PROGESTIN
LOW ANDROGENIC ACTIVITY*		
Monophasic		
Brevicon (Searle)	EE 35 μg	Norethindrone 0.5 mg
Modicon (Ortho)	EE 35 μg	Norethindrone 0.5 mg
Ovcon 35 (Bristol-Myers)	EE 35 μg	Norethindrone 0.4 mg
OrthoCyclen (Ortho)	EE 35 μg	Norgestimate 0.25 mg
OrthoCept (Ortho)	EE 30 μg	Desogestrel 0.15 mg
Desogen (Organon)	EE 30 μg	Desogestrel 0.15 mg
Triphasic		
Ortho Tri-Cyclen (Ortho)	EE 35 μg	Norgestimate 0.18/0.22/0.25 mg
MODERATE ANDROGENIC ACTIVITY†		
Monophasic		
Ovcon 50 (Bristol-Myers)	EE 50 μg	Norethindrone 1.0 mg
Ortho-Novum 1/50 (Ortho)	ME 50 μg	Norethindrone 1.0 mg
Ortho-Novum 1/35 (Ortho)	EE 35 μg	Norethindrone 1.0 mg
Demulen 1/50 (Searle)	EE 50 μg	Ethynodiol diacetate 1.0 mg
Demulen 1/35 (Searle)	EE 35 μg	Ethynodiol diacetate 1.0 mg
Loestrin 1/20 (Parke-Davis)	EE 20 μg	Norethindrone acetate 1.0 mg
Triphasic		
Ortho-Novum 7-7-7 (Ortho)	EE 35 μg	Norethindrone 0.5/0.75/1.0 mg
Triphasil (Wyeth-Ayerst)	EE 30/40/30 μg	LNG 0.05/0.075/0.125 mg
Tri-Levlen (Berlex)	EE 30/40/30 μg	LNG 0.05/0.075/0.125 mg
HIGH ANDROGENIC ACTIVITY‡		
Monophasic		
Ovral (Wyeth-Ayerst)	EE 50 μg	Norgestrel 0.5 mg
Loestrin 1.5/30 (Parke-Davis)	EE 30 μg	Norethindrone acetate 1.5 mg
Lo-Ovral (Wyeth-Ayerst)	EE 30 μg	Norgestrel 0.3 mg
Nordette (Wyeth-Ayerst)	EE 30 μg	LNG 0.15
Levlen (Berlex)	EE 30 μg	LNG 0.15

*Low-androgen progestins: norgestimate, desogestrel; norethindrone in the 0.4- 0.5-mg range.
†Moderate-androgen progestins: LNG (triphasic doses); norethindrone 1.0 mg (monophasic or triphasic); norethindrone acetate 1.0 mg; ethynodiol diacetate 1.0 mg.
‡High-androgen progestins: norgestrel (0.3 mg), norethindrone acetate (1.5–2.5 mg); LNG 0.15.
EE, ethinyl estradiol; LNG, levonorgestrel; ME, mestranol.

tives are probably not the best choice for diabetic patients who are also hypertensive, because type 1 diabetes associated with hypertension is almost invariably associated with vascular disease, and both hypertension and the constellation of metabolic abnormalities linked to type 2 diabetes are likely to be worsened by oral contraceptive use.

The two long-acting progestins available for contraception include depot medroxyprogesterone acetate (Depo-Provera) and Norplant, which is a system of six levonorgestrel-containing capsules implanted under the skin. Users of both of these agents exhibit increased insulin levels and deterioration in glucose tolerance, although glucose tolerance test results do not exceed the limits of normal.[82, 104, 105] Weight gain is to be expected among users of Depo-Provera,[82] which also worsens insulin resistance and hypertension. There are no studies of either method in diabetic women, and these methods cannot be recommended without reservation. Their ease of use, contraceptive efficacy, and long duration of action do make them attractive; however, if a progestin-only method is desired, the progestin-only pill is a better choice for the diabetic woman, because of longer experience and because of greater ease of reversibility of any adverse metabolic effects that may occur.

Diabetes and Pregnancy

Among the important benefits of contraception for the diabetic woman is the ability to plan pregnancies at a time when she is in optimal metabolic control. This contributes not only to her health but also to the health of her offspring, inasmuch as hyperglycemia during organogenesis is associated with a strikingly high incidence of congenital abnormalities.

The frequency of congenital abnormalities among infants born to women with pregestational diabetes is 6% to 10%, compared with the background population risk of 2% to 5%.[106] These abnormalities include malformations of the heart and great vessels, central nervous system, vertebrae and limbs, and genitourinary system. Spontaneous abortion rates among diabetic women are also high, at least among that subgroup of women with poor early glucose control (Fig. 9–4).[107]

It is now clear that preconceptional diabetes management and control of hyperglycemia in the first trimester is the most important factor influencing the rate of congenital abnormalities in this population. Glycosylated hemoglobin (HbA1c) provides a convenient marker for diabetic control. When HbA1c levels are normal at less than 14 weeks' gestation (<8.5%), malformation rates are approximately 3%, whereas with levels above 9.5%, the rate of malformations exceeds 20%.[106] When diabetic women are enrolled in preconception programs, the prevalence of major malformations among their infants is decreased by as much as

90%.[108–111] Because diabetes care in general has been influenced by the findings of the DCCT and glucose control overall has been tightened, we may see a decrease in malformation rates even among offspring of women who were not enrolled in a specific preconception program.

The metabolic pathways by which hyperglycemia promotes teratogenesis are not clearly elucidated. Ketone bodies, somatomedin inhibitors, increased free oxgen radicals, and decreased *myo*-inositol or arachidonic acid concentrations all have been evaluated for a contributory role.[112] In the absence of a definite mechanism, no specific recommendations can be made as to prophylaxis against diabetic embryopathy, other than to reiterate that glucose control should be optimal prior to pregnancy. There is also a role for periconceptional supplementation with folic acid in preventing neural tube defects.[113]

During preconception planning, the patient's general medical status is assessed and the degree of vascular complications, if any, is quantified. Ophthalmologic evaluation is carried out so that if significant retinopathy exists, laser coagulation can be performed. Tests of renal function are completed. Historical or electrocardiographic evidence of coronary artery disease implies profound risks to maternal health, and the patient should be counseled to avoid pregnancy.[106]

If a type 2 diabetic woman has been taking oral hypoglycemic agents, she should discontinue them and achieve control with insulin. Hypertensive diabetic women should discontinue ACE-I therapy, which has been associated not only with birth defects but also with intrauterine growth restriction (IUGR), perinatal renal failure, and fetal death.[114] β-Blockers, calcium blockers, α_1-receptor blockers, α-methyldopa, and hydralazine all have been used successfully in pregnancy. Diuretics are not recommended.[115, 116]

Glucose control is achieved by two or three injections of insulin daily, aiming for fasting plasma glucose levels of 60 to 80 mg/ dL, with postprandial values below 120.[117] Human insulin is recommended for use preconceptionally and during pregnancy. Blood glucose levels are monitored at least four times daily. Glycosylated hemoglobin should be normal before pregnancy is attempted and should be monitored in each trimester. Hypoglycemic reactions often oc-

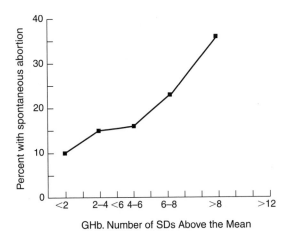

FIGURE 9–4. Rate of spontaneous abortion in pregestational diabetes mellitus as a function of HbA1c (glycosylated hemoglobin [GHb]). SDs, standard deviations. (Adapted from data published in Mills JL, Simpson JL, Driscoll SG. The Diabetes in Early Pregnancy Study: Incidence of spontaneous abortion among normal and insulin-dependent diabetic women whose pregnancies were identified within 21 days of conception. N Engl J Med 1988;319:1617–1623.)

cur, but are not associated with obvious fetal compromise.[118]

Once conception has occurred, glucose must be strictly controlled. Maternal serum screening for α-fetoprotein should be offered at 16 weeks' gestation. First-trimester ultrasonography is important in establishing accurate gestational dating. Detailed ultrasonographic survey of fetal anatomy should be performed at 20 weeks' gestation, including fetal echocardiography.[106] The physician should be prepared to offer counseling if malformations are detected, and the patient's wishes should be respected regarding termination or continuation of a pregnancy with a known fetal anomaly.

Intrauterine fetal demise has become less prevalent among diabetic women but is still seen at high rates among women with poor glycemic control or with disturbances of fetal growth.[119] In the past, efforts to prevent third-trimester stillbirth sometimes led to a policy of routine preterm delivery, usually by cesarean section, with a high prevalence of infant respiratory distress syndrome and neonatal death from the complications of prematurity. These policies have since been replaced by techniques of antepartum assessment of fetal well-being, with early delivery only for clear fetal compromise. With good maternal metabolic control and reassuring findings on fetal testing, elective induction of labor is planned at or near term. If delivery is contemplated before 39 weeks' gestation, amniocentesis may be considered to document fetal lung maturity, which is frequently delayed among fetuses of diabetic mothers.[119] Cesarean section need not be performed if fetal macrosomia is not an issue.

Fetal growth is commonly deranged in diabetic pregnancies. In the absence of maternal vascular disease, hyperglycemia in the mother leads to fetal hyperglycemia, and the unaffected fetal pancreas produces high levels of insulin, which promotes fetal growth. With maternal vascular disease, however, such as hypertension, placental blood flow is impaired and fetal growth is restricted.

The incidence of hypertensive disorders of pregnancy among 175 patients with type 1 diabetes was 15% in a study by Siddiqi and colleagues,[120] which represents a doubling of the incidence among the general pregnancy population. Patients with preexisting vascular disease of any type were at 50% greater risk than those without preexisting disease.[120] Poor glycemic control, as reflected by glycosylated hemoglobin (glycohemoglobin) concentrations, was more likely to be associated with hypertensive disorders of pregnancy. There was no significant difference in neonatal outcome among babies born to hypertensive women or normotensive diabetic women.

In another study by the same group, women with type 1 diabetes and retinopathy at the start of pregnancy were more likely to experience progression of retinopathy if they were also hypertensive.[121] More than twice as many of the diabetics with chronic hypertension in this study experienced progression of retinopathy, compared with those who remained normotensive (61% versus 25%). For women with pregnancy-induced hypertension, 50% showed progression. Worsening of retinopathy during pregnancy was also associated with both poor first-trimester glucose control, as measured by glycohemoglobin testing, and with the magnitude of the decrease in glycohemoglobin from first to second trimester.

The diabetic woman with nephropathy is at added risk for complications. The risk of IUGR is estimated at 17% to 25% (compared with 5%–10% of controls), and fetal distress complicates nearly 25% of such pregnancies. The risk of preterm delivery is well above 50%, compared with a preterm birth rate in the general population of 7% to 10%.[116] Of maternal complications, preeclampsia is the most frequent, occurring in at least 40%. Higher degrees of proteinuria at baseline evaluation are associated with higher preeclampsia risk.[116]

The distinction between true preeclampsia and worsening of nephropathy cannot always be made; increases in blood pressure and proteinuria characterize both. Unfortunately, the treatment is quite different: The former is best treated by bringing about delivery, the latter by bed rest and an increase in drug therapy.

Other maternal complications in diabetic pregnancy include diabetic ketoacidosis, hypoglycemia, and pyelonephritis. Maternal death is rare unless diabetes is complicated by myocardial infarction, in which case mortality may be as high as 50%.[122] Unfortunately, nearly 90% of pregestational diabetic women who sustain a myocardial infarction during pregnancy have had no previous diagnosis of coronary artery disease.

Gestational Diabetes

Gestational diabetes (GDM) is defined as carbohydrate intolerance of varying severity with its onset or recognition during the index pregnancy.[123] GDM is believed to affect approximately 3% to 5% of all pregnancies in the United States[106] and accounts for about 90% of all diabetic pregnancies.

In normal pregnancy, circulating insulin is increased and insulin sensitivity is decreased. Women with GDM manifest an exaggerated glycemic response to mixed-meal feeding, a diminished peak insulin response, and a further decrement in insulin sensitivity.[124] Women who had gestational diabetes often have persistent defects in insulin secretion and sensitivity months after delivery, which puts them at risk for development of type 2 diabetes. Persistent maternal hyperglycemia puts the fetus at risk for macrosomia and the neonate at risk for several metabolic complications as well as the possibility of delayed pulmonary maturation.[125] Glucose control, however, may not be sufficient.

A 1991 case-control study in Israel confirmed higher rates of neonatal macrosomia, hypoglycemia, hyperbilirubinemia, hypocalcemia, and polycythemia when mothers had GDM than when glucose tolerance testing was normal.[126] These differences were found, interestingly enough, despite stringent metabolic control and the maintenance of euglycemia. Severe perinatal morbidity and perinatal mortality, however, are not increased among infants born to mothers with GDM.[127]

The greatest significance of GDM may be its efficacy as a marker for the eventual development of type 2 diabetes. In 1990, O'Sullivan summarized studies evaluating the relationship between GDM and later development of overt diabetes, and found a wide range of incidence rates.[128] Commonly accepted figures put the likelihood of type 2 diabetes at approximately 20% 8 to 10 years after a diagnosis of GDM, with the lifetime risk at 50%.

Screening for GDM is somewhat controversial. The Third International Conference on Gestational Diabetes Mellitus recommended continued universal screening at 24 to 28 weeks of pregnancy, using a 50-g glucose challenge.[129] A venous plasma glucose level of 140 mg/dL should be followed by a full 100-g, 3-hour glucose tolerance test

TABLE 9–9. CRITERIA FOR THE DIAGNOSIS OF GESTATIONAL DIABETES USING 100-GRAM ORAL GLUCOSE TOLERANCE TEST

Any two of the following (all are plasma glucose values in mg/dL):
    Fasting $\geq$ 105
      1 h $\geq$ 190
      2 h $\geq$ 165
      3 h $\geq$ 145

Data from Metzger BE, Organizing Committee. Summary and recommendations of the Third International Workshop: Conference on Gestational Diabetes Mellitus. Diabetes 1991;40(suppl 2):197–201.

performed in the fasting state. Criteria for the diagnosis of gestational diabetes are given in Table 9–9.

The 1997 report of the Expert Committee on the Diagnosis and Classification of Diabetes Mellitus departs from these recommendations in stating that pregnant women who are younger than 25 years old, of normal body weight, have no first-degree relatives with diabetes, and are not members of a high-risk ethnic group (e.g., Hispanic, Native American, African American) need not be screened for GDM.[9]

The Fourth International Workshop-Conference on Gestational Diabetes Mellitus recommended continued universal screening for GDM among women in high-risk groups but retreated from this stance in women who are low risk.[130] This panel also called for a change in the values of the 3-hour glucose tolerance test to the levels advocated by Carpenter and Coustan (Table 9–10).[130, 131]

In sum, all three bodies state that use of

TABLE 9–10. MODIFIED CRITERIA FOR GLUCOSE TOLERANCE TESTING IN GESTATIONAL DIABETES

TIME	WHOLE BLOOD (SOMOGYI-NELSON)	PLASMA (GLUCOSE OXIDASE)
Fasting	90 mg/dL	95 mg/dL
1 h	165 mg/dL	180 mg/dL
2 h	143 mg/dL	155 mg/dL
3 h	127 mg/dL	140 mg/dL

*If two threshold values are met or exceeded, gestational diabetes mellitus is the diagnosis.

Modified from Carpenter MW, Coustan DR. Criteria for screening tests for gestational diabetes. Am J Obstet Gynecol 1982;144:768–783; reprinted in Ellenberg and Rifkin: Diabetes Mellitus, 5th ed. Stamford, CT: Appleton & Lange, 1997.

the 75-g glucose tolerance test, as employed in the diagnosis of diabetes in nonpregnant individuals, may eventually become standard practice in testing for GDM as well.[9, 129, 130]

Lactation in Diabetes

The issue of lactation and breast-feeding management among diabetic women must be addressed. Breast milk is, of course, the optimal food for newborns, and this is no less true among the offspring of diabetic mothers.

One study has addressed the incidence of breast-feeding among diabetic women.[132] In this small case-control study, 53% of pregestational insulin-dependent diabetic women planned to breast-feed, which was no different from the percentage in the control population. Initiation of breast-feeding was, however, delayed among the diabetic women: By the third postpartum day, only 12% had initiated breast-feeding, compared with 100% of the control subjects. No doubt this difference related to the unavailability of the first group of infants, all of whom were placed in the neonatal intensive care unit for at least 8 hours after birth. Early mother-infant separation resulted in an average delay of breast-feeding initiation of 36 hours among diabetic women, compared with 12 hours among nondiabetic women. In addition, all babies born to diabetic mothers were offered artificial formula on their second day of life, whereas no baby born to a control breast-feeding mother was given formula. These two factors—early mother-infant separation and the offering of a bottle—are detrimental to the establishment of effective breast-feeding.[133]

Breast-feeding may be even more important for children born to type 1 diabetic mothers than for other children, inasmuch as breast-feeding may protect the genetically susceptible child against the later development of diabetes.[133, 134] Breast-feeding of less than 3 months' duration, or not at all, is associated with an up to 50% increase in the odds of development of type 1 diabetes.[135–138] Speculation as to the cause of the increased risk associated with artificial infant feeding centers on the role of early exposure to cow's milk proteins. Patients with type 1 diabetes have humoral and cellular immune responses to cow's milk antigens, and the antibody directed against bovine serum albumin cross-reacts with human β-cell proteins.[139] Thus, exposure to cow's milk proteins may provoke an antibody response in genetically susceptible children, which then cross-reacts with β-cell antigens, either causing or accelerating autoimmune pancreatic destruction.

Women with type 1 diabetes should be encouraged to breast-feed. Lactogenesis may be somewhat delayed in these women,[140] an effect that can be offset by good metabolic control and by avoidance of mother-infant separation. Preliminary work among Pima Indians seems to suggest a higher risk for type 2 diabetes among adults who were not breast-fed in infancy, an effect that would have to be mediated by some other mechanism.[141]

In managing the diabetic who is breast-feeding, the physician must factor in the metabolic cost of lactation into diet and drug therapy. Lactation requires an additional 300 to 500 kcal/day,[133] which can be provided as additional intake in thin or normal-weight women; in obese women, it can be incorporated into a weight-maintenance or gradual weight-loss program. Insulin doses may be adjusted downward accordingly. Some type 2 diabetic women who had been receiving oral agents before pregnancy may require no drug therapy at all while breast-feeding.

For the patient who is both diabetic and hypertensive, the choice of pharmacologic agent may be influenced by the decision to breast-feed. The American Academy of Pediatrics has published a list of drugs that are transferred into breast milk.[142] Such transfer of drugs and chemicals depends on multiple factors, including (1) the degree of protein binding (only free drug can pass from maternal plasma into milk), (2) the volume of distribution in the mother, and (3) the pH difference between maternal plasma and breast milk. When a drug can be found in breast milk, it is typically found in low concentrations and may or may not have clinical effects on the newborn. Insulin does not pass into breast milk.

Of the oral antidiabetic agents, acarbose is probably the best choice, because absorption from the gastrointestinal tract is poor, ranging from 0.5% to 1.7%. Both glipizide and glyburide, though highly protein-bound, have small volumes of distribution and, therefore, somewhat higher potential for passage into milk. They are, however, better choices than chlorpropamide, which has been used in the past. Metformin is probably the least desirable of the oral hypoglycemics for the nursing mother, given its low protein binding.[143]

No large studies are available regarding these drugs, and if doubt exists, the nursing infant may undergo capillary blood glucose testing. Captopril, enalapril, atenolol, clonidine, diltiazem, hydralazine, methyldopa, metoprolol, minoxidil, nifedipine, prazosin, and most of the diuretics are compatible with breast-feeding, although diuretics may result in diminished milk production.[133, 142]

Diabetes and Cancer

Shifting gears into the realm of the pathologic, we now briefly discuss cancers of the breast and reproductive tract. Diabetes has been linked with an increased risk of both endometrial and breast cancer. In a case-control study of 5000 Italian women with cancer of the breast, ovary, or endometrium,[144] the relative risk (RR) for ovarian cancer was decreased slightly but not significantly among diabetic patients (RR, 0.7, 95%; confidence interval [CI] 0.5–1.0), as was the breast cancer risk (RR, 0.8, 95%; CI 0.6–1.0), but the relative risk of endometrial cancer was 3.4 (RR, 3.4, 95%; CI 2.7–4.3). Adjustment for BMI reduced the risk only slightly, to 2.8. Other epidemiologic studies have repeatedly documented an increase in the endometrial cancer risk among diabetic women, usually about twofold.[145] An association has also been found between endometrial cancer and hypertension, although of lesser magnitude, about a 50% increase in risk.[145] Both relationships remain even after adjustment for confounding factors such as obesity and socioeconomic status. It is not clear whether the presence of both diabetes and hypertension further increases endometrial cancer risk.

A Finnish group[146] performed screening endometrial biopsies in nearly 600 women with diabetes or hypertension, or with both, and found that 13% of the premenopausal and 3.9% of the postmenopausal women with diabetes had preinvasive histopathologic lesions (atypical or adenomatous hyperplasia or carcinoma in situ), compared with 4.8% of premenopausal women with hypertension and 0.8% of postmenopausal

women with hypertension. Women who had both diabetes and hypertension were not at any increased risk compared with women with diabetes alone.

The relationship between breast cancer and diabetes is not as strong, although there does appear to be a relative risk of 1.2 to 1.5.[147, 148] Demographically, obesity and increased waist-hip ratios are associated with a higher rate of breast cancer.[149] These are clearly a feature of type 2 diabetes (see earlier). Furthermore, nondiabetic postmenopausal women with early breast cancer are more insulin-resistant than controls.[151] Human breast cancers have insulin receptors.[152] An intriguing hypothesis has been proposed that hyperinsulinemia, as seen in many women with type 2 diabetes and hypertension, may predispose to breast cancer either by suppressing sex hormone–binding globulin, thus making available more free estradiol and androgens, or by increasing effective circulating levels of insulin-like growth factor-1 (IGF-1), a mitogen.[150]

Hormone Replacement Therapy in Diabetes

As a woman passes into menopause, other issues come to the fore. In these years, women begin to lose their protection against coronary artery disease,[153] and as we have seen, rates of hypertension and diabetes increase. The loss of endogenous estrogen has also been implicated in osteoporosis and in the development of Alzheimer's disease.[154] The decision whether to begin hormone replacement therapy must be made.

Hormone replacement therapy (HRT) in some studies has been shown to reduce cardiovascular mortality by as much as 50%.[149] Women with other risk factors for coronary artery disease, such as smoking, obesity, hypertension, or diabetes, enjoy the greatest reduction in cardiovascular mortality when taking HRT. The benefits appear to diminish after 10 years of use, however, at which time breast cancer mortality among long-term HRT users increases by as much as 40%.[155] However, coronary artery disease is responsible for 30% of deaths among women aged 50 to 94 years, compared with fewer than 3% of deaths attributed to breast cancer.[156] HRT does not worsen hypertension or insulin resistance; in fact, the estrogen moiety may improve insulin sensitivity somewhat, an effect that can nonetheless be offset by the progestin component.[157] Orally administered estrogen appears to increase HDL cholesterol, whereas transdermal preparations do not[157]; again, the relatively androgenic effect of the progestin moiety may obviate this beneficial effect. Micronized progesterone or, to a lesser degree, medroxyprogesterone acetate, is preferred as HRT.

After hysterectomy, unopposed estrogen is a valid alternative. There are no specific studies examining metabolic effects of various HRT regimens among women with type 2 diabetes. The inferences drawn from studies in other populations are that the metabolic profile of type 2 diabetics need not be worsened, and in fact may be improved, with the use of appropriately designed hormone replacement regimens. The physician caring for diabetic women with or without hypertension should consider HRT an important option in their care.

References

1. Harris, MI. Summary. Classification, diagnostic criteria, and screening for diabetes. *In* National Diabetes Data Group. Diabetes in America, 2nd ed. Bethesda: National Institutes of Health, Pub No. 95-1468, 1995, pp 1–36.
2. Reiber GE, Boyko EJ, Smith DG. Lower extremity foot ulcers and amputations in diabetes. *In* National Diabetes Data Group. Diabetes in America, 2nd ed. Bethesda: National Institutes of Health, Pub No. 95-1468, 1995, pp 409–428.
3. Nelson RG, Knowler WC, Pettitt DJ, Bennett PH. Kidney diseases in diabetics. *In* National Diabetes Data Group. Diabetes in America, 2nd ed. Bethesda: National Institutes of Health, Pub No. 95-1468, 1995, pp 349–400.
4. Klein R, Klein BEK. Vision disorders in diabetes. *In* National Diabetes Data Group. Diabetes in America, 2nd ed. Bethesda: National Institutes of Health, Pub No. 95-1468, 1995, pp 293–338.
5. Wingard DL, Barrett-Connor E. Heart disease and diabetes. *In* National Diabetes Data Group. Diabetes in America, 2nd ed. Bethesda: National Institutes of Health, Pub No. 95-1468, 1995, pp 429–448.
6. National Diabetes Data Group. Classification and diagnosis of diabetes mellitus and other categories of glucose intolerance. Diabetes 1979;28:1039–1057.
7. World Health Organization (WHO). Report of the Expert Committee on Diabetes. Geneva: WHO, 1980. Technical Report Series, No. 646.
8. World Health Organization (WHO) Diabetes mellitus: Report of a WHO study group. Geneva: WHO, 1985. Technical Report Series, No. 727.
9. American Diabetes Association. Report of the Expert Committee on the Diagnosis and Classification of Diabetes Mellitus. Diabetes Care 1997; 20:1183–1197.
10. LaPorte RE, Matsushima M, Chang Y-F. Prevalence and incidence of insulin-dependent diabetes mellitus. *In* National Diabetes Data Group. Diabetes in America, 2nd ed. Bethesda: National Institutes of Health, Pub No. 95-1468, 1995, pp 37–46.
11. Fishbein H, Palumbo PJ. Acute metabolic complications in diabetes. *In* National Diabetes Data Group. Diabetes in America, 2nd ed. Bethesda: National Institutes of Health, Pub No. 95-1468, 1995, pp 283–292.
12. Dorman JS, McCarthy BJ, O'Leary LA, Koehler AN. Risk factors for insulin-dependent diabetes. *In* National Diabetes Data Group. Diabetes in America, 2nd ed. Bethesda: National Institutes of Health, Pub No. 95-1468, 1995, pp 165–178.
13. Olmos P, Ahearn R, Heaton DA, et al. The significance of concordance rate for type I (insulin-dependent) diabetes in identical twins. Diabetologia 1988;31:747–750.
14. Dahlquist GG, Blom LG, Persson L, et al. Dietary factors and the risk of developing insulin dependent diabetes in childhood. BMJ 1990;300:1302–1306.
15. Kostraba JN, Cruickshanks KJ, Lawler-Heavner J, et al. Early exposure to cow's milk and solid foods in infancy, genetic predisposition, and risk of IDDM. Diabetes 1993;42:288–295.
16. Savilahti E, Tuomilehto J, Savkkonen TT, et al. Increased levels of cow's milk and beta-lactoglobulin antibodies in young children with newly diagnosed IDDM. Diabetes Care 1993;16:984–89.
17. Reaven GM. Role of insulin resistance in human disease. Diabetes 1988;37:1595–1607.
18. DeFronzo RA, Bonadonna RC, Ferrannini E. Pathogenesis of NIDDM: A balanced overview. Diabetes Care 1992;15:318–368.
19. Kenny SJ, Aubert RE, Geiss LS. Prevalence and incidence of non–insulin-dependent diabetes. *In* National Diabetes Data Group. Diabetes in America, 2nd ed. Bethesda: National Institutes of Health, Pub No. 95-1468, 1995, pp 47–68.
20. Harris MI, Hadden WC, Knowler WC, Bennett PH. Prevalence of diabetes and impaired glucose tolerance and plasma glucose levels in US population aged 20–74 yr. Diabetes 1987;36:523–534.
21. Hamman RF. Genetic and environmental determinants of non–insulin-dependent diabetes mellitus (NIDDM). Diabetes Metab Rev 1992;8:287–338.
22. Rewers M, Hamman RF. Risk factors for non-insulin-dependent diabetes. *In* National Diabetes Data Group, Diabetes in America, 2nd ed. Bethesda: National Institutes of Health, Pub No. 95-1468, 1995, pp 179–220.
23. Kahn SE, Porte D. The pathophysiology of type II (non–insulin-dependent) diabetes mellitus: Implications for treatment. *In* Porte D, Sherwin RS (eds). Ellenberg and Rifkin's Diabetes Mellitus, 5th ed. Stamford, CT: Appleton & Lange, 1997, pp 487–512.
24. Saad MF, Knowler WC, Pettitt DJ, et al. The natural history of impaired glucose tolerance in the Pima Indians. N Engl J Med 1988;319:1500–1506.
25. Haffner SM, Stern MP Hazuda HP, et al. Hyperinsulinemia in a population at high risk for non–insulin-dependent diabetes mellitus. N Engl J Med 1986;315:220–224.
26. Martin BC, Warram JH, Krolewski AS, et al. Role of glucose and insulin resistance in development

of type II diabetes mellitus: Results of a 25-year follow-up study. Lancet 1992;340:925–929.

27. Semplicini A, Ceolotto G, Massimino M, et al. Interactions between insulin and sodium homeostasis in essential hypertension. Am J Med Sci 1994;307(suppl 1):S43–46.

28. Rocchini AP. The relationship of sodium sensitivity to insulin resistance. Am J Med Sci 1994;307 (suppl 1):S75–S80.

29. Barbagallo M, Resnick LM. The role of glucose in diabetic hypertension: Effects on intracellular calcium metabolism. Am J Med Sci 1994;307 (suppl 1): S60–S65.

30. Sowers JR, Sowers PS, Peuler JD. Role of insulin resistance and hyperinsulinemia in development of hypertension and atherosclerosis. J Lab Clin Med 1994;123:647–652.

31. Epstein M, Sowers JR. Diabetes mellitus and hypertension. Hypertension 1992;19:403–418.

32. Bennet PH, Haffner S, Kasiske BL, et al. Screening and management of microalbuminuria in patients with diabetes mellitus: Recommendations to the Scientific Advisory Board of the National Kidney Foundation from an ad hoc committee of the Council on Diabetes Mellitus of the National Kidney Foundation. Am J Kidney Dis 1995;25:107–112.

33. Alzaid AA. Microalbuminuria in patients with NIDDM: An overview. Diabetes Care 1996;19:79–89.

34. Rabkin R, Fervenza FC. Renal hypertrophy and kidney disease in diabetes. Diabetes Metab Rev 1996;12:217–241.

35. Mogensen CE, Hansen KW, Osterby R, Damsgaard EM. Blood pressure elevation versus abnormal albuminuria in the genesis and prediction of renal disease in diabetes. Diabetes Care 1992;15:1192–1204.

36. Mogensen CE, Christensen CK. Predicting diabetic nephropathy in insulin-dependent patients. N Engl J Med 1984;31:89–93.

37. Parving HH, Smidt UM, Friesberg B, et al. A prospective study of glomerular filtration rate and arterial blood pressure in insulin-dependent diabetics with diabetic nephropathy. Diabetologia 1981;20:457–461.

38. Leese GP, Vora JP. The management of hypertension in diabetes: With special reference to diabetic kidney disease. Diabetes Med 1996;13:401–410.

39. Cowie CC, Harris MI. Physical and metabolic characteristics of persons with diabetes. In National Diabetes Data Group. Diabetes in America, 2nd ed. Bethesda: National Institutes of Health, Pub No. 95-1468, 1995; pp 117–164.

40. Sowers JR, Epstein M. Diabetes mellitus and associated hypertension, vascular disease, and nephropathy: An update. Hypertension 1995;26(pt 1):869–879.

41. Haffner S, Valdez R, Morales PA, et al. Greater effect of glycemia on hypertension in women than in men. Diabetes Care 1992;15:1277–1284.

42. Morris AD, Connell JMC. Insulin resistance and essential hypertension: Mechanisms and clinical implications. Am J Med Sci 1994;304(suppl 1):S47–S52.

43. Mitchell BD, Stern MP, Haffner SM, et al. Risk factors for cardiovascular mortality in Mexican-Americans and non-Hispanic whites: The San Antonio Heart Study. Am J Epidemiol 1990;131:423–433.

44. Modan M, Halkin H, Alm S, et al. Hyperinsulinemia: A link between hypertension, obesity and glucose intolerance. J Clin Invest 1985;75:809–817.

45. Ferrannini E, Haffner SM, Mitchell BD, Stern MP. Hyperinsulinaemia: The key feature of a cardiovascular and metabolic syndrome. Diabetologia 1991;34:416–422.

46. Viberti G, Yip-Messent J, Morocutti A. Diabetic nephropathy: Future avenue. Diabetes Care 1992;15:1216–1225.

47. Hostetter TH. Diabetic nephropathy: Metabolic versus hemodynamic considerations. Diabetes Care 1992;15:1205–1215.

48. Wilson PWF, Cupples AD, Kannel WB. Is hyperglycemia associated with cardiovascular disease? The Framingham Study. Am Heart J 1991;121:586–590.

49. Manson JE, Colditz GA, Stampfer MJ, et al. A prospective study of maturity-onset diabetes mellitus and risk of coronary heart disease and stroke in women. Arch Intern Med 1991;151:1141–1147.

50. Reis SE, Zell KA, Holubkov R. Women's hearts are different. Curr Probl Obstet Gynecol Fertil 1997;20:69–92.

51. The National High Blood Pressure Working Group. National High Blood Pressure Education Program Working Group Report on Hypertension in Diabetes. Hypertension 1994;23:145–158.

52. Assman G, Schulte H. The Prospective Cardiovascular Munster (PROCAM) Study: Prevalence of hyperlipidemia in persons with hypertension and/or diabetes mellitus and the relationship to coronary heart disease. Am Heart J 1988;116(6 pt 2):1713–1724.

53. The Fifth Report of the Joint National Committee on Detection, Evaluation, and Treatment of High Blood Pressure (JNC V). Arch Intern Med 1993;153:154–183.

54. Christlieb AR. Treatment selection considerations for the hypertensive diabetic patient. Arch Intern Med 1990;150:1167–1174.

55. Breyer JA, Hunsicker LG, Bain RP, et al. Angiotensin-converting enzyme inhibition in diabetic nephropathy. Kidney Int 1994;45(suppl 45):S156–S160.

56. Ravid M, Savin H, Jutrin I, et al. Long-term effect of ACE inhibition on development of nephropathy in diabetes mellitus type II. Kidney Int 1994;45(suppl 45):S161–S164.

57. Ravid M, Savin H, Jutrin I, et al. Long-term stabilizing effect of angiotensin-converting enzyme inhibition on plasma creatinine and on proteinuria in normotensive type II diabetic patients. Ann Intern Med 1993;118:577–581.

58. Dawson KG, McKenzie JK, Ross SA, et al. Report of the Canadian Hypertension Society Consensus Conference: 5. Hypertension and diabetes. Can Med Assoc J 1993;149:821–826.

59. American Diabetes Association. Clinical Practice Guidelines 1996. Treatment of hypertension in diabetes. Diabetes Care 1996;19(suppl 1):S107–113.

60. American Diabetes Association. Clinical Practice Guidelines 1996. Nutritional recommendations and principles for individuals with diabetes mellitus. Diabetes Care 1996;19(suppl 1):S16–S19.

61. American Diabetes Association. Clinical Practice Guidelines 1996. Diabetes mellitus and exercise. Diabetes Care 119:19(suppl 1):S30.

62. Kasiske BL, Kalil RSN, Ma JZ, et al. Effect of antihypertensive therapy on the kidney in patients with diabetes: A meta-regression analysis. Ann Intern Med 1993;118:129–138.
63. Veenstra J, van der Hulst JP, Wildenborg IH, et al. Effect of antihypertensive drugs on insulin absorption. Diabetes Care 1991;14:1089–1092.
64. The Treatment of Mild Hypertension Study Group. Treatment of Mild Hypertension study: Final results. JAMA 1993;270:713–724.
65. The Diabetes Control and Complications Research Group. The effect of intensive treatment of diabetes on the development and progression of long-term complications in insulin-dependent diabetes mellitus. N Engl J Med 1993;329:977–986.
66. Nathan DM. Insulin treatment of noninsulin-dependent diabetes mellitus. In Porte D, Sherwin RJ (eds). Ellenberg and Rifkin's Diabetes Mellitus, 5th ed. Stamford, CT: Appleton & Lange, 1997.
67. Bressler R, Johnson DG. Pharmacologic regulation of blood glucose levels in non–insulin-dependent diabetes mellitus. Arch Intern Med 1997;157:836–848.
68. Nolan JJ, Ludvik B, Beerdsen P, et al. Improvement in glucose tolerance and insulin resistance in obese subjects treated with troglitazone. N Engl J Med 1994;331:1188–1193.
69. Berkowitz K, Peters R, Kjos SL, et al. Effect of troglitazone on insulin sensitivity and pancreatic beta-cell function in women at high risk for NIDDM. Diabetes 1996;45:1572–1579.
70. Antonucci T, Whitcomb R, McLain R, Lockwood D. Impaired glucose tolerance is normalized by treatment with the thiazolidinedione troglitazone. Diabetes Care 1997;20:188–193.
71. Iwamoto Y, Kosaka K, Kuzuya T, et al. Effects of troglitazone: A new hypoglycemic agent in patients with NIDDM poorly controlled with diet therapy. Diabetes Care 1996;19:151–156.
72. Johnson JL, Wolf SL, Kabadi UM. Efficacy of insulin and sulfonylurea combination therapy in type II diabetes. Arch Intern Med 1996;156:259–264
73. Golay A, Guillet-Dauphine N, Fendel A, et al. The insulin-sparing effect of metformin in insulin-treated diabetic patients. Diabetes Metab Rev 1995;11(suppl 1):S63–S67.
74. Chiasson JL, Josse RG, Hunt JA. The efficacy of acarbose in the treatment of paptients with non–insulin-dependent diabetes mellitus: A multi-center controlled clinical trial. Ann Intern Med 1994;121:928–935.
75. Poretsky L, Kalin MF. The gonadotropic function of insulin. Endocr Rev 1987;8:132–141.
76. Djursing H, Nyholm HC, Hagen C, et al. Clinical and hormonal characteristics in women with anovulation and insulin-treated diabetes mellitus. Am J Obstet Gynecol 1982;143:876–882.
77. Joslin EP, Root HF, White P. The growth, development and prognosis of diabetic children. JAMA 1925;85:420–422.
78. Dunaif A. Hyperandrogenic anovulation (polycystic ovary syndrome): A unique disorder of insulin action associated with an increased risk of non–insulin-dependent diabetes mellitus. Am J Med 1995;98(suppl 1):S33–S39.
79. Dunaif A, Futterweit W, Segal KR, Dobrjansky A. Profound peripheral insulin resistance, independent of obesity, in the polycystic ovary syndrome. Diabetes 1989;38:1165–1174.
80. Dunaif A, Segal KR, Shelley DR, et al. Evidence for distinctive and intrinsic defects in insulin action in the polycystic ovary syndrome. Diabetes 1992;41:1257–1266.
81. Dunaif E, Johansson S, Lindstedt G, et al. Women with polycystic ovary syndrome wedge resected in 1956 to 1965: A long-term follow-up focusing on natural history and circulating hormones. Fertil Steril 1992;57:505–513.
82. Hatcher RA, Trussell J, Stewart F, et al. Contraceptive Technology, 16th ed. New York: Irvington Publishers, 1994.
83. Farley TMM, Rosenberg MJ, Rowe PJ, et al. Intrauterine devices and pelvic inflammatory disease: An international perspective. Lancet 1992;339:785–788.
84. Lee NC, Rubin GL. The intrauterine device and pelvic inflammatory disease. Obstet Gynecol 1983;62:1–6.
85. Lee NC, Rubin GL. The intrauterine device and pelvic inflammatory disease revisited: New results from the Women's Health Study. Obstet Gynecol 1988;72:1–6.
86. Kjos SL. Contraception in diabetic women. Obstet Gynecol Clin North Am 1996;23:243–258.
87. Kjos SL, Ballagh SA, LaCour M, et al. The copper T380A intrauterine device in women with type II diabetes mellitus. Obstet Gynecol 1994;84:1006–1009.
88. Skouby SO, Molsted-Pedersen L, Kosonen A. Consequences of intrauterine contraception in diabetic women. Fertil Steril 1984;42:568–572.
89. Layde PM, Feral V. Further analysis of mortality in oral contraceptive users: Royal College of General Practicioners' oral contraceptive study. Lancet 1981;1:541–546.
90. Stampfer MJ, Willer WC, Colditz GA, et al. A prospective study of past use of oral contraceptive agents and risk of cardiovascular diseases. N Engl J Med 1988;319:1313–1319.
91. Porter JB, Hunter JR, Jick H, et al. Oral contraceptives and nonfatal vascular disease. Obstet Gynecol 1985;66:1–4.
92. Porter JB, Jick H, Walker AM. Mortality among oral contraceptive users. Obstet Gynecol 1987;70:29–32.
93. Rosenberg L, Palmer JR, Lesko SM, et al. Oral contraceptive use and the risk of myocardial infarction. Am J Epidemiol 1990;131:1009–1016.
94. Wilson ES, Cruickshank J, McMaster M, et al. A prospective controlled study of the effect on blood pressure of contraceptive preparations containing different types of dosages and progestogen. Br J Obstet Gynecol 1984;91:1254–1260.
95. Godsland IF, Crook D, Simpson R, et al. The effects of different formulations of oral contraceptive agents on lipid and carbohydrate metabolism. N Engl J Med 1990;323:1375–1381.
96. Perlman JA, Russell-Briefel R, Ezzati T, et al. Oral glucose tolerance and the potency of contraceptive progestins. J Chron Dis 1985;38:857–864.
97. Godsland IF, Walton C, Felton C. Insulin resistance, secretion and metabolism in users of oral contraceptives. J Clin Endocrinol Metab 1992;74:64–70.
98. Lim KG, Isles CG, Hodsman GP, et al. Malignant hypertension in women of childbearing age and its relation to the oral contraceptive pill. Br Med J 1987;294:1057–1059.

99. Cook NR, Scherr PA, Evans DA, et al. Regression analysis on blood pressure with oral contraceptive use. Am J Epidemiol 1985;121:530–540.

100. Radberg T, Gustafson A, Skryten A, et al. Oral contraception in diabetic women: Diabetes control, serum and high-density lipoprotein lipids during low-dose progestogen, combined oestrogen-progestogen and non-hormonal contraception. Acta Endocrinol 1981;98:246–251.

101. Skouby SO, Molsted-Pedersen, Kuhl C, et al. Oral contraceptives in diabetic women: Metabolic effects of four compounds with different estrogen-progestogen profiles. Fertil Steril 1986;46:858–864.

102. Klein BEK, Moss SE, Klein R. Oral contraceptives in women with diabetes. Diabetes Care 1990; 13:895–898.

103. Lidegaard O. Oral contraceptives, pregnancy and the risk of cerebral thromboembolism: The influence of diabetes, hypertension, migraine and previous thrombotic disease. Br J Obstet Gynaecol 1995;102:153–159.

104. Fahmy K, Abdel-Razik M, Shaaraway M, et al. Effect of long-acting progestogen-only injectable contraceptives on carbohydrate metabolism and its hormonal profile. Contraception 1991;44:419–429.

105. Konje JC, Otolorin EO, Ladipo AO. The effect of continuous subdermal levonorgestrel (Norplant) on carbohydrate metabolism. Am J Obstet Gynecol 1992;166 (1 pt 1):15–19.

106. Miller E, Hare JW, Cloherty JP, et al. Elevated maternal hemoglobin A1c in early pregnancy and major congenital anomalies in infants of diabetic mothers. N Engl J Med 1981;304:1331–1334.

107. Mills JL, Simpson JL, Driscoll SG. The Diabetes in Early Pregnancy Study: Incidence of spontaneous abortion among normal and insulin-dependent diabetic women whose pregnancies were identified within 21 days of conception. N Engl J Med 1988;319:1617–1623.

108. Fuhrman K, Reiher H, Semmler K, et al. Prevention of congenital malformations in infants of diabetic mothers. Diabetes Care 1983;6;219–223.

109. Goldman JA, Dicker D, Feldberg D. Pregnancy outcome in patients with insulin-dependent diabetes mellitus and preconceptional diabetes control: A comparative study. Am J Obstet Gynecol 1986;155:293–297.

110. Steel JM, Johnstone FD, Hepburn DA, Smith AF. Can prepregnancy care of diabetic women reduce the risk of anomalous babies? BMJ 1990;301:1070–1074.

111. Kitzmiller JL, Gavin LA, Ginn GD, et al. Preconception care of diabetes. Glycemic control prevents congenital malformations. JAMA 1991; 265:731–736.

112. Reece EA, Eriksson UJ. The pathogenesis of diabetes-associated congenital malformations. Obstet Gynecol Clin North Am 1996;23:29–45.

113. Centers for Disease Control. Recommendations for the use of folic acid to reduce the number of cases of spina bifida and other neural tube defects. MMWR Morb Mortal Wkly Rep 1992;41 (No. RR-14):1–7.

114. Shotan A, Widerhorn J, Hurst A, Elkayam U. Risks of angiotensin-converting enzyme inhibition during pregnancy: Experimental and clinical evidence, potential mechanisms, and recommendations for use. Am J Med 1994;96:451–456.

115. Fairlie FM, Sibai BM. Hypertensive disorders in pregnancy. In Reece EA, Hobbins JC, Mahoney MJ, Petrie RH (eds). Medicine of the Fetus and Mother. Philadelphia: JB Lippincott, 1992.

116. Kitzmiller JL, Combs CA. Diabetic nephropathy and pregnancy. Obstet Gynecol Clin North Am 1996;23:173–203.

117. Homko CJ, Khandelwal M. Glucose monitoring and insulin therapy during pregnancy. Obstet Gynecol Clin North Am 1996;23:47–74.

118. Reece EA, Hagay Z, Roberts AB, et al. Fetal behavioral responses during induced hypoglycemia in pregnant women using the insulin clamp technique. Am J Obstet Gynecol 1995;172:151–155.

119. Landon MB, Gabbe SG. Fetal surveillance and timing of delivery in pregnancy complicated by diabetes mellitus. Obstet Gynecol Clin North Am 1996;23:109–123.

120. Siddiqi T, Rosenn B, Mimouni F, Khoury J, Miodovnik M. Hypertension during pregnancy in insulin-dependent diabetic women. Obstet Gynecol 1991;7:514–519.

121. Rosenn B, Miodovnik M, Kranias G, et al. Progression of diabetic retinopathy in pregnancy: Association with hypertension in pregnancy. Am J Obstet Gynecol 1992;166:1214–1218.

122. Gordon MC, Landon MB, Boyle J, et al. Coronary artery disease in insulin-dependent diabetes mellitus of pregnancy (class H): A review of the literature. Obstet Gynecol Surv 1996;51:437–444.

123. American College of Obstetricians and Gynecologists (ACOG). Technical Bulletin No. 200. Diabetes and Pregnancy. Washington, DC: ACOG, 1994.

124. Lesser KB, Carpenter MW. Metabolic changes associated with normal pregnancy and pregnancy complicated by diabetes mellitus. Semin Perinatol 1994;18:399–406.

125. Langer O, Hod M. Management of gestational diabetes mellitus. Clin Obstet Gynecol North Am 1996;23:137–160.

126. Hod M, Merlob P, Fiedman S, et al. Gestational diabetes mellitus: A survey of perinatal complications in the 1980s. Diabetes 1991;40(suppl 2):74–78.

127. Coustan DR. Diagnosis of gestational diabetes: What are our objectives? Diabetes 1990;40(suppl 2):14–17.

128. O'Sullivan JB. Diabetes mellitus after GDM. Diabetes 1990;40(suppl 2):131–135.

129. Metzger BE, Organizing Committee. Summary and recommendations of the Third International Workshop: Conference on Gestational Diabetes Mellitus. Diabetes 1991;40(suppl 2):197–201.

130. Proceedings of the Fourth International Workshop: Conference on Gestational Diabetes Mellitus. Diabetes Care 21(suppl 2):81–167, 1998.

131. Carpenter MW, Coustan DR. Criteria for screening tests for gestational diabetes. Am J Obstet Gynecol 1982;144:768–783.

132. Ferris AM, Dalidowitz CK, Ingardia CM, et al. Lactation outcome among insulin-dependent women. J Am Diet Assoc 1988;88:317–322.

133. Lawrence RA. Breastfeeding: A Guide for the Medical Profession, 4th ed. St. Louis: Mosby–Year Book, 1994.

134. Mayer EJ, Hamman RF, Gay EC, et al. Reduced risk of IDDM among breast-fed children. The Colorado IDDM Registry. Diabetes 1988;37:1625–1632.

135. Virtanen SM, Rasanen L, Aro A, et al. Feeding in

infancy and the risk of type I diabetes mellitus in Finnish children. Diabet Med 1992;9:815–819.

136. Gerstein H. Cow's milk exposure and type I diabetes mellitus? A critical overview of the clinical literature. Diabetes Care 1994;17:13–19.

137. Kostraba JN. What can epidemiology tell us about the role of infant diet in the etiology of IDDM? Diabetes Care 1994;17:87–91.

138. Verge CF, Howard NJ, Irwig L, et al. Environmental factors in childhood IDDM. Diabetes Care 1994;17:1381–1389.

139. Gerstein HC, van der Meulen J. The relationship between cow's milk exposure and type I diabetes. Diabet Med 1996;13:23–29.

140. Neubauer SH, Ferris AM, Chase CG, et al. Delayed lactogenesis in women with insulin-dependent diabetes mellitus. Am J Clin Nutr 1993;58:54–60.

141. Pettitt DJ, Forman MR, Hanson RL, et al. Breastfeeding and incidence of non–insulin-dependent diabetes mellitus among Pima Indians. Lancet 1997;350:166–168.

142. The Committee on Drugs, American Academy of Pediatrics. The transfer of drugs and other chemicals into breast milk. Pediatrics 1994;93:137–150.

143. Friedman L, Lawrence R, Lactation Study Center, University of Rochester, personal communication, 1997.

144. LaVecchia C, Negri E, Franceschi S, et al. A case-control study of diabetes and cancer risk. Br J Cancer 1994;70:950–953.

145. Parazzini F, LaVecchia C, Bocciolone L, Franceschi S. The epidemiology of endometrial cancer. Gynecol Oncol 1991;41:1–16.

146. Gronroos M, Salmi TA, Vuenta MH, et al. Mass screening for endometrial cancer directed in groups of patients with diabetes and/or hypertension. Cancer 1993;71:1279–1282.

147. Weiderpass E, Gridley G, Persson I, et al. Risk of endometrial and breast cancer risk in patients with diabetes mellitus. Int J Cancer 1997;71:360–363.

148. Talamini R, Franceschi S, Favero A, et al. Selected medical conditions and risk of breast cancer. Br J Cancer 1997;75:1699–1703.

149. The Writing Group for the PEPI Trial. Effects of estrogen or estrogen-progestin regimens on heart disease risk factors in post-menopausal women. JAMA 1996;273;199–208.

150. Kazer RR. Insulin resistance, insulin-like growth factor I and breast cancer: A hypothesis. Int J Cancer 1995;62:403–406.

151. Bruning PF, Bonfrer JMG, van Noord PAH, et al. Insulin resistance and breast cancer risk. Int J Cancer 1992;52:511–516.

152. Papa V, Pezzino V, Costantino A, et al. Elevated insulin receptor content in human breast cancer. J Clin Invest 1990;86:1503–1510.

153. Grodstein F, Stampfer MJ. The epidemiology of coronary heart disease and estrogen replacement in postmenopausal women. Prog Cardiovasc Dis 1995;38:199–210.

154. Tang MX, Jacobs D, Stern Y, et al. Effect of oestrogen during menopause on risk and age at onset of Alzheimer's disease. Lancet 1996;348:429–432.

155. Grodstein F, Stampfer MJ, Colditz GA, et al. Postmenopausal hormone therapy and mortality. N Engl J Med 1997;336:1769–1775.

156. Brinton LA, Schairer C. Postmenopausal hormone-replacement therapy— time for a reappraisal? N Engl J Med 1997;336:1821–1822.

157. Sattar N, Jaap AJ, MacCuish AC. Hormone replacement therapy and cardiovascular risk in postmenopausal women with NIDDM. Diabet Med 1996;13:782–788.

10 LIFE-THREATENING COMPLICATIONS of HYPERTENSION in PREGNANCY

William C. Mabie

Maternal mortality in the United States has been reduced to 7.8 per 100,000 live births, with pulmonary embolism being the most common cause; however, the triad of hemorrhage, infection, and toxemia (HIT) still is a major contributor to maternal mortality. Hypertension is the second leading cause of maternal death.[1] In addition, many "near-miss" patients may require treatment in an intensive care unit but do survive (0.04%–0.9% of deliveries).[2] In this chapter I discuss the life-threatening complications associated with hypertension in pregnancy.

PULMONARY EDEMA

Clinical manifestations of pulmonary edema include:

- Dyspnea
- Anxiety
- Restlessness

Physical signs include:

- Rales
- Wheezing
- Use of accessory respiratory muscles
- Expectoration of pink, frothy sputum
- Decreased peripheral perfusion

Radiographic abnormalities include:

- Cardiomegaly
- Interstitial and perihilar vascular engorgement
- Kerley B lines
- Airspace opacification
- Pleural effusions

The radiographic abnormalities may follow development of symptoms by several hours, and their resolution may be out of phase with clinical improvement.

As shown in Table 10–1, pulmonary edema in pregnancy may be *cardiogenic* (pulmonary artery wedge pressure [PAWP] > 18 mmHg) or *noncardiogenic* (PAWP < 18 mmHg).

Cardiogenic Pulmonary Edema

Cardiogenic pulmonary edema may result from systolic dysfunction or impaired myocardial contractility (e.g., peripartum cardiomyopathy); it may also result from diastolic dysfunction or impaired myocardial relaxation. Patients with left ventricular hypertrophy due to chronic hypertension develop diastolic dysfunction, which precedes the onset of systolic dysfunction by several years. These patients, who have thick walls and stiff ventricles, require high filling pressures and are thus predisposed to hydrostatic pulmonary edema if they retain excess sodium and water during late pregnancy or receive an iatrogenic fluid overload.[3] Com-

---

TABLE 10–1. CAUSES OF PULMONARY EDEMA IN PREECLAMPSIA

Cardiogenic
   Systolic dysfunction
   Diastolic dysfunction
   Combined
Noncardiogenic
   Increased capillary permeability
Narrowed COP–wedge pressure gradient
   Decreased COP
   Delayed mobilization of extravascular fluid
   Iatrogenic fluid overload

COP, colloid osmotic pressure.

165

bined systolic and diastolic dysfunction usually occurs in elderly multiparas with long-standing, severe hypertension.

Echocardiography is a readily available, noninvasive method of accessing ventricular dimensions, mass, and function as well as valve morphology and function. It may be used to define subgroups and to tailor therapy according to cardiac structure and function.[4]

Noncardiogenic Pulmonary Edema

Noncardiogenic pulmonary edema results either from a pulmonary capillary leak or from narrowing of the colloid osmotic pressure (COP)–wedge pressure gradient. Plasma proteins (e.g., albumin, globulins, fibrinogen) exert osmotic pressure to hold water in the vasculature and counteract hydrostatic pressure that pushes water out of the vasculature. Interstitial COP and interstitial hydrostatic pressure have similar antagonist effects on the other side of the membrane.

Normal intravascular COP in the nonpregnant state is 25.4 ± 2.3 mmHg, whereas normal PAWP (a measure of pulmonary vascular hydrostatic pressure) is 6 to 12 mmHg. Therefore, the normal COP–wedge pressure gradient is about 12 mmHg. A COP–wedge pressure gradient of 4 mmHg or less has been associated with an increased risk of pulmonary edema. The normal COP in pregnancy at term is 22.4 ± 0.5 mmHg. With delivery accompanied by blood loss and crystalloid replacement, COP decreases to 15.4 ± 2.1 mmHg. With preeclampsia, COP has been reported to fall from 17.9 ± 0.7 mmHg to 13.7 ± 0.05 mmHg post partum. This narrowing of the COP–wedge pressure gradient reflects predisposition to pulmonary edema.[5]

Pulmonary edema associated with preeclampsia-eclampsia usually occurs post partum. Serum albumin decreases due to renal losses, impaired liver synthesis, and blood loss with crystalloid replacement. PAWP increases as a result of delayed mobilization of extravascular fluid. Beginning 24 to 72 hours post partum, edema fluid is mobilized and returned to the intravascular space more quickly than the diseased kidneys can excrete it. Iatrogenic fluid overload may also contribute to raising the wedge pressure; however, elevations in filling pressures may not be significant enough to account for pulmonary edema without simultaneous lowering of the intravascular colloid osmotic pressure.

In a study of 37 patients, the incidence of pulmonary edema in hypertensive disorders of pregnancy was reported by Sibai and associates to be 2.3%.[6] The incidence was higher in older patients and in multigravid patients. In 30%, pulmonary edema occurred before delivery; in 70%, onset was after delivery. In the postpartum group, the average onset was at 71 hours after delivery. There were four maternal deaths in this series of 37 patients, and the perinatal mortality was 530/1000. There were a number of maternal complications, including disseminated intravascular coagulation (DIC) in 48%, acute renal failure in 27%, abruptio placentae (placental abruption) in 32%, sepsis in 46%, and cardiopulmonary arrest in 14%. The Sibai investigators suggested that pulmonary edema was infrequent in women with preeclampsia-eclampsia unless there were associated medical, surgical, or obstetric complications.[6]

Using echocardiography, Mabie and colleagues prospectively studied 45 pregnant women with pulmonary edema.[4] Only 18% had known preexisting heart disease. Figure 10–1 shows both the clinical and the echocardiographic diagnoses. There was no valvular heart disease. Patients could be categorized into three groups according to echocardiographic findings:

- Systolic dysfunction
- Diastolic dysfunction
- Normal heart

Treatment

The acute episode of pulmonary edema usually responds to oxygen, morphine, and furosemide. Digitalis, nitroglycerin, sodium nitroprusside, dopamine, dobutamine, amrinone, intra-aortic balloon counterpulsation, mechanical ventilation, hemodialysis, hemofiltration, or a ventricular assist device may be needed in special situations.

Initial management involves sitting the patient upright, which improves pulmonary function and assists in venous pooling, and administering oxygen by nasal cannula or face mask to produce an arterial oxygen saturation of greater than 90%. Morphine sulfate is given 2 to 5 mg intravenously (IV)

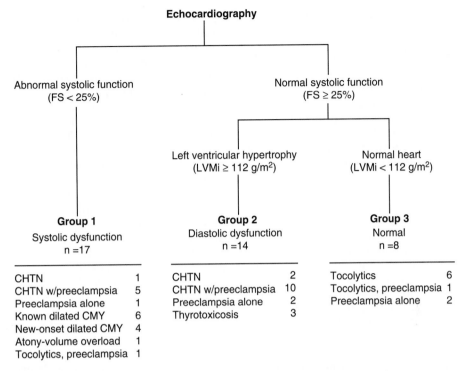

FIGURE 10–1. Echocardiographic classification of patients with pulmonary edema and the accompanying primary clinical diagnosis. CHTN, chronic hypertension; CMY, cardiomyopathy; FS, fractional shortening; LVMi, left ventricular mass index. (From Mabie WC, Hackman BB, Sibai BM. Pulmonary edema associated with pregnancy: Echocardiographic insights and implications for treatment. Obstet Gynecol 1993;81:227–234. Reprinted with permission from the American College of Obstetricians and Gynecologists.)

every 10 minutes as needed to reduce anxiety and to dilate the pulmonary and systemic veins. Furosemide, given in an initial dose of 40 mg intravenously, causes venodilation and diuresis and decreases pulmonary congestion. After diuresis of approximately 1800 to 2000 mL, the pulmonary edema usually clears.

For patients needing chronic care, an echocardiogram is useful for individualizing therapy according to cardiac structure and function. In patients with normal hearts (e.g., "pure" preeclampsia or tocolytic-induced pulmonary edema), no chronic therapy is indicated. For patients with dilated cardiomyopathy and decreased systolic function, postpartum treatment usually includes digoxin, diuretics, and an angiotensin-converting enzyme (ACE) inhibitor. Patients with left ventricular hypertrophy and predominantly diastolic dysfunction require long-term antihypertensive therapy and control of heart rate with β-blockers or rate-limiting calcium channel blockers. The goal of the long-term antihypertensive therapy is to produce regression of left ventricular hypertrophy. Virtually all of the antihypertensive drugs can accomplish this except vasodilators such as hydralazine and minoxidil.[4]

HYPERTENSIVE ENCEPHALOPATHY

Hypertensive encephalopathy is a complication of malignant hypertension. A diastolic blood pressure of 130 mmHg is often seen; however, there are no rigid blood pressure criteria. Some patients experience vascular damage at lower levels of pressure, whereas others withstand even higher levels without apparent harm.

In this acute syndrome, severe hypertension is associated with headache, visual disturbances, nausea, vomiting, seizures, confusion, stupor, and coma. Focal or lateralizing neurologic signs, either transient or lasting, may occur but are uncommon and therefore suggest some other vascular disease, such as hemorrhage, embolism, or atherosclerotic thrombosis. Retinal hemorrhages, exudates, papilledema, and evidence of renal or cardiac disease may be present. In most cases, cerebrospinal fluid (CSF) pressure and protein levels are elevated. Lowering the blood pressure reverses the process, but permanent damage may have occurred. Neuropathologic examination reveals multifocal or diffuse cerebral edema with hemorrhages that vary in size from petechiae to massive. Microscopically, necrosis of arterioles, minute cerebral infarcts, and hemorrhages are noted.[7, 8]

Incidence

Hypertensive encephalopathy develops in fewer than 1% of nonpregnant hypertensive patients. In a 10-year review of cerebrovascular disorders complicating pregnancy, published in 1997, only three cases of hypertensive encephalopathy were found among 79,301 deliveries.[9] During the same time period, there were more than 250 cases of eclampsia at the same institution. Differentiating women with hypertensive encephalopathy from women with eclampsia is problematic.[9]

Pathophysiology

Patients with eclampsia and hypertensive encephalopathy exhibit similar neuropathologic findings and have similar computed tomographic (CT) and magnetic resonance imaging (MRI) scans. There has been controversy for many years about the pathophysiology of eclampsia. Some argue that eclampsia is a form of hypertensive encephalopathy,[10] whereas others claim that most patients with eclampsia do not have severe hypertension. Twenty per cent of eclamptic patients have blood pressure below 140/90 mmHg. Furthermore, papilledema and retinal hemorrhages (common findings in hypertensive encephalopathy) are rarely seen in severe preeclampsia or eclampsia.[11] Nevertheless, there is a growing consensus outside of obstetrics that eclampsia and hypertensive encephalopathy have similar pathophysiologic mechanisms.[12–17]

One mechanism is loss of autoregulation, producing generalized vasodilatation. This "breakthrough" of cerebral blood flow hyperperfuses the brain, causing leakage of fluid into the perivascular tissue and resulting in vasogenic cerebral edema. The upper limit of autoregulation of cerebral blood flow varies.[18] Normotensive patients autoregulate or maintain constant cerebral blood flow between mean arterial pressures for 60 to 130 mmHg. In hypertensive patients there is a "shift to the right" caused by structural thickening of the arterioles with autoregulation occurring between 110 and 180 mmHg mean arterial pressure. This explains why previously normotensive persons, such as children with acute glomerulonephritis or women with eclampsia, have convulsions with blood pressures as low as 150/100 mmHg.[19] Altered vascular reactivity to normally circulating pressor substances, a deficiency of vasodilating prostaglandins, endothelial cell dysfunction, and activation of the coagulation cascade may contribute to the brain–capillary leak syndrome of eclampsia and hypertensive encephalopathy.[13]

MRI of the brain in eclampsia most commonly shows foci of hyperintense signal on T2-weighted images in the subcortical white matter of the occipital lobes. Blurred vision and cortical blindness are associated with these lesions. Lesions are less often seen in the cerebellum, brain stem, parieto-occipital region, basal ganglia, and frontal lobes. Strikingly similar findings are seen with hypertensive encephalopathy.[12–17, 20]

Both hypertensive encephalopathy and eclampsia are part of an increasingly recognized brain disorder known as *reversible posterior leukoencephalopathy syndrome*. First described in 1996, patients usually had renal insufficiency and hypertension or were receiving immunosuppressive therapy.[13] The predilection for cerebral edema development in the posterior circulation is curious. Some evidence suggests that sympathetic innervation of the anterior circulation may be protective, allowing sustained vasoconstriction. The vertebrobasilar vessels are relatively devoid of sympathetic innervation. Thus, acute elevations of blood pressure might be expected to preferentially transmit pressure to the vertebrobasilar circulation. The protective sympathetic mechanism of the anterior circulation may be overcome, accounting for the diffuse distribution of cerebral edema seen in some cases.[17]

Treatment

Because it is difficult to distinguish eclampsia from hypertensive encephalopathy, magnesium sulfate ($MgSO_4$) should be given for seizure prophylaxis. A 6-g loading dose intravenously over 20 minutes is followed by 2 to 3 g/h. It is important to check the serum creatinine level because $MgSO_4$ is excreted renally.

A list of potential antihypertensive medications is shown in Table 10–2. Before therapy is selected, it is important to address how quickly and to what level blood pressure must be lowered. For women with hypertensive encephalopathy, blood pressure should be lowered by 20% in 1 hour. The most reliable medication for achieving this is sodium nitroprusside. Because of the risk of fetal cyanide toxicity, hydralazine or labetalol is sometimes chosen instead. These drugs are less powerful but may contribute to hypotension after large doses have failed to control blood pressure and sodium nitroprusside is given.

Hydralazine is a direct arteriolar vasodilator that causes a secondary baroreceptor-mediated sympathetic discharge resulting in tachycardia and increased cardiac output. This latter effect increases uterine blood flow and blunts the hypotensive response. If late decelerations of the fetal heart rate do occur after hydralazine administration, they usually respond to fluid loading, administration of oxygen, turning the patient on her side, and discontinuing oxytocin. Hydralazine is metabolized in the liver; in patients with a slow acetylating mechanism, its duration of action is longer. Hydralazine is somewhat erratic in its onset of action and peak effect. It should be started at 5 mg intravenously, and a second dose of 5 to 10 mg should be given every 20 to 30 minutes. If a total dose of 30 mg intravenously does not control blood pressure, another agent should be used. Because of its long duration

of action, constant intravenous infusion of hydralazine is not advised.[21]

The second commonly used agent for severe hypertension is labetalol, a nonselective β-blocker and a postsynaptic $α_1$-blocker. Because it slows heart rate and because it is only a moderately powerful agent, labetalol is a good choice in patients who do not respond to hydralazine. It is unlikely to cause overshoot hypotension. Labetalol decreases systemic vascular resistance with little or no change in cardiac output. Uteroplacental blood flow appears to be unaffected by intravenous labetalol. Onset of action is in 5 minutes, peak effect is in 10 to 20 minutes, and duration of action ranges from 45 minutes to 6 hours. It is usually given in escalating doses of 20, 40, 80, 80, and 80 mg every 10 minutes to a maximum cumulative dose of 300 mg or until the diastolic blood pressure is below 100 mmHg.[22]

Sodium nitroprusside is an equal arteriolar and venular vasodilator acting directly on the vessel wall. It is the most potent antihypertensive drug on the market. Nitroprusside crosses the placenta. It has no effect on uterine contractility. Uterine blood flow has been reported to increase, to decrease, and to remain unchanged. Because of its potency and rapid onset of action, monitoring blood pressure by indwelling arterial catheter is advised. Additionally, the drug must be shielded from light. The usual dosage is 0.25 to 5 µg/kg/min. Thiocyanate and cyanide toxicity occurs when infusion rates exceed 5 µg/kg/min and in patients with renal dysfunction. Early manifestations of cyanide toxicity include metabolic acidosis and rising mixed venous oxygen saturation. Antidotes are amyl nitrite, sodium nitrite, sodium thiosulfate, and cyanocobalamin. It has been recommended that sodium

TABLE 10–2. PARENTERAL DRUGS FOR TREATMENT OF SEVERE HYPERTENSION IN PREGNANCY

DRUG	DOSE	ONSET OF ACTION	DURATION OF ACTION	ADVERSE EFFECTS
Hydralazine	5–10 mg IV q 20 min	10–20 min	3–6 h	Tachycardia, headache, flushing, exacerbation of angina
Labetalol	20–80 mg IV q 10 min	5–10 min	3–6 h	Scalp tingling, vomiting, heart block
Sodium nitroprusside	0.25–10 µg/kg/min IV	immediate	1–2 min	Nausea, vomiting, muscle twitching, thiocyanate and cyanide intoxication
Nicardipine	5–15 mg/h IV	5–10 min	1–4 h	Tachycardia, headache, phlebitis

IV, intravenously.

nitroprusside not be used during pregnancy for longer than 30 minutes because of the risk of fetal cyanide toxicity, although some reports have described its longer use.[23, 24] Other adverse effects of the drug include hypotension, undesired vasodilatation in some vascular beds (increased intracranial pressure and intrapulmonary shunting), and a hyperdynamic response. In this latter situation, the fall in systemic vascular resistance is offset by a reflex catecholamine-mediated increase in cardiac output so that blood pressure remains unchanged. This situation can be resolved by decreasing nitroprusside and adding a β-blocker or by switching to another antihypertensive agent (e.g., nicardipine).

Nicardipine is a dihydropyridine calcium channel blocker available for oral and intravenous therapy of hypertension. It is considered a drug of choice in hypertensive emergencies in the nonpregnant patient.[25, 26] Nicardipine is a pregnancy category C drug. Its advantage over nifedipine is that it acts more selectively on the blood vessels than on the myocardium, causing less negative inotropic effect and less reflex tachycardia.[27] Animal experiments, however, suggest that the hemodynamic effects of nicardipine may be responsible for fetal acidosis and death.[28, 29] Furthermore, little has been published about this agent in human pregnancy.[27, 30]

INTRACRANIAL HEMORRHAGE

Intracranial hemorrhage (ICH) in pregnancy can be caused by hypertension or by a structural malformation of the brain such as an aneurysm or an arteriovenous (A-V) malformation. In a large population-based study on stroke in pregnancy, there were 17 cerebral infarctions and 14 intracranial hemorrhages during 8,011,852 weeks of pregnancy exposure.[31] The causes of cerebral infarction were preeclampsia-eclampsia in four, primary central nervous system vasculopathy in two, thrombotic thrombocytopenic purpura in one, cortical vein thrombosis in one, postherpetic vasculitis in one, and indeterminate cause in six. For cerebral hemorrhage, the causes were A-V malformation in three, preeclampsia-eclampsia in two, cocaine use in two, primary central nervous system vasculopathy in one, sarcoid vasculitis in one, and indeterminate cause in four.

The risks of both cerebral infarction and intracerebral hemorrhage were increased in the 6 weeks after delivery but not during the pregnancy itself.

In a study from Dallas, the incidence of ICH was one in 15,000 pregnancies.[32] Intracerebral hemorrhage is the most common cause of death in eclampsia (60%). This discussion focuses on hypertensive ICH only.

The most common sites of hemorrhage in nonpregnant, hypertensive patients are:

- Basal ganglia (putamen, thalamus, and adjacent white matter)
- Cerebellum
- Pons

With eclampsia, the cerebral lesions can be categorized into five groups[33]:

- Patches of petechial hemorrhages in the cerebral cortex
- Multiple 3- to 5-mm areas of ischemic softening
- Small hemorrhages in the subcortical white matter
- Single, large hemorrhages in the white matter separate from the basal ganglia
- Hemorrhage into the basal ganglia or pons, often rupturing into the ventricles and producing subarachnoid hemorrhage

Signs and Symptoms

Intracerebral hemorrhage usually presents as the acute onset of focal neurologic deficits that reflect the location and size of the hemorrhage. Headache, vomiting, and altered mental status reflect increased intracranial pressure. Brain herniation and death may occur rapidly. With cerebral hemorrhage associated with eclampsia, focal deficits may not be manifested for 6 hours after the onset of convulsions.

Diagnosis

Aggressive workup is indicated for the hypertensive pregnant woman with nuchal rigidity, papilledema, lateralizing signs, seizures while receiving MgSO$_4$, seizures later than 48 hours post partum, or seizures with prolonged coma. CT scan without contrast reliably detects acute hemorrhages of 1 cm or more in diameter. MRI is more sensitive for delineating associated abnormalities such as aneurysms, A-V malformations, and neo-plasms. Lumbar puncture may be needed to rule out subarachnoid hemorrhage if there is no evidence of midline shift or other in-tracranial mass effect. Cerebral angiography may be needed to rule out aneurysm or A-V malformation when the cause of hemorrhage is uncertain.[34]

Treatment

Neurosurgical consultation should be ob-tained to assist in the evaluation. Evacuation of a cerebellar hematoma may be lifesaving, but most ICHs in pregnancy do not involve the cerebellum. Evacuation of deep cerebral hematomas is rarely helpful. Removal of the hematoma does not necessarily correct the problem of intracranial hypertension, and intracranial pressure often returns to pre-evacuation levels soon after surgery.[35]

Much of the morbidity and mortality of intracerebral hemorrhage can be ascribed to primary tissue destruction from the initial hemorrhage, but secondary injury results from ischemia, rebleeding, and edema. The management of blood pressure in the acute period after ICH as a potential means of modifying the secondary injury is controver-sial. Proponents of lowering blood pressure believe that doing so decreases the risk of rebleeding, edema formation, and acute sys-temic complications. Opponents favor not treating hypertension as a means of preserv-ing, or at least not decreasing, cerebral per-fusion pressure to areas of low cerebral blood flow at risk for ischemic damage.

During the early period after ICH, autoreg-ulation is impaired and a hypertensive re-sponse is commonly seen. The cause of this hypertensive response is unknown, but ma-jor contributors may be the Cushing reflex or catecholamine discharge. In general, the balance of data does not suggest that it is imperative to treat hypertension unless it is very severe. Moderate reductions of blood pressure are probably safe. The drug of choice is the α/β-blocker labetalol because it does not increase intracranial pressure and it preserves cerebral blood flow. Use of hydralazine or nicardipine is probably also safe. Vasodilators (e.g., sodium nitroprus-side, nitroglycerin, diazoxide) raise intra-cranial pressure and decrease cerebral blood flow in patients with intracranial hyperten-sion and should be avoided, as should tri-methaphan, a ganglionic blocker that causes mydriasis and bronchospasm.[35]

Other aspects of management include (1) correcting any coagulopathy; (2) administer-ing anticonvulsants; and (3) monitoring in-tracranial pressure, jugular venous oxygen saturation, arterial blood gases, and intake and output. Intracranial pressure may be lowered by elevating the head of the bed, by intubation and mechanical ventilation to reduce arterial pCO_2 to 25 mmHg, and by administration of furosemide.[36]

Mannitol should be used cautiously be-cause it crosses the placenta and may accu-mulate in the fetus. Maternal infusion of mannitol in rabbits shifts free water from the fetus to the mother, resulting in fetal dehydration, bradycardia, and cyanosis. Similar changes have been seen in hu-mans.[34]

DISSEMINATED INTRAVASCULAR COAGULATION

In obstetrics, DIC may be seen in associa-tion with:

- Abruptio placentae
- Amniotic fluid embolism
- Septic abortion
- Severe preeclampsia
- HELLP (*h*emolysis, *e*levated *l*iver en-zymes, *l*ow *p*latelets) syndrome
- Acute fatty liver of pregnancy
- Retained dead fetus
- Saline abortion

The pathophysiology involves consumption of clotting factors and platelets and genera-tion of fibrin degradation products that in-terfere with clot formation. Fibrin degrada-tion products are formed by intense secondary fibrinolysis of polymerized fibrin monomers. Microangiopathic hemolytic anemia secondary to red blood cell fragmen-tation is also seen.

The diagnosis is based on finding a pro-longed prothrombin time and partial throm-boplastin time, low fibrinogen level, and low platelet count as well as the presence of fibrin degradation products. D-dimer immu-noassay specifically measures cross-linked fibrin derivatives. The peripheral smear re-veals schistocytes and thrombocytopenia. Plasma fibrinogen levels correlate most closely with clinical bleeding; low fibrinogen levels are associated with more bleeding.

Management of DIC depends on the progression of the illness. For this reason, it is useful to place the patient into one of two categories:

1. "Fast" DIC is an acute, fulminating, uncompensated, consumptive coagulopathy with bleeding (e.g., amniotic fluid embolism, abruptio placentae).

2. "Slow" DIC is a more chronic, indolent, compensated course in which there is little bleeding (e.g., retained dead fetus syndrome, saline abortion, and certain malignancies).[37]

The focus of therapy is to treat the underlying cause of DIC and to provide replacement of red blood cells, coagulation factors, and platelets. The theoretical concern of "adding fuel to the fire" and causing obstruction of the microcirculation is not supported by any good evidence.

The primary cause of DIC in hypertensive disorders of pregnancy is abruptio placentae. Abruption causes consumption of clotting factors in the retroplacental clot and releases placental tissue thromboplastin into the bloodstream. A correlation has been found between the alteration in hemostasis and the percentage of the placental surface that is separated.[38] Hypofibrinogenemia is a prominent manifestation of this syndrome. The main danger with hypertension, abruption, and DIC is acute renal failure. The mechanism of the renal failure is poorly understood.

Treatment of abruption involves delivery of the fetus and correction of the coagulopathy with cryoprecipitate or fresh-frozen plasma. Close attention should be paid to blood volume and urine output. The hematocrit should be maintained at 30% and urine output at a minimum of 30 mL/h. Cesarean section may be required for fetal distress or other obstetric indications. There is no evidence for an arbitrary time limit for delivery after severe abruption.

ACUTE RENAL FAILURE

Acute renal failure is a syndrome characterized by:

- A rapid decline in glomerular filtration rate (GFR)
- Retention of nitrogenous wastes

- Perturbation of extracellular fluid volume
- Electrolyte and acid-base disturbances

Renal failure may be oliguric (urine output < 500 mL/day) or nonoliguric. As shown in Table 10–3, the causes of acute renal failure are classified into three categories:

- *Prerenal* (renal hypoperfusion, ≈55%)
- *Renal* (directly involving renal parenchyma, ≈40%)
- *Postrenal* (urinary tract obstruction, ≈5%)

Acute renal failure is reversible, the kidney being relatively unique among major organs in its ability to recover from almost complete loss of function. In addition, the kidney is one of the few organs whose function can be replaced artificially (e.g., by dialysis) for protracted periods of time. Nevertheless, acute renal failure is an extremely costly disorder that carries great morbidity.[39]

Pathophysiology

Prerenal azotemia is a functional disorder that results from a decrease in effective arterial blood volume. Stretch receptors in the carotid sinus and cardiac baroreceptors trigger neural and humoral responses designed to restore blood volume and arterial pressure. These include activation of the sympathetic nervous system and renin-angiotensin-aldosterone system as well as release of arginine vasopressin (AVP), which was formerly called antidiuretic hormone. In an attempt to preserve cardiac and cerebral per-

---

TABLE 10–3. DIFFERENTIAL DIAGNOSIS OF ACUTE AZOTEMIA

Prerenal
    Decreased extracellular fluid
    Decreased "effective" blood
      volume
    "Third space" fluids
Renal
    Glomerular disease
    Interstitial disease
    Vascular disease
    Acute tubular necrosis
Postrenal
    Urethral obstruction
    Neurogenic bladder
    Ureteral stone, tumor, stricture
    Retroperitoneal tumor, fibrosis
    Gravid uterus, uterine
      incarceration, polyhydramnios

fusion, norepinephrine, angiotensin II, and AVP stimulate vasoconstriction in the skin, skeletal muscle, and splanchnic circulation.

Glomerular function is preserved during mild hypoperfusion by several compensatory mechanisms. Stretch receptors in the afferent arterioles, in response to a reduction in perfusion pressure, trigger afferent arteriolar vasodilatation through a local myogenic reflex (autoregulation). Biosynthesis of vasodilator prostaglandins (e.g., prostacyclin [PGI_2], PGE_2) and, possibly, nitric oxide enhance dilatation of afferent arterioles. In addition, angiotensin II induces preferential vasoconstriction in efferent arterioles. As a result, intraglomerular pressure, filtration fraction, and GFR are preserved.

Autoregulatory dilation of afferent arterioles is maximal at a mean arterial pressure of about 80 mmHg, and hypotension below this level is associated with a precipitous decline in GFR. Pharmacologic inhibitors of renal prostaglandin synthesis (e.g., nonsteroidal anti-inflammatory drugs [NSAIDs]) and angiotensin-converting enzyme inhibitors are thus major culprits in worsening prerenal azotemia and should be avoided in the setting of renal hypoperfusion.[39]

The kidney contains glomeruli, tubules, blood vessels, and interstitium, any of which may be involved in producing acute renal failure; however, most intrinsic renal azotemia results from acute tubular necrosis triggered by ischemia or nephrotoxins (Table 10–4).

Postrenal azotemia may be due to upper or lower urinary tract obstruction. Early diagnosis and relief of obstruction is essential to prevent permanent renal damage. Renal ultrasonography and a Foley catheter aid in the diagnosis of this condition. If postobstructive diuresis appears, replacement of fluids and electrolytes should be guided by

TABLE 10–4. CAUSES OF ACUTE TUBULAR NECROSIS

Toxic
  Aminoglycoside
  Cisplatin
  Radiographic contrast agents
  Solvents (ethylene glycol)
  Rhabdomyolysis
Ischemic
  Hemorrhage
  Hypotension and shock
  Sepsis

TABLE 10–5. CAUSES OF ACUTE RENAL FAILURE IN PREGNANCY

Preeclampsia-eclampsia
HELLP (*h*emolysis, *e*levated *l*iver enzymes, *l*ow *p*latelets) syndrome
Hemorrhage (abruptio placentae, placenta previa, ectopic pregnancy)
Puerperal sepsis
Septic abortion
Thrombotic thrombocytopenic purpura/hemolytic uremic syndrome
Acute fatty liver of pregnancy

daily weights, urine output, orthostatic blood pressure changes, and serum and urine electrolyte concentration.[39]

Etiology

Table 10–5 shows the causes of acute renal failure in pregnancy.[40] Sibai and coworkers studied acute renal failure in 30 hypertensive patients between 1977 and 1989, during which time 1684 women with preeclampsia-eclampsia delivered at their referral center.[41] Sixteen patients (52%) had abruptio placentae; 18 patients had "pure" preeclampsia. Of these 18 women, nine (50%) required dialysis and two died (one of a massive pulmonary embolism in the setting of congenital heart disease, the other of cardiac arrest with hypoxic encephalopathy). All 16 survivors had normal renal function on follow-up. Twelve of the 30 patients had chronic hypertension or chronic renal disease or both. Nine of these had acute tubular necrosis, and three had cortical necrosis. Nine of 11 survivors required chronic dialysis (one died of unknown causes after termination of pregnancy at 16 weeks' gestation). Four women died during follow-up with end-stage renal disease. The authors concluded that with proper management of acute renal failure, "pure" preeclampsia does not result in residual functional impairment.

In a study of 435 patients with HELLP syndrome occurring between 1977 and 1992, another Sibai study involved 32 patients (7.4%) with acute renal failure.[42] Twenty-six had preeclampsia; six had chronic hypertension. There were four maternal deaths (13%). DIC occurred in 27 (84%) pulmonary edema in 14 (44%), and dialysis in 10 (31%) of the cases. Twenty-three women with preeclampsia survived;

none had residual kidney damage. Five chronic hypertensive patients survived, two of whom required chronic dialysis.

Table 10–6 depicts 37 years of data on acute renal failure in pregnancy collected by Stratta and colleagues in Torino, Italy.[43] The table shows that pregnancy-related acute renal failure has nearly disappeared. The incidence has fallen from 43% to 0.5% with respect to the total number of cases of renal failure and from 1/3000 to 1/18,000 with respect to the total number of pregnancies. Maternal mortality has fallen from 31% to 0. The worst maternal and renal prognosis was in the group with preeclampsia and abruption, with irreversible renal damage recorded in 18.7% of cases. The main causes of maternal death were sepsis, hepatic failure, and adult respiratory distress syndrome. Reasons given for the decline in incidence of acute renal failure were (1) legalized abortion and (2) earlier, more aggressive management of obstetric complications (e.g., timely cesarean section and immediate hysterectomy in cases of serious uterine atony with hemorrhage).

Thrombotic thrombocytopenic purpura (TTP) and hemolytic uremic syndrome (HUS) also produce acute renal failure in pregnancy. Egerman and associates reviewed 11 cases from the years 1988 to 1996.[44] Eight women had TTP; three had HUS. Eight cases occurred at greater than 20 weeks' gestation. Plasma transfusions were used in all 11 cases; plasmapheresis was used in nine. Other treatment included packed red blood cell transfusions in nine, platelet transfusions in five, and splenectomy in one. There were two maternal deaths. Four of the nine survivors had chronic renal disease, one of whom had re-

sidual neurologic deficit. Preterm delivery occurred in five of eight pregnancies continuing beyond 20 weeks' gestation, and there was one stillbirth.

Dashe and coworkers reviewed 13 pregnancies in 11 women with TTP-HUS at Parkland Hospital from the years 1972 to 1997.[45] The incidence was 1/25,000 births. In three pregnancies (23%), severe and refractory disease occurred before 20 weeks' gestation. In 10 other pregnancies, disease developed either in the peripartum period (62%) or several weeks post partum (15%). In general, there was a prompt response to therapy, although one woman died. The disease recurred in 50% during a mean follow-up of 8.7 years. Long-term sequelae were present in eight of 10 survivors. The authors concluded that TTP and HUS are rare. The diseases are not easily confused with preeclampsia. The likelihood of immediate survival is high; however, long-term morbidity and mortality are common.

Management

The approach to the patient with acute renal failure should begin with a review of the patient's chart to determine the clinical events and medications that preceded the onset of renal failure. This should be followed by a history and physical examination. Laboratory studies should include urinalysis; blood urea nitrogen; electrolytes; complete blood count; and serum calcium, phosphorus, creatinine, and uric acid levels. A 24-hour urine sample should be obtained to determine creatinine clearance and total protein. Renal ultrasonography, iodohippurate (Hippuran) scan, or renal biopsy may

---

TABLE 10–6. CAUSES OF PREGNANCY-RELATED ACUTE RENAL FAILURE

	1958–1967	1968–1977	1978–1987	1988–1994	TOTAL
Acute renal failure	60	298	535	562	1455
Pregnancy-related	26 (43%)	40 (13.4%)	15 (2.8%)	3 (0.5%)	84 (5.7%)
Postabortion	14	16	1	0	31
Preeclampsia	4	8	7	1	20
Obstetric complications	6	10	6	1	23
Hemolytic uremic syndrome	0	1	1	0	2
Other	2	5	0	1	8

Data from Stratta P, Besso L, Canavese C, et al. Is pregnancy-related acute renal failure a disappearing clinical entity? Ren Fail 1996;18:575–584.

also be needed. Calculation of the fractional excretion of sodium is useful, although not always diagnostic.[46] The formula is as follows:

$$FE_{Na} = \frac{U_{Na}}{P_{Na}} \times \frac{P_{Cr}}{U_{Cr}}$$

$FE_{Na} < 1$ = prerenal

$FE_{Na} > 1$ = acute tubular necrosis

where U = urine, P = plasma, Na = sodium, and Cr = creatinine.

Early treatment goals are to rule out hypovolemia and urinary obstruction. It is desirable to convert oliguric to nonoliguric renal failure to simplify patient management. The patient can receive a more liberal fluid intake, and it is easier to administer drugs and parenteral nutrition. After determining vital signs and orthostatic change in blood pressure and pulse, as well as reviewing intake and output, one may give a fluid challenge of normal saline. If the volume status is unclear, central venous pressure or PAWP monitoring can be employed. After euvolemia is established, a 200-mg dose of intravenous furosemide may be given. This increases renal blood flow and may wash out debris obstructing the tubules. Renal-dose dopamine is controversial. It may be given at 1 to 3 μg/kg/min to increase renal blood flow; however, an editorial from 1996 emphasized the striking paucity of scientific data to support this treatment.[47]

General management of the patient with acute renal failure should emphasize prevention of infection, which is the leading cause of death in these patients. Foley catheters should be avoided in oliguric patients. Urinary output can be monitored with daily intermittent bladder catheterization, with a lower risk of infection. Attention should be paid on a daily basis to the points outlined in Table 10–7.

Indications for dialysis include hyperkalemia, volume overload, acidosis, and uremia. Hemodialysis is a risky procedure because of the possibility of bleeding, hypotension, arrhythmias, and seizures.[48] Dialysis may delay recovery of renal function with acute renal failure, possibly by hypotension or activation of inflammatory cascades by the blood-dialyzer interface.[49] Cellulose acetate membranes cause more complement activation than the newer,

TABLE 10–7. CONSERVATIVE MANAGEMENT OF ACUTE RENAL FAILURE

Attention should be paid to the following areas:
Fluids
Diet
Weight
Blood pressure
Calcium and phosphorus
Drug dosage
Infection
Gastrointestinal bleeding
Anemia

more expensive, polysulfone membranes. Prospective studies have shown that dialysis with biocompatible membranes shortens the course of acute renal failure.[50]

Although the traditional method of dialysis is intermittent hemodialysis, alternatives include peritoneal dialysis and continuous renal replacement therapy. The latter is now frequently used for patients in intensive care units. Continuous arteriovenous hemofiltration and hemodiafiltration were introduced in the 1980s, but it was difficult to maintain a catheter in a peripheral artery. These methods have now been supplanted by pump-driven continuous venovenous hemofiltration or hemodiafiltration. As experience with continuous renal replacement therapy has grown, it is clear that this therapy achieves metabolic control as good as, or better than, conventional dialysis. Clearances are up to 40 L/day with continuous venovenous hemodiafiltration. This is in contrast to every-other-day hemodialysis, with its clearance rate of about 20 L/day, and peritoneal dialysis, with its rate of 5 to 10 L/day.[51] Whether these advantages translate into better outcomes is unclear.

PHEOCHROMOCYTOMA

Pheochromocytomas produce, store, and release catecholamines. They are rare and may cause death, but they also may be incidental findings at autopsy. Pheochromocytomas manifest clinically as paroxysms or crises. During an attack, the patient may experience a headache, profuse sweating, palpitations, apprehension, chest or abdominal pain, nausea, vomiting, pallor or flushing. Blood pressure is often strikingly elevated, and the elevation is usually accompanied by tachycardia. Other cardiac manifestations of pheochromocytoma include supraventricular arrhythmias, premature ventricular contractions, angina, myocardial infarction, and cardiomyopathy. Other distinctive features include diminished plasma volume, elevated hematocrit, carbohydrate intolerance, and seizures. Paroxysms may be precipitated by activity that displaces the abdominal contents. Associated diseases include multiple endocrine neoplasia, neurofibromatosis, and von Hippel–Lindau disease.

In one series of 41 patients reported between 1988 and 1997, maternal mortality was 2% and 83% of the cases were diagnosed ante partum.[52] Fetal mortality was 11%. Before 1969, only 25% of cases associated with pregnancy had been diagnosed ante partum. From 1969 to 1979, the rate was 52%; from 1980 to 1987, it was 53%. When the diagnosis is made ante partum, maternal and fetal mortality are reduced.

Diagnosis

The most important aid to early diagnosis is to think of pheochromocytoma. The diagnostic workup is summarized in Figure 10–2. The diagnosis can usually be confirmed on the basis of a single 24-hour urine sample, provided that the patient is hypertensive or symptomatic at the time of collection. The 24-hour urine sample should be tested for vanillylmandelic acid, metanephrine, and unconjugated or free catecholamines. The creatinine level should be determined as well to assess the adequacy of the collection.

Provocative tests using phentolamine are potentially dangerous and are rarely indicated. When catecholamine levels are borderline, a clonidine suppression test may be used. Clonidine, a centrally acting α_2 agonist, inhibits neurally mediated catecholamine release such as occurs in stress or anxiety. It has no influence on the autonomously and peripherally driven catecholamine production of pheochromocytoma.

After the tumor has been diagnosed, it is localized, commonly by ultrasound, CT, or MRI. Probably the best technique is MRI because no radiation is involved. Ninety per cent of pheochromocytomas are in the adrenal gland, and 98% are in the abdomen; 10% are bilateral, particularly in association with multiple endocrine neoplasia. Other locations are the thorax, neck, and urinary

bladder. Fewer than 10% of the tumors are malignant; however, local invasion into the surrounding tissues is seen with both benign and malignant tumors, and the main criterion for malignancy is distant metastasis.

The fetus is protected from catecholamine surges by an enzymatic barrier at the placental interface, which consists of catechol-O-methyltransferase and monoamine oxidase. Injury to the fetus is not produced directly by the catecholamines but rather through alpha stimulation, causing vasoconstriction and resulting in decreased uterine blood flow. Spontaneous abortion, intrauterine growth retardation, hypoxia, and fetal death may result. Paroxysmal elevations in blood pressure may also lead to abruptio placentae.

Treament

Management of pheochromocytoma can be medical or surgical. The drug of choice for control of hypertension in these patients is phenoxybenzamine, a noncompetitive α-receptor blocker. β-Blockade should not be used without prior α-blockade because of the risk of unopposed α-adrenergic activity. The β-blockers most commonly used in pregnancy are propranolol and atenolol.

If pheochromocytoma is diagnosed in the first two trimesters, the patient should be prepared with phenoxybenzamine and the tumor removed as soon as the diagnosis is confirmed. The pregnancy need not be terminated, but the operative procedure may itself result in spontaneous abortion. In the third trimester, treatment with phenoxybenzamine should be continued until the fetus is sufficiently grown and pulmonary maturity is documented. A cesarean section may then be performed with extirpation of the tumor during the same operation or later. Vaginal delivery has also been accomplished successfully in women with pheochromocytoma, and treatment may be individualized.

Follow-up requires measurement of urinary vanillylmandelic acid and catecholamines, which return to normal levels in about a week. Recurrences can occur for up to 20 years. The 5-year survival rate after surgery is above 95%. For malignant pheochromocytoma, the 5-year survival rate is less than 50%.[52]

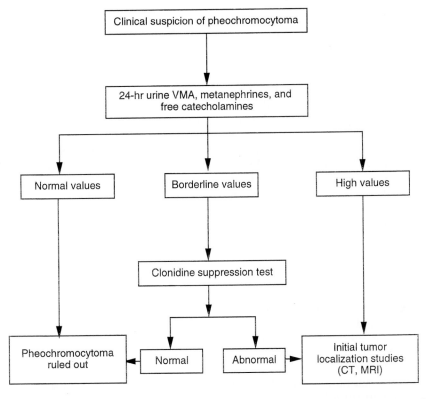

FIGURE 10–2. An approach to the diagnosis of pheochromocytoma during pregnancy. CT, computed tomography; MRI, magnetic resonance imaging; VMA, vanillylmandelic acid. (Modified from Ahlawat SK, Jain S, Kumari S, et al. Pheochromocytoma associated with pregnancy: Case report and review of the literature. Obstet Gynecol Surv 1999;54:728–737.)

AORTIC DISSECTION

Aortic dissection is uncommon in women younger than 40 years of age. Nevertheless, pregnancy increases the risk of dissection. In one study, 50% of dissections in women of childbearing age occurred during pregnancy.[53] The cause of dissection during pregnancy is unclear, but hemodynamic and hormonal changes are often named. The increase in cardiac output, as manifested by increased heart rate and stroke volume, may increase shear stress in the aorta. Hypertension, if it occurs during pregnancy, is a risk factor. Biochemical alterations occur in the connective tissue of blood vessels during pregnancy. Aneurysms are more likely to rupture during pregnancy. Other risk factors associated with aortic dissection in pregnancy areas follows[54]:

- Advanced age
- Multiparity
- Marfan syndrome
- Ehlers-Danlos syndrome
- Trauma
- Coarctation of the aorta
- Bicuspid aortic valve

Aortic dissection occurs most commonly in the third trimester. It is often described as a tearing pain in the interscapular area. Associated symptoms depend on the arteries involved. If the dissection involves the aortic root, aortic insufficiency or cardiac tamponade can result. Stroke, myocardial infarction, paralysis, or limb and visceral ischemia can occur. Pulse asymmetry or an aortic insufficiency murmur may be present on physical examination. The chest radiograph can reveal widening of the mediastinum. The most sensitive and specific diagnostic tests are transesophageal echocardiography and MRI. CT scanning and aortography are more widely available and have reasonable sensitivity and specificity in achieving a diagnosis.

Marfan syndrome is an important risk factor for aortic dissection during pregnancy. In one study, however, no predisposing causes were found in 63% of dissections.[55] In the literature of the past, maternal mortality with Marfan syndrome in pregnancy was quoted as 50%. This high value is attributed to selective reporting of poor-outcome cases.[56] The critical aortic root diameter above which pregnancy should be discouraged is 40 mm; this measurement is determined echocardiographically.[56] An aortic diameter of 55 mm or greater is an indication for surgical repair.[57] Patients with Marfan syndrome are encouraged to complete their childbearing early because aortic dilatation increases with age.

Marfan syndrome is caused by one of 20 or more different missense mutations in the fibrillin gene located on chromosome band 15q21.1. Fibrillin is a structural protein that is the main component of extracellular microfibrils.[58] Inheritance is autosomal dominant, with 50% of the offspring affected.

Prophylactic β-blockade with propranolol or atenolol is recommended for adolescent and adult patients to slow the progress of aortic dilatation.[59] Serial echocardiography every 6 to 8 weeks can be performed during pregnancy to maintain adequate surveillance of the aortic root diameter. Cesarean delivery is considered if the aortic root is dilated. If vaginal delivery is elected, epidural anesthesia should be used to minimize pain and the second stage of labor should be shortened by forceps or vacuum extraction.

Aortic dissection has been classified into three groups by DeBakey and associates[54]:

Type I begins at the ascending aorta and extends to the descending aorta.
Type II begins at the ascending aorta and does not extend beyond.
Type III involves the descending thoracic aorta distal to the origin of the left subclavian artery.

Type III was further divided into *type IIIA*, which is limited to the thoracic aorta, and type *IIIB*, where the dissection extends below the diaphragm. Later, the classification was simplified to ascending dissection (types I and II) and descending dissection (type III).[54]

When chest pain leads to the discovery of aortic dissection during pregnancy, the patient should be moved to an intensive care unit. Oxygen, intravenous fluid, an arterial line, and continuous maternal and fetal heart rate monitoring should be started. Pain should be relieved by narcotics such as mor-

phine. Medical therapy is aimed at decreasing the force and velocity of myocardial contractility.

A β-blocker such as propranolol 1 mg IV should be given every 5 minutes to produce a 20% reduction in maternal heart rate. Systolic blood pressure should be lowered to 100 to 120 mmHg with hydralazine 2.5 to 5 mg IV every 15 minutes.

Labetalol, a combined α- and β-blocker, has been used in aortic dissection and would be an excellent alternative to hydralazine in pregnancy.[54] Sodium nitroprusside is the antihypertensive agent of choice outside of pregnancy; however, because of possible fetal cyanide and thiocyanate toxicity, it should be used only in cases refractory to treatment.[23]

Immediate delivery by cesarean section under epidural anesthesia generally is indicated if the fetus can survive. If the fetus is too premature for delivery, surgical repair can be attempted. There is a paucity of information about maternal and fetal outcome following surgical correction of aortic dissection in pregnancy. In general, fetuses tolerate cardiopulmonary bypass poorly, even with short bypass times and high flow rates.

Indications for surgical management of aortic dissection include proximal dissection (types I and II) and complicated distal dissection (e.g., compromise of renal or mesenteric perfusion, rupture, or impending rupture). Thus, surgery can be avoided in patients with distal aortic dissection. Surgery can involve excision of the intimal tear, oversewing the aortic layers, reapproximation of the aorta with synthetic material, or complete replacement of the ascending aorta. If the aortic root is involved, replacement of the aortic valve may be necessary.[54]

References

1. Centers for Disease Control and Prevention. Mortality patterns—United States, 1992. JAMA 1995;273:100.
2. Baskett TF, Sternadel J. Maternal intensive care and near-miss mortality in obstetrics. Br J Obstet Gynaecol 1998;105:981–984.
3. Mabie WC, Ratts TE, Ramanathan KB, Sibai BM. Circulatory congestion in obese hypertensive women: A subset of pulmonary edema in pregnancy. Obstet Gynecol 1988;72:553–558.
4. Mabie WC, Hackman BB, Sibai BM. Pulmonary edema associated with pregnancy: Echocardiographic insights and implications for treatment. Obstet Gynecol 1993;81:227–234.

5. Moise KJ Jr, Cotton DB. The use of colloid osmotic pressure in pregnancy. Clin Perinatol 1986;13:827–842.

6. Sibai BM, Mabie BC, Harvey CT, Gonzalez AR. Pulmonary edema in severe preeclampsia-eclampsia: Analysis of thirty-seven consecutive cases. Am J Obstet Gynecol 1987;156:1174–1179.

7. Easton JD, Hauser SL, Martin JB. Cerebrovascular diseases. *In* Fauci AS, Braunwald E, Isselbacher KJ, et al (eds). Harrison's Principles of Internal Medicine, 14th ed. New York: McGraw-Hill, 1998, pp 2, 325–348.

8. Healton EB, Brust JC, Feinfeld DA, Thomson GE. Hypertensive encephalopathy and the neurologic manifestations of malignant hypertension. Neurology 1982;32:127–132.

9. Witlin AG, Friedman SA, Egerman RS, et al. Cerebrovascular disorders complicating pregnancy—beyond eclampsia. Am J Obstet Gynecol 1997;176:1139–1148.

10. Donaldson JO. The brain in eclampsia. Hypertens Pregn 1994;13:115–133.

11. Sibai BM. On the brain in eclampsia. Hypertens Pregn 1994;13:111–112.

12. Bakshi R, Bates VE, Mechtler LL, et al. Occipital lobe seizures as the major clinical manifestation of reversible posterior leukoencephalopathy syndrome: Magnetic resonance imaging findings. Epilepsia 1998;39:295–299.

13. Hinchey J, Chaves C, Appignani B, et al. A reversible posterior leukoencephalopathy syndrome. N Engl J Med 1996;334:494–500.

14. Sanders TG, Clayman DA, Sanchez-Ramos L, et al. Brain in eclampsia: MR imaging with clinical correlation. Radiology 1991;180:475–478.

15. Schaefer PW, Buonanno FS, Gonzalez RG, Schwann LH. Diffusion-weighted imaging discriminates between cytotoxic and vasogenic edema in a patient with eclampsia. Stroke 1997;28:1082–1085.

16. Schwartz RB, Mulkern RV, Gudbjartsson H, Jolesz F. Diffusion-weighted MR imaging in hypertensive encephalopathy: Clues to pathogenesis. AJNR Am J Neuroradiol 1998;19:859–862.

17. Sheth RD, Riggs JE, Bodensteiner JB, et al. Parietal occipital edema in hypertensive encephalopathy: A pathogenic mechanism. Eur Neurol 1996;36:25–28.

18. Strandgaard S, Paulson OB. Cerebral autoregulation. Stroke 1984;15:413–416.

19. Jones BV, Egelhoff JC, Patterson RJ. Hypertensive encephalopathy in children. AJNR Am J Neuroradiol 1997;18:101–106.

20. Dahmus MA, Barton JR, Sibai BM. Cerebral imaging in eclampsia: Magnetic resonance imaging versus computed tomography. Am J Obstet Gynecol 1992;167:935–941.

21. National High Blood Pressure Education Program Working Group on High Blood Pressure in Pregnancy. Am J Obstet Gynecol 1990;163:1689–1712.

22. Mabie WC, Gonzalez AR, Sibai BM, Amon E. A comparative trial of labetalol and hydralazine in the acute management of severe hypertension complicating pregnancy. Obstet Gynecol 1987;70:328–333.

23. Naulty J, Cefalo RC, Lewis PE. Fetal toxicity of nitroprusside in the pregnant ewe. Am J Obstet Gynecol 1981;139:708–711.

24. Stempel JE, O'Grady JP, Morton MJ, Johnson KA. Use of sodium nitroprusside in complications of gestational hypertension. Obstet Gynecol 1982; 60:533–538.

25. Kaplan NM. Management of hypertensive emergencies. Lancet 1994;334:1335–1338.

26. Wallin JD. Intravenous nicardipine hydrochloride: Treatment of patients with severe hypertension. Am Heart J 1990;119:434–437.

27. Carbonne B, Jannet D, Touboul C, et al. Nicardipine treatment of hypertension during pregnancy. Obstet Gynecol 1993;81:908–914.

28. Ducsay CA, Thomson JS, Wu AT, Novy MJ. Effects of calcium entry blocker (nicardipine) tocolysis in rhesus macaques: Fetal plasma concentrations and cardiorespiratory changes. Am J Obstet Gynecol 1987;157:428–436.

29. Parisi VM, Salinas J, Stockmar E. Fetal vascular responses to maternal nicardipine administration in the hypertensive ewe. Am J Obstet Gynecol 1989;161:1035–1039.

30. Jannet D, Carbonne B, Sebban E, Milliez J. Nicardipine versus metoprolol in the treatment of hypertension during pregnancy: A randomized comparative trial. Obstet Gynecol 1994;84:354–359.

31. Kittner SJ, Stern BJ, Feeser BR, et al. Pregnancy and the risk of stroke. N Engl J Med 1996;335:768–774.

32. Simolke GA, Cox SM, Cunningham FG. Cerebrovascular accidents complicating pregnancy and the puerperium. Obstet Gynecol 1991;78:37–42.

33. Barton JR, Sibai BM. Cerebral pathology in eclampsia. Clin Perinatol 1991;18:891–910.

34. Das MS, Sekhar LN. Intracranial hemorrhage from aneurysms and arteriovenous malformations during pregnancy and the puerperium. Neurosurgery 1990;27:855–866.

35. Adams RE, Powers WJ. Management of hypertension in acute intracerebral hemorrhage. Crit Care Clin 1997;13:131–161.

36. Tuttelman RM, Gleicher N. Central nervous system hemorrhage complicating pregnancy. Obstet Gynecol 1981;58:651–656.

37. Goodnough LT. Management of disseminated intravascular coagulation. *In* Rossi EC, Simon TL, Moss GS, Gould SA (eds). Principles of Transfusion Medicine, 2nd ed. Baltimore: Williams & Wilkins, 1996, pp 443–452.

38. Gilabert J, Estelles A, Aznar J, Galbis M. Abruptio placentae and disseminated intravascular coagulation. Acta Obstet Gynecol Scand 1985;64:35–39.

39. Brady HR, Brenner BM. Acute renal failure. *In* Fauci AS, Braunwald E, Isselbacher KJ (eds). Harrison's Principles of Internal Medicine, 14th ed. New York: McGraw-Hill, 1998, pp 1504–1513.

40. Krane NK. Acute renal failure in pregnancy. Arch Intern Med 1988;148:2347–2357.

41. Sibai BM, Villar MA, Mabie BC. Acute renal failure in hypertensive disorders of pregnancy. Am J Obstet Gynecol 1990;162:777–783.

42. Sibai BM, Ramadan MK. Acute renal failure in pregnancies complicated by hemolysis, elevated liver enzymes, and low platelets. Am J Obstet Gynecol 1993;168:1682–1690.

43. Stratta P, Besso L, Canavese C, et al. Is pregnancy-related acute renal failure a disappearing clinical entity? Ren Fail 1996;18:575–584.

44. Egerman RS, Witlin AG, Friedman SA, Sibai BM. Thrombotic thrombocytopenic purpura and hemolytic uremic syndrome in pregnancy: Review of 11 cases. Am J Obstet Gynecol 1996;175:950–956.

45. Dashe JS, Ramin SM, Cunningham FG. The long-term consequences of thrombotic microangiopathy

(thrombotic thrombocytopenic purpura and hemolytic uremic syndrome) in pregnancy. Obstet Gynecol 1998;91:662–668.

46. Miller TR, Anderson RJ, Linas SL, et al. Urinary diagnostic indices in acute renal failure. Ann Intern Med 1978;89:47–50.

47. Denton MD, Chertow GM, Brady HR. "Renal-dose" dopamine for the treatment of acute renal failure: Scientific rational, experimental studies, and clinical trials. Kidney Int 1996;49:4–14.

48. Star RA. Treatment of acute renal failure. Kidney Int 1998;14:1817–1831.

49. Pastan S, Bailey J. Dialysis therapy. N Engl J Med 1998;338:1428–1437.

50. Hakim RM, Wingard RL, Parker RA. Effect of the dialysis membrane in the treatment of patients with acute renal failure. N Engl J Med 1994; 331:1338–1342.

51. Bellomo R, Farmer M, Parkin G, et al. Severe acute renal failure: A comparison of acute hemodiafiltration and conventional dialytic therapy. Nephron 1995;71:59–64.

52. Ahlawat SK, Jain S, Kumari S, et al. Pheochromocytoma associated with pregnancy: Case report and review of the literature. Obstet Gynecol Surv 1999;54:728–737.

53. Pumphrey CW, Fay T, Weir I. Aortic dissection during pregnancy. Br Heart J 1986;55:106–108.

54. James KB. Heart disease arising during pregnancy. *In* Douglas PS (ed). Cardiovascular Health and Disease in Women. Philadelphia: WB Saunders, 1993, pp 337–359.

55. Konishi Y, Tatsuta N, Kumada K, et al. Dissecting aneurysm during pregnancy and the puerperium. Jpn Circ J 1980;44:726–733.

56. Pyeritz RE. Maternal and fetal complications of pregnancy in the Marfan's syndrome. Am J Med 1981;71:784–790.

57. Treasure T. Elective replacement of the aortic root in Marfan's syndrome. Br Heart J 1993;69:101–103.

58. Francke U, Furthmayr H. Marfan's syndrome and other disorders of fibrillin. N Engl J Med 1994;330:1384–1385.

59. Shores J, Berger KP, Murphy EA, Pyeritz RE. Progression of aortic dilatation and the benefit of long-term beta-adrenergic blockade in Marfan's syndrome. N Engl J Med 1994;330:1335–1341.

11

ANTIHYPERTENSIVE DRUGS in PREGNANCY

James J. Walker

Eclampsia, first described by the ancient Greeks, remains the main presentation of preeclampsia-eclampsia in many parts of the world. It is not surprising that in most countries treatment regimens are directed primarily toward anticonvulsant therapy rather than toward antihypertensive treatment. In the United Kingdom (U.K.), however, there has been a dramatic fall in incidence of eclampsia,[1] to 4.9/10,000 deliveries.[2] Maternal mortality and morbidity from both eclampsia and preeclampsia have also declined, although hypertensive disorders remain one of the main causes of death.[3] In those who die, there has been a change in the cause of death, with a steady drop in the mortality from cerebrovascular accident, which has coincided with a greatly increased use of antihypertensive drugs[4]; pulmonary edema now accounts for 50% of the mortality rate.

WHY USE ANTIHYPERTENSIVE DRUGS IN PREGNANCY?

Antihypertensive drugs are used to reduce blood pressure. Although there are many different modes of action, the end results are the same. All antihypertensive drugs have side effects, some of which may produce further benefits and others harmful results. Because they are powerful cardiovascular agents, it would be surprising if they did not have some potential adverse maternal or fetal effects. The obstetrician must balance any desired benefit of antihypertensive therapy against any possible side effects.

Although there is no consensus about therapy for pregnancy hypertension and the role of antihypertensive drugs, many clinicians think that their use during pregnancy helps protect the mother and may reduce fetal mortality and morbidity by allowing

the prolongation of pregnancy.[5, 6] Although it is agreed that antihypertensive drugs do protect the mother from the dangers of severe hypertension ($\geq$170/110 mmHg), particularly cerebral hemorrhage, it is still debatable whether treatment of a lower level of hypertension confers any benefit,[7] although it appears to allow a more controlled management protocol to be implemented.[6]

When a diastolic blood pressure (DBP) of 90 mmHg is taken as the level for intervention, many pregnant women fall into this range, particularly at term.[8] Women with mild hypertension in pregnancy do not require antihypertensive therapy if they are closely observed during pregnancy and delivery, especially if there has been no hypertension before pregnancy and no proteinuria develops.[9–11] Delaying the treatment of hypertension of pregnancy until DBP is 100 mmHg is not associated with additional maternal or fetal risk and reduces the number of patients requiring treatment by more than 50%.[12]

If antihypertensive drugs are to be used, they can have only two benefits:

- Reducing the risk of the hypertension to the mother, stabilizing the clinical situation, and allowing well-planned management.
- Improving fetal outcome by prolonging pregnancy to allow the use of prophylactic steroids or to delay the delivery to a more optimal time.

Stabilization before delivery probably is sensible at all times, but prolongation of the pregnancy is of less value as gestation advances. It is when the disease develops far from term that antihypertensive therapy is potentially at its most valuable.[6, 13] Pregnancies can be prolonged for an average of 15 days from acute admission, with a reduction in neonatal complications and length of neonatal stay in the newborn intensive care unit. Close monitoring of the mother and fetus is required at a perinatal center.[13, 14]

WHEN SHOULD ANTIHYPERTENSIVE AGENTS BE USED?

Decisions regarding the need for antihypertensive treatment during pregnancy and selection of a specific antihypertensive agent should be based on an assessment of the relative risks and benefits for each patient. The effects of antihypertensive agents on the underlying pathophysiologic processes involved in preeclampsia may help therapeutic decision making[15, 16]; however, because this information may not be available in most settings, the "best bet" drug therapy must be used. A number of agents have a favorable risk-benefit profile for use in this condition, such as centrally acting drugs, β-blockers, and vasodilators. However, angiotensin-converting enzyme (ACE) inhibitors should be used only in exceptional circumstances because they pose an unacceptable risk to the fetus.[5, 17–19]

In North America, hydralazine and methyldopa have been the drugs of choice for the acute hypertensive crisis and management of chronic hypertension, although calcium channel blockers and labetalol came to the fore in the 1990s.[7, 16, 20–26] Parenteral magnesium sulfate ($MgSO_4$) remains the preferred immediate therapeutic approach in preeclampsia for prevention of eclampsia.[27–29] In the U.K., the antihypertensive drugs most commonly used are labetalol (35%), methyldopa (23%), and parenteral hydralazine (29%).

Although diuretics are not used routinely, they have a place in women with a fluid overload.[6] In 1992, anticonvulsants were prescribed by 85% of U.K. consultants to prevent seizures; the drugs used were diazepam (41%), phenytoin (30%), and chlormethiazole (24%). Very few consultants in the U.K. had used $MgSO_4$ (2%).[4] This intervention changed dramatically in the late 1990s, when the study by the Eclampsia Collaborative Group showed that $MgSO_4$ is superior to both phenytoin and diazepam for prevention of recurrent convulsions.[30, 31] This revelation led to the widespread acceptance of $MgSO_4$ by clinicians in the U.K.[6, 29, 32]

Although the conversion to the use of $MgSO_4$ in established eclampsia has taken place, there still is a reluctance to use it in women with preeclampsia as prophylaxis before convulsion has occurred. The reason is the relative rarity of eclampsia[1] and the consensus that treatment with antihypertensive drugs alone is all that is required.[6] The only controlled trials comparing the use and nonuse of $MgSO_4$ have been small and inconclusive.[33, 34] Although $MgSO_4$ appears to be superior to other therapies,[28, 34] no study has shown it to be necessary in women with preeclampsia alone.[35] Therefore, in the U.K., antihypertensive drugs are the first-line therapy in women who have not had convulsions; they are used in combination with $MgSO_4$ in women with eclampsia.[6]

If the benefits of the use of antihypertensive agents are accepted, clinicians caring for pregnancies complicated by hypertension must have a well-formulated management plan and guidelines to assess the need for antihypertensive drugs.[6] In general, antihypertensive medications should be reserved for patients considered having high-risk hypertension.[7, 13] An individualized management plan and referral to a tertiary care center will improve maternal and perinatal outcome in women who are remote from term and in those with the HELLP (*he*molysis, *e*levated *l*iver enzymes, *l*ow *p*latelets) syndrome.[13]

WHICH ANTIHYPERTENSIVE DRUGS CAN BE USED?

Drugs exist that can alter the responses of every known blood pressure control system. They can be divided into five main groups (Table 11–1):

- Centrally acting drugs
- Agents that alter cardiac output
- Drugs that affect the peripheral vascular resistance
- ACE inhibitors
- Diuretics

Other medications that have been used in pregnant women with hypertension include (1) low-dose aspirin, (2) $MgSO_4$, and (3) antioxidants.

Centrally Acting Drugs

Although many new drugs have proved useful in the management of hypertension in

TABLE 11–1. ANTIHYPERTENSIVE DRUGS FOR USE IN PREGNANCY

	BENEFITS	SIDE EFFECTS
CENTRALLY ACTING DRUGS		
Methyldopa	Proven	Tiredness/dry mouth; not good in the acute situation
Clonidine	None	Little experience
DRUGS THAT AFFECT CARDIAC OUTPUT		
Atenolol	Simple	Neonatal hypoglycemia; IUGR
Oxprenolol	Fewer side effects; ISA	Neonatal hypoglycemia
Metoprolol	Fewer side effects	Neonatal hypoglycemia
Labetalol	α-blockade IV and oral use	Neonatal hypoglycemia; tremor
DRUGS THAT AFFECT THE PERIPHERAL VASCULAR RESISTANCE		
Hydralazine	Proven	Headache/tremor; IV only of value; fetal distress
Nifedipine	Oral	Headache; tachycardia
Nicardipine	Oral	Little experience
Nimodipine	Cerebral vasodilator	Little experience
ANGIOTENSIN-CONVERTING ENZYME INHIBITORS		
Captopril	Contraindicated	Fetal loss, neonatal renal failure
Enalapril	Contraindicated	Postpartum only; little experience
DIURETICS		
Furosemide	Potent	Postpartum only

ISA, intrinsic sympathomimetic activity; IUGR, intrauterine growth restriction; IV, intravenous.

pregnancy and preeclampsia, methyldopa has continued to be used particularly for the long-term treatment of chronic hypertension.[36] Methyldopa acts by central inhibition of the sympathetic drive.[37] Although it is very effective, it is associated with troublesome side effects that have led to the move away from its use in the nonpregnant patient.[38] However, methyldopa is still the most widely used drug for pregnancy hypertension throughout the world. This is partly due to its relative low cost but also its apparent safety.[39–41]

For long-term therapy, methyldopa is the only drug that has been fully assessed and shown to be safe for the neonate and infant.[42] Its use in lowering maternal blood pressure does not appear to affect fetal well-being in utero, and fetal heart rate characteristics are not significantly influenced by treatment with methyldopa.[43] After 48 hours of methyldopa therapy, middle cerebral artery velocities are decreased significantly but to a lesser degree than changes induced by nifedipine. This reduction is independent of changes in the blood pressure or heart rate. Therefore, maternal cerebral hemodynamics are influenced by antihypertensive treatment. This suggests that methyldopa, along with other antihypertensive drugs, can reduce the cerebral vasospasm associated with preeclampsia, and this appears to be a direct effect of the medication on the cerebral arteries.[44]

Drugs That Alter Cardiac Output

Preeclampsia is thought to be a state of sympathetic overactivity.[45] This leads to increased systemic vascular resistance, maternal heart rate, and, potentially, cardiac output. The consistent hemodynamic action of β-adrenergic blockade is a reduction in the cardiac output, with varying effects on the peripheral vessels.[46] Although this is attractive in the nonpregnant hypertensive patient, in whom increased cardiac output is the main pathologic finding and the peripheral resistance is normal, it may be less successful in preeclampsia, where the main finding in severe disease is the increased systemic vascular resistance with varying changes in cardiac function. β-Blockers can be subdivided into (1) those that are blockers to both β₁ and β₂ receptors, (2) those that are selective β₁-receptor blockers, (3) those with intrinsic sympathomimetic activity, and (4) different lipid solubility and membrane-stabilizing effects. These different properties can alter both the beneficial and harmful effects of these drugs.

Adrenoceptor antagonists are now widely used in the treatment of preeclampsia in Europe, Australia, and North America.[6, 47–49] They are generally considered safe to use, although some concerns exist.[50] Antagonists without intrinsic sympathomimetic activity may increase the chance of intrauterine growth restriction (retardation).[51, 52] Intrauterine growth retardation is one of the main contributory factors in the increased perinatal morbidity and mortality associated with preeclampsia. Doppler flow changes have been studied during therapy with atenolol, such as an increase in the fetal aortic pulsatility index (PI) and the resistance index of the uterine artery after 7 days. These results suggest that atenolol may not be the best drug to use in women with hypertensive pregnancies.[53]

There is also concern that very-low-birth-weight (≤1500 g) infants born to mothers with preeclampsia who have been given β-blockers are at particular danger for side effects from the therapy. In one study, it was found that during the first year of life, seven of 19 infants died when the mothers' antihypertensive regimen included β-blockers. Four of the deaths occurred within 15 days. There were no deaths in 16 infants whose mothers received other antihypertensive treatment. These results suggest that some β-blocker therapy may have adverse effects on the very-low-birth-weight infants.[54]

The most studied drugs are the nonselective blockers pindolol and oxprenolol, the selective β-blockers atenolol and metoprolol, and the combined α/β-blocker labetalol.[5] Labetalol is a unique adrenoceptor antagonist because it has both α₁-adrenoceptor antagonist and nonselective β-adrenoceptor antagonist properties. The β-blocking effect of labetalol is four times less potent than that of propranolol. It appears to exert its hypotensive effects without compromising the maternal cardiovascular system by producing peripheral vasodilatation and maintaining cardiac output.[55] These changes help maintain renal and uterine blood flow. Acute administration of labetalol causes a reduction in blood pressure, heart rate, and peripheral resistance, but there is no change

in the cardiac output in standing and supine positions.[55]

In a comparison of maternal therapy with labetalol versus hydralazine, the median pH of the umbilical cord was lower and the number of infants with a cord pH below 7.20 was higher in the hydralazine group. However, as with other β-blockers, blood glucose levels were lower in the labetalol infants at 6 hours of age ($P < .05$), but no clinical sign of adrenergic blockade was found at 24 hours of age.[56] Some evidence suggests that labetalol may diminish the amount of proteinuria in patients who already have proteinuric preeclampsia.[57, 58] Labetalol therapy appears to reduce the aggregability of platelets,[59] which may be beneficial in maintaining placental function, but despite its vasodilator properties and platelet effects, it also may contribute to intrauterine growth retardation.[60]

One advantage of labetalol is that it can be used for both acute and chronic management. Acute hypertension can be managed by repeated oral labetalol therapy, which compares favorably with hydralazine and is more predictable.[61] If oral therapy is not successful, intravenous (IV) labetalol 50 mg, given by slow bolus followed by labetalol infusion, reduces blood pressure in most patients.[49]

In St. James University Hospital, Leeds, the antihypertensive regimen used is oral labetalol with a starting dose of 200 mg three times a day. This can be increased steadily to a maximum of 300 mg four times a day. In some patients, monotherapy does not control the hypertension, and 10 mg oral sustained-release nifedipine is added twice a day, which is increased to a maximum of 60 mg a day.

Drugs That Affect Peripheral Vascular Resistance

Drugs acting on the vascular wall to reduce peripheral resistance are among the oldest and the newest antihypertensive agents. Because preeclampsia is associated with increased peripheral vascular resistance, drugs that cause vasodilation appear to be potentially beneficial. However, their effects depend on other aspects of the cardiovascular system that affect the woman's ability to respond to the vasodilation, such as cardiac output and plasma volume.

Diazoxide, a benzothiadiazine derivative that is closely related to the thiazide diuretics, is now rarely used. In large doses, it is associated with acute fetal distress and intrauterine death.[62]

Hydralazine is the oldest antihypertensive drug still in regular clinical use. It acts directly on the vascular wall, requiring an intact endothelium to produce its effect, and works best with the patient lying flat in bed. The fall in blood pressure results from vasodilatation.

Used as monotherapy, hydralazine produces side effects such as tachycardia, flushing, nasal congestion, tremors, headaches, nausea, and vomiting,[63] and studies suggest that if it is going to be used as chronic therapy, it should be in combination with a β-blocker.[47] A few patients may be unusually sensitive to hydralazine because of a reduced capacity to metabolize the drug. Its use is usually restricted to single or short-term use, because prolonged use leads to both the stimulation of the renin-angiotensin-aldosterone system and reduction in renal perfusion pressure causing fluid retention, blunting of the drug's hypotensive effect, and increasing the chances of cardiac failure.

After IV dihydralazine, mean arterial blood pressure decreases significantly but diastolic blood pressure is affected more than systolic blood pressure. The Doppler PI in the uterine artery increases, implying alteration in the uteroplacental circulation.[64] This has been confirmed in animal studies, in which placental blood flow is reduced,[65] and may explain the acute fetal distress seen with acute use.[66, 67] These changes may be due to a combination of acute vasodilatation in women with a reduced plasma volume. Although hydralazine has been used successfully combined with plasma expansion, the results are no better than with antihypertensive therapy alone.[68] The effect of a single dose of hydralazine wears off in about 2 to 3 hours. Orally, its effect is minimal but it can be used as an adjunct to β-blocker therapy.[47]

Cadralazine, a 6-substituted derivative of 3-hydrazinopyridoxine structurally related to hydralazine, is effective in lowering blood pressure levels in pregnant hypertensive women. In one report, no adverse effects from the drug were observed on fetal development or immediate postnatal adaptation to stress during labor, and only mild maternal side effects such as headache were detected.[69] With the increased usage of the calcium antagonists, this drug may not gain widespread use.

Sodium nitroprusside is an effective IV drug for the management of acute hypertension in the nonpregnant patient. It has been used in pregnancy but there is concern about the effects on the placental blood flow and the potential toxic effects.[70] Because it is light sensitive, it is difficult to administer, and there are now easier and equally effective drugs that are preferable to use.

Calcium channel blockers act primarily by inhibiting extracellular calcium influx into cells through slow calcium channels. They reduce peripheral resistance, and their action is proportional to the amount of vasoconstriction.[71] They are antagonistic against any form of vasoconstrictor and have a mild tocolytic effect.

The drugs that are most commonly used in primary hypertension are nifedipine, nicardipine, and verapamil, but newer ones are constantly appearing on the scene. They are potent orally and are used alone or in combination with β-adrenergic blockers.[5] They can be used in the acute situation or chronically. The half-life of nifedipine in pregnancy appears to be shorter than in the nonpregnant woman, and studies indicate that it may achieve greater antihypertensive efficacy in pregnant women if administered at shorter intervals. Nifedipine can be detected in samples of fetal cord blood and amniotic fluid at concentrations approximately 93% and 53% of those of simultaneous maternal vein samples, respectively.[22, 72]

Studies have suggested that calcium antagonists may have beneficial effects on maternal blood flow in preeclampsia. Transcranial Doppler ultrasound examinations of maternal middle cerebral arteries were performed before and 45 minutes after administration of nifedipine. Blood pressure and middle cerebral artery velocities decreased significantly following short-acting antihypertensive therapy. The middle cerebral artery mean velocity decrease was independent of changes in the blood pressure or heart rate. The reduction of middle cerebral artery flow velocities following administration of nifedipine may suggest that cerebral vasodilatation is occurring, which is consistent with the concept that cerebral vasospasm is present in women with preeclampsia. The cerebral vasodilatation may result from a direct effect of the medication on the arteries in question.[44]

Similarly, after acute administration of nimodipine, another calcium antagonist, there was a significant reduction in the PI in the maternal ophthalmic and central retinal arteries and in the fetal middle cerebral artery, suggesting vasodilatation of the cerebral vessels of both mother and fetus.[16] The umbilical artery systolic-diastolic ratio was also significantly reduced. Maternal blood pressure was controlled without the need for other antihypertensive medication, and nimodipine was well tolerated, although heart rate was increased.

In another study, no significant differences were found in umbilical and uterine circulation in patients receiving nifedipine; however, there was a short-term significant increase in PI in the maternal middle cerebral artery at 60 minutes that had returned to normal at 120 minutes and 48 hours.[53] After acute treatment with nicardipine in patients with preeclampsia, diastolic blood pressure fell at 30, 45, and 60 minutes. The uteroplacental systolic-diastolic ratio rose significantly at 30 minutes, but this change was no longer apparent at 60 minutes. Umbilical artery and maternal brachial artery systolic-diastolic ratios were unchanged.[73]

Animal studies have suggested that placental blood flow is reduced by nicardipine, with an increase in fetal hypoxia.[74, 75] Other studies do not support this finding,[76] and human experience suggests that with therapeutic dosages, calcium channel blockers are safe.[36] Use of nifedipine results in a steady decrease in mean arterial pressure and systemic vascular resistance without fetal heart rate changes.[26]

Calcium antagonists may have other cellular effects. Nifedipine therapy restores erythrocyte aggregation to the normal state. Increased erythrocyte aggregation may be caused either by changes of the cell membrane occurring during hypertension or by a redistribution of the ionic charges on the two surfaces of the membrane. The effect of nifedipine may be due to restoring the ionic charges and might explain some of the other physiologic effects seen.[77]

Both hydralazine and calcium antagonists can be used for rapid reduction of severely elevated blood pressure,[36] and newer preparations, such as isradipine[78] and nimodipine,[79] compare favorably with dihydralazine in the treatment of severe hypertension

of pregnancy. In North America, hydralazine is still the most common used antihypertensive medication, usually in combination with MgSO$_4$.[80, 81] However, because oral labetalol and nifedipine appear to be at least as good as hydralazine,[61, 67] hydralazine has largely been superseded in many other parts of the world[6] and nifedipine is now commonly used in preeclampsia, often in combination with labetalol.[82]

Care should be taken because sudden falls in blood pressure may occur,[83] especially with sublingual usage, which has led to the recommendation that this form of therapy should not be used.[6] The combination of nifedipine and MgSO$_4$ was thought to be potentially dangerous because of synergism, but many centers have used this combination extensively without problems.[6]

Other vasodilators have been used. Urapidil is an antagonist of postsynaptic α_1 receptors, which leads to a diminution of the increased blood pressure by reducing the peripheral vascular resistance. When used post partum, blood pressure was reduced in all treated women without any tachycardia or serious side effects.[84] Similarly, isosorbide spray has been successfully used for preeclampsia.[85] Neither appears to have advantages over calcium antagonists.

Angiotensin-Converting Enzyme Inhibitors

ACE inhibitors are relatively new, very effective drugs for treatment of hypertension in the nonpregnant patient. They act by inhibiting the action of the ACE, causing reduced production of angiotensin II and reduced peripheral vascular resistance.[86] There is no reflex tachycardia. This action may seem attractive for use in preeclampsia with its abnormalities of angiotensin II sensitivity. However, the original ACE inhibitor, *captopril*, has produced unacceptable side effects in both animal experiments and clinical practice.[17] Fetal deformity, neonatal renal failure, intrauterine death, and a significant reduction in placental blood flow have all been reported. When captopril was given to pregnant sheep and rabbits, there was an appallingly high fetal and neonatal death rate in both species. It was concluded that this treatment should not be used in humans.[17]

Enalapril is a newer drug with fewer side

effects, but adverse reports have begun to appear in the literature. For these reasons, the use of either drug in pregnancy must be restricted. However, either drug may be used in the postpartum period when blood pressure control is difficult to achieve. Enalapril is effective in lowering blood pressure in all grades of essential and renovascular hypertension. It is at least as effective as other established and newer ACE inhibitors. This favorable profile of efficacy and tolerability and the substantial weight of clinical experience explain the increasing acceptance of enalapril as a major antihypertensive treatment in the immediate postpartum period.[87] Its use in pregnancy can be justified only in women for whom there is no alternative to control the blood pressure.

Diuretics

Diuretics probably act by exerting a mild vasodilator action and by reducing plasma volume by altering sodium balance. The thiazides are the most commonly used, often in combination with other drugs. Thiazides are not very effective in lowering blood pressure in pregnancy and have dangerous side effects of severe hyponatremia and acute pancreatitis in the mother and the fetus. A rise in blood urea and uric acid levels, neonatal thrombocytopenia, and hyperglycemia and glycosuria in diabetic or prediabetic patients can all be produced by the use of thiazide diuretics. There is some evidence to indicate that they can interfere with placental function. However, Sibai and colleagues[88] showed that patients with chronic hypertension taking diuretics can have the normal blood volume changes of pregnancy.

In general, diuretics have a relatively weak action and their de nouveau use in pregnancy cannot be recommended. Patients already receiving diuretic therapy will probably have chronic hypertension mild enough to allow cessation of therapy for the duration of the pregnancy. The main use of diuretics in preeclampsia should be restricted to the use of furosemide in the postpartum period to help treat fluid overload and pulmonary edema.[6]

OTHER DRUGS

Other drugs and medications have been used in the management of hypertension in pregnancy. Some agents have a degree of antihypertensive action, but others have a different mode of action and may alter the pathophysiology of the disease process.

Magnesium Sulfate

$MgSO_4$ is not an antihypertensive agent. In an in vivo rat study, $MgSO_4$ alone had no significant effect on mean arterial pressure but attenuated the pressor response to both noradrenaline and angiotensin II.[89] After discontinuation of the $MgSO_4$ infusion, the pressor responses returned to normal.

Although $MgSO_4$ is not an efficient primary antihypertensive agent, it may affect blood pressure by attenuating the actions of circulating vasoconstrictors. It has been used for more than 70 years in the treatment of preeclampsia, largely in North America.[90] In other parts of the world, different sedation agents have been used, including diazepam and phenytoin.[4] Now this has changed.[29, 32]

A large multicenter study showed $MgSO_4$ to be superior to both phenytoin and diazepam in the management of eclampsia.[30] The rate of both subsequent convulsions and maternal death was found to be significantly reduced compared with use of either diazepam or phenytoin. Although there is now no doubt about what preparation to use, no treatment will completely prevent seizures with rates of subsequent convulsions varying between 5% and 20%.[30] Both the IV and intramuscular (IM) regimens used in the study were similar to those previously published.[91, 92] There is no evidence that one route is superior to any other. Both regimens use a slow IV loading dose of 4 to 6 g $MgSO_4$, which can be used to treat the convulsion. This dose should be given over 20 minutes because a faster bolus may produce cardiac arrest. There is no need to use diazepam initially to stop the seizure.

Whether the IM or the IV maintenance dosage is used depends on the preference and facilities of the center. The IM route has the advantage of ease of use, although IV therapy may provide better blood levels.[93] One of the concerns many obstetricians have is the fear of magnesium toxicity. The collaborative study used clinical evaluation alone and showed that toxicity did not occur and the side effects from magnesium were no worse than from diazepam and significantly less than those found with pheny-toin.[30] Therefore, with these dose regimens, there is no need to check magnesium levels or to have this facility available at all times. Magnesium levels are useful in the management of treatment failures.

The role of prophylactic MgSO$_4$ in women with preeclampsia is less clear. If in doubt, it is probably safer to give it than not, but magnesium is not without its own risks; in some series, the only deaths have come from magnesium toxicity. Although studies have demonstrated that MgSO$_4$ is a superior drug for seizure prophylaxis in preeclampsia,[31, 94] small studies have found no evidence that magnesium is superior to antihypertensive drugs alone.[33]

In the U.K., the incidence of eclampsia is now only 1/2000,[2] a dramatic fall over the last 50 years.[1] The risk of eclampsia occurring in women with preeclampsia is probably between 1/100 and 1/200, and the use of MgSO$_4$ as a prophylactic therapy would have a low impact in U.K. practice. However, if a prophylactic anticonvulsant is to be used, MgSO$_4$ is the drug of choice.[28, 29, 32]

Aspirin

Although the theory behind the use of low-dose aspirin is attractive,[95] there is mixed evidence of its value.[96] The large multicenter study on high-risk women (Collaborative Low-dose Aspirin Study in Pregnancy [CLASP]) failed to show an overall difference in the treated group, although it was suggested that those with early-onset disease may gain some delay in the onset of disease.[97] Other studies have yielded similar results.[99]

Although it has been suggested that there is an increase in placental abruption in women taking aspirin, the available data do not support this.[98] If any women do benefit, it is those with a history of early-onset preeclampsia or intrauterine growth retardation, pathologic results of a Doppler examination of the uterus, pathologic results of the angiotensin test, or antiphospholipid syndrome.[99, 100] Use of aspirin must be made only after careful consideration of each individual case.

Antioxidant Therapy

Most therapies in preeclampsia are based on correcting abnormalities as they occur.

Antihypertensive drugs are the best example of this concept, in which blood pressure is controlled with little effect on the disease process. Evidence indicates that there is an increase in the free radical activity in preeclampsia,[101] perhaps because of an oxidant-antioxidant imbalance among the pathogenic factors involved in preeclampsia.[102] Endothelial dysfunction is the final common pathway in the pathogenesis of preeclampsia.

Future therapeutic modalities aimed at preventing or treating preeclampsia should either reduce the extent of (or even prevent) endothelial cell dysfunction (primary prevention) or reduce the consequences of endothelial cell dysfunction (secondary and tertiary prevention). If lipid peroxidation and reactive oxygen activity are part of the disease process, alteration of these systems may moderate disease progression. This might be done using exogenous antioxidants.

A nonrandomized controlled trial showed that vitamin E supplementation did not improve fetal outcome in women with established severe preeclampsia or show favorable effects on maternal hypertension and proteinuria.[103] Combined antioxidant therapy with vitamin E, vitamin C, and allopurinol did not result in measurable changes in placental lipid peroxide levels, suggesting the local nature of both the damage and the necessary protective measures.[104]

Another study of a similar antioxidant cocktail did reduce the proportion of women delivering within 14 days to 52%, compared with 76% in the placebo group, but did not result in altered lipid peroxide levels, although serum uric acid levels were reduced.[105] Although these results were encouraging, the authors did not recommend routine use of antioxidants in preeclampsia at that time. However, further research with modified strategies, such as earlier initiation of therapy or different combinations, seems worthwhile. Indeed, a recent randomized trial of a limited number of women considered at risk for preeclampsia revealed a significant reduction in preeclampsia in women receiving 1000 mg of vitamin C and 400 IU of vitamin E, starting at 16 to 18 weeks' gestation.[105a]

Although the results of studies on the role of nitric oxide in preeclampsia are inconclusive, the effect of the nitric oxide donor S-nitrosoglutathione on women with severe preeclampsia demonstrates that uterine artery resistance, blood pressure, and platelet activation are all reduced, suggesting that platelet-specific nitric oxide donors may prove beneficial in the management of severe preeclampsia in the future.[106]

GUIDELINES FOR THE USE OF ANTIHYPERTENSIVE THERAPY

Severe Hypertension

No randomized study has evaluated antihypertensive therapy (Table 11–2) in severe hypertension in pregnancy, although most agree about starting hypotensive treatment when diastolic blood pressure is above 110 mmHg.[5] When a woman presents with severe preeclampsia, high blood pressure is the primary risk to her life. The potential vascular, renal, hepatic, and neurologic damage is mostly secondary to the hypertension. Therefore, control of blood pressure using antihypertensive therapy should be the initial aim, especially during labor or before intubation for general anesthetic for cesarean section, because an acute rise in blood pressure can occur.[107]

The fetus is at risk because of placental damage leading to intrauterine growth retardation and intrauterine death. The placental

---

TABLE 11–2. THE STEP-WISE MANAGEMENT OF PREGNANCY HYPERTENSION

SCREENING

Screen women for the risk or signs of hypertension in pregnancy.
Monitor women at risk in an antenatal day unit.

BEFORE DELIVERY

Regularly update management protocols.
Involve senior medical staff early.
Stabilize patient with antihypertensive drugs if required.
Administer prophylactic steroids if the pregnancy is under 34 weeks' gestation.
Consider the need for magnesium sulfate.
Continue monitoring for signs of disease progression.
Induce delivery on the best day, the best way, and in the best place.

AFTER DELIVERY

Maintain vigilance.
Stop magnesium sulfate therapy after 24 hours of stability.
Reduce antihypertensive therapy gradually.

---

pathology is not directly related to the hypertension, and lowering blood pressure is unlikely to improve placental function; it may even be detrimental. Any benefit to the baby is brought from prolongation of the pregnancy sufficiently to reduce the complications of prematurity without increasing the risk to the mother. As with all therapies, there must be a balance between the benefits of treatment and any potential harm that might occur.

If antihypertensive drugs are to be used, hydralazine is still the most commonly used in acute hypertension, given intravenously by injection or infusion.[108] Satisfactory control of blood pressure can also be easily achieved with an IV infusion of labetalol in severe hypertension in pregnancy.[49, 109, 110] Oral labetalol has also been found to be effective.[61] There are fewer maternal side effects or hypotensive episodes with labetalol than with hydralazine. Nifedipine has also proved effective in pregnancy and in the puerperium.[111, 112] In comparison with hydralazine, nifedipine has been as effective in lowering blood pressure and has the advantage of being an oral therapy. One potential serious problem is the possible interaction between calcium channel blockers and $MgSO_4$, which can result in a sudden excessive drop in blood pressure, although this risk may have been overstated.

The aim of therapy is not to normalize the blood pressure but to stop the rise and achieve a moderate fall. The therapeutic dose should be increased until a fall of around 10 mmHg in diastolic blood pressure is achieved. Once control is adequate, increasing dosage may be required in the future to maintain this.

Because patients with severe preeclampsia-eclampsia can present acutely, often outside of office hours, it is important that all staff be familiar with the management guidelines and the aims of therapy. In the absence of convulsions, prolongation of the pregnancy is possible, in most cases, for an average of 15 days.[5] This may improve the outcome for the baby without detriment to the mother. Rushing the delivery in the maternal interest is not of benefit to the mother and can lead to increased morbidity for the baby because it is the length of gestation that influences the outcome of the baby more than any other parameter.[113] It is important that the mother's condition be stable so that prolongation of pregnancy does not jeopardize her life. The situation should be constantly reassessed because a woman who is stable may not remain so. The plan of management is more along the lines of "not needing delivery now" rather than "let's deliver her next week."

If the gestation is less than 34 weeks and delivery within the next few days is thought to be a possibility, prophylactic steroids (dexamethasone 12 mg given IM twice, 12 hours apart) should be given to enhance fetal lung maturity. The aim is to prolong the pregnancy for at least 48 hours to achieve maximum effect, although even if the delivery is earlier, some benefit would be gained. Delivery before this time should be carried out if there are strong maternal or fetal reasons. After 48 hours, if further prolongation for more than a week is not thought to be achievable, delivery should be instituted when the mother is stable and the baby is well and has received maximum benefit from prophylactic steroids. Transfer of the mother to a tertiary care facility before delivery may be necessary for the optimal care for mother or her newly born, possibly premature baby.

Because antihypertensive drugs have varying modes of action, beneficial results achieved with one preparation may not be seen with another, and failure of action of one antihypertensive drug does not mean that all will be unsuccessful. Side effects seen with some medications are not seen with others. Before giving any patient antihypertensive therapy, the obstetrician must assess whether the patient would benefit from the medication and which drug would be best to use. As in the nonpregnant patient, the potential benefits are balanced against the potential risks of therapy. In pregnancy, the situation is complicated by the presence of the fetus. Although the benefits of therapy may be directed at the mother, the side effects may be experienced by both the mother and her unborn child. The fear of teratogenicity and other fetal complications has meant that most new drugs are contraindicated for use in pregnancy, although there is no evidence of their harm. With the increasing cost of litigation and the relatively low profits from the use of drugs in pregnancy, few companies support or fund antihypertensive studies in pregnancy. This has led to a relative paucity of information concerning the overall benefits and, equally, the possible harm of antihypertensive therapy for the pregnant woman.

Mild to Moderate Hypertension

Most of the studies of the use of antihypertensive drugs in pregnancy (see Table 11–2) have been conducted in women with mild to moderate disease. Many of the women have had a mixture of mild preeclampsia and chronic hypertension. Methyldopa was first assessed in pregnancy more than 30 years ago.[40] The most comprehensive study of methyldopa was performed by Redman and associates,[39, 114] who concluded that it was safe and that it appeared to reduce fetal loss from second-trimester abortions. There was no difference in perinatal mortality rate or the incidence of superimposed preeclampsia. The children of the women who took part in this study were monitored for 7 years, and there was no obvious difference between the children from the treatment group and those from the control group in terms of physical and mental handicaps, behavior, vision, hearing, and intellectual ability, thus emphasizing not only the drug's safety but also the lack of measurable benefit.[41] These results have led the authors to state that methyldopa should be the drug of choice in pregnancy because it is proven to be safe. Yet the other drugs have not been shown to be unsafe. Maternal side effects were troublesome enough to cause 15% of the women to be withdrawn from the study.

In the 1970s, studies were carried out on the use of β-blockers. Initially, studies with propranolol demonstrated fetal side effects, but later work showed increasing safety. With evidence that preeclampsia is associated with sympathetic overactivity,[45] the role of β-blockers appears to be more established. The first randomized controlled study of an adrenoceptor antagonist in preeclampsia was performed with atenolol, a selective β-receptor antagonist.[115] This was a study of 120 women. Atenolol effectively controlled blood pressure and reduced the subsequent development of proteinuria, suggesting a possible beneficial effect on the disease process. It is not a surprise, however, if antihypertensive therapy reduces the incidence of proteinuria, because this is probably a result of the reduction in the perfusion pressure to the kidney. There was no difference in fetal and neonatal complications, such as intrauterine growth retardation, neonatal hypoglycemia, and hyperbilirubinemia between the two groups. Respiratory distress was seen only in the control group. However, neonatal bradycardia was more common in the atenolol group, although there was no effect on neonatal blood pressure. The children from this study were monitored for 1 year, and atenolol did not appear to have any adverse effects on their development. Other studies have confirmed these findings, although long-term therapy in chronic hypertension may be associated with growth retardation.[116] Some clinicians recommend the use of a vasodilator, such as hydralazine or nifedipine, as concomitant or second-line therapy to overcome the vasoconstriction of preeclampsia and to counteract some of the side effects of β-blockers.[117, 118]

From these studies, it seems that adrenoceptor antagonists are both safe and effective in the treatment of mild preeclampsia and may have some beneficial effects on the disease process. Whether any particular adrenoceptor antagonist is more effective than the others is not certain. Labetalol has been shown to be as good as or superior to methyldopa, whereas both labetalol and pindolol appear to have advantages over atenolol.[5, 119]

In a prospective double-blind randomized placebo-controlled study of labetalol in 144 women who developed mild preeclampsia after 20 weeks' gestation, labetalol significantly lowered blood pressure and reduced the incidence of proteinuria. The placebo-treated group included more patients who developed severe hypertension (>150/110 mmHg) and had a greater requirement for additional antihypertensive therapy before labor than the group treated with labetalol. Therefore, the maximum blood pressure before labor and the incidence of proteinuria were reduced in women given labetalol therapy. However, because late-onset disease did not appear to benefit, the appropriateness of pharmacologic therapy for late-onset mild preeclampsia may be questioned.[120]

Labetalol controls the blood pressure in most women within 24 hours of commencement of therapy. This control is often short-lived, requiring dose escalation after 3 to 5 days in most cases. Labetalol is well tolerated, and no significant maternal toxicity has been noted.[121] In various studies, labetalol-treated patients had a reduction in hospital inpatient antenatal stay. There is a trend suggesting a possible prolongation of pregnancy, a reduction in emergency cesarean sections, and an increase in spontaneous vaginal deliveries in women given labetalol.

In a double-blind study of pindolol in 60 women presenting with a diastolic blood pressure of 85 to 99 mmHg before the 35th week of pregnancy, early treatment of the hypertension was not associated with adverse effects in either mother or newborn. However, 15 patients receiving placebo required additional treatment compared with six in the pindolol group. Therefore, it appears that 50% of pregnant women with mild to moderate hypertension would have a progressive disease eventually requiring antihypertensive therapy, whereas the remainder would be able to complete the pregnancy without treatment.[12]

Hydralazine is frequently used as a second-line drug to augment the effects of adrenoceptor antagonists and methyldopa when satisfactory control is not achieved with a single agent.[15] Erratic metabolism can yield unpredictable responses by the oral route, and nifedipine has largely superseded hydralazine for this indication.[14]

Although blood pressure control is usually easily achieved in pregnancy, few individual studies have shown any measurable benefit to the mother or baby.[5] However, a meta-analysis of all the available studies of antihypertensive therapy in pregnancy has shown that early treatment reduces the incidence not only of hypertensive crisis but also of neonatal complications such as respiratory distress syndrome.[122] Therefore, there is now abundant evidence that early aggressive use of antihypertensive therapy benefits both mother and baby. The meta-analysis did not compare different drugs. It probably does not matter which drugs are used as long as attendant staff are experienced in their use and the drugs are thought to be safe. No one therapy can control all patients, and increasing doses of drug and additive therapies are often required.[6]

The aim of any therapy is to stabilize the mother and to allow delivery at the best time in the best place. Whenever the delivery takes place, recovery of the mother follows, but not immediately, and there is a continuing need for vigilance and usually antihypertensive therapy.

Postpartum Care

Continued close monitoring (see Table 11–2) is required in a suitable environment. An initial improvement may be seen, but most women worsen again within 48 hours to some degree. Women with severe disease should be kept in an obstetric intensive care area and should not be transferred to the postnatal wards until parameters begin to return to normal.

The main cause of mortality in mothers with this condition is now pulmonary edema,[3] probably attributable to various underlying mechanisms associated with the preeclamptic woman, including a low albumin level and increased capillary leak. After delivery, a relative oliguria is not uncommon, occurring in about 30% of patients with severe disease. Therapy is not required because urine output recovers in its own time. Renal impairment is a rare complication and can usually be managed conservatively. Fluid challenges are potentially dangerous in preeclampsia because much of the fluid is lost from the vessels into the pulmonary interstitial fluid, exacerbating the existing tissue edema.

One of the best methods of assessing pulmonary edema is continuous measurement of oxygen saturation with a pulse oximeter. It is far safer and more sensible to run a patient "dry" and restrict IV fluids than to run the risk of pulmonary overload. If the patient is in positive balance or if there is evidence of pulmonary edema, 40 mg of furosemide is given, usually producing a good response. This measure helps minimize the probability of pulmonary edema, increases oxygen saturation, reduces cerebral edema, and improves blood pressure control.

Therefore, after delivery, management should be aimed at maintaining blood pressure control and carefully monitoring the fluid balance. If convulsions occur, anticonvulsant therapy can be added. Because the majority of postnatal convulsions occur within the first 24 hours, anticonvulsant therapy is usually continued for 48 hours after delivery. If the patient is well, especially if prophylactic anticonvulsant therapy is being used in the absence of any convulsions, this therapy can be stopped within 24 hours.

Antihypertensive therapy needs to be reduced after delivery, depending on the blood pressure. There may be a significant drop within the first 24 hours, with a rise again after 48 hours. Antihypertensive drugs may be necessary for some weeks after delivery.

References

1. Leitch CR, Cameron AD, Walker JJ. The changing pattern of eclampsia over a 60-year period. Br J Obstet Gynaecol 1997;104:917–922.
2. Douglas KA, Redman CWG. Eclampsia in the United Kingdom. BMJ 1994;309:1395–1400.
3. Department of Health Welsh Office, Scottish Home and Health Department, Department of Health and Social Security, Northern Ireland. Report on Confidential Inquiries into Maternal Deaths in the United Kingdom 1991–1993. London: Her Majesty's Stationery Office, 1996.
4. Hutton JD, James DK, Stirrat GM, et al. Management of severe preeclampsia and eclampsia by U.K. consultants. Br J Obstet Gynaecol 1992;99:554–556.
5. Walker JJ. Hypertensive drugs in pregnancy: Antihypertension therapy in pregnancy, preeclampsia, and eclampsia. Clin Perinatol 1991;18:845–873.
6. Walker JJ. Care of the patient with severe pregnancy induced hypertension. Eur J Obstet Gynecol Reprod Biol 1996;65:127–135.
7. Sibai B. Drug-therapy: Treatment of hypertension in pregnant women. N Engl J Med 1996;335:257–265.
8. Stone P, Cook D, Hutton J, et al. Measurements of blood pressure, edema and proteinuria in a pregnant population of New Zealand. Aust N Z J Obstet Gynaecol 1995;35:32–37.
9. Walker JJ. Day-care obstetrics. Br J Hosp Med 1993;50:225–226.
10. Walker JJ. The case for early recognition and intervention in pregnancy induced hypertension. *In* Sharp F, Symonds EM (eds). Hypertension in Pregnancy. Proceedings of the Sixteenth Study Group of the Royal College of Obstetricians and Gynaecologists. New York: Perinatology Press, 1987, pp 289–299.
11. Hjertberg R, Belfrage P, Hanson U. Conservative treatment of mild and moderate hypertension in pregnancy. Acta Obstet Gynecol Scand 1992;71:439–446.
12. Bott Kanner G, Hirsch M, Friedman S, et al. Antihypertensive therapy in the management of hypertension in pregnancy—a clinical double-blind study of pindolol. Part B. Hypertension in pregnancy. Clin Exp Hypertens 1992;11:207–220.
13. Sibai BM, Mercer BM, Schiff E, Friedman SA. Aggressive versus expectant management of severe preeclampsia at 28 to 32 weeks gestation: A randomized controlled trial. Am J Obstet Gynecol 1994;171:818–822.
14. Witlin AG, Sibai BM. Hypertension in pregnancy: Current concepts of preeclampsia. Annu Rev Med 1997;48:115–127.
15. Easterling TR, Benedetti TJ, Schmucker BC, Carlson KL. Antihypertensive therapy in pregnancy directed by noninvasive hemodynamic monitoring. Am J Perinatol 1989;6:86–89.
16. Belfort MA, Saade GR, Moise KJ, et al. Nimodipine in the management of preeclampsia—maternal and fetal effects. Am J Obstet Gynecol 1994;171:417–424.
17. Broughton Pipkin F, Turber SR, Symonds EM. Possible risk with captopril in pregnancy. Lancet 1980;1:1256–1260.
18. Broughton Pipkin F, Symonds EM, Turner SR. The effect of captopril (SQ14,225) upon mother and

fetus in the chronically cannulated ewe and in the pregnant rabbit. J Physiol (Lond) 1982; 323:415–422.

19. Lindheimer MD, Barron WM. Enalapril and pregnancy-induced hypertension. Ann Intern Med 1988;108:911.

20. Sibai BM, Gonzalez AR, Mabie WC, Moretti M. A comparison of labetalol plus hospitalization versus hospitalization alone in the management of preeclampsia remote from term. Obstet Gynecol 1987;70:323–327.

21. Belfort MA, Moore PJ. Verapamil in the treatment of severe postpartum hypertension. S Afr Med J 1988;74:265–267.

22. Barton JR, Prevost RR, Wilson DA, et al. Nifedipine pharmacokinetics and pharmacodynamics during the immediate postpartum period in patients with preeclampsia. Am J Obstet Gynecol 1991;165:951–954.

23. Belfort MA, Kirshon B. Nisoldipine—a new orally administered calcium antagonist used in the treatment of severe postpartum pregnancy-induced hypertension: Preliminary results. S Afr Med J 1992;81:267–270.

24. Belfort M, Akovic K, Anthony J, et al. The effect of acute volume expansion and vasodilatation with verapamil on uterine and umbilical artery Doppler indexes in severe preeclampsia. J Clin Ultrasound 1994;22:317–325.

25. Sibai BM, Barton JR, Akl S, et al. A randomized prospective comparison of nifedipine and bed rest versus bed rest alone in the management of preeclampsia remote from term. Am J Obstet Gynecol 1992;167:879–884.

26. Scardo JA, Vermillion ST, Hogg BB, Newman RB. Hemodynamic effects of oral nifedipine in preeclamptic hypertensive emergencies. Am J Obstet Gynecol 1996;175:336–339.

27. Roberts JM. Magnesium for preeclampsia and eclampsia. N Engl J Med 1995;333:250–251.

28. Lucas MJ, Leveno KJ, Cunningham FG. A comparison of magnesium-sulfate with phenytoin for the prevention of eclampsia. N Engl J Med 1995; 333:201–205.

29. Walker JJ. Magnesium-sulfate is the drug of choice for the treatment of eclampsia. Hypertens Pregn 1996;15:1–6.

30. Duley L, Carroli G, Belizan J, et al. Which anticonvulsant for women with eclampsia? Evidence from the collaborative eclampsia trial. Lancet 1995;345:1455–1463.

31. Chien PFW, Khan KS, Arnott N. Magnesium-sulfate in the treatment of eclampsia and preeclampsia—an overview of the evidence from randomized trials. Br J Obstet Gynaecol 1996; 103:1085–1091.

32. Robson SC. Magnesium-sulfate—the time of reckoning. Br J Obstet Gynaecol 1996;103:99–102.

33. Moodley J, Moodley VV. Prophylactic anticonvulsant therapy in hypertensive crises of pregnancy—the need for a large, randomized trial. Hypertens Pregn 1994;13:245–252.

34. Chen FP, Chang SD, Chu KK. Expectant management in severe preeclampsia: Does magnesium-sulfate prevent the development of eclampsia? Acta Obstet Gynecol Scand 1995;74:181–185.

35. Burrows RF, Burrows EA. The feasibility of a control population for a randomized control trial of seizure prophylaxis in the hypertensive disorders of pregnancy. Am J Obstet Gynecol 1995;173:929–935.

36. Khedun SM, Moodley J, Naicker T, Maharaj B. Drug management of hypertensive disorders of pregnancy. Pharmacol Ther 1997;74:221–258.

37. Frolich ED. Methyldopa mechanisms and treatment 25 years on. Arch Intern Med 1980;140:954–957.

38. Reid JL, Elliot HL. Methyldopa. In Doyle A (ed). Handbook of Hypertension. Vol 5. Clinical Pharmacology of Antihypertensive Drugs. Amsterdam: Elsevier, 1984, pp 92–112.

39. Redman CW. Fetal outcome in trial of antihypertensive treatment in pregnancy. Lancet 1976; 2:753–756.

40. Leather HM, Humphries DM, Baker P, Chadd MA. A control trial of hypotensive agents in hypertension in pregnancy. Lancet 1968;2:488–492.

41. Ounsted M, Moar V, Redman CW. Infant growth and development following treatment of maternal hypertension. Lancet 1980;1:705.

42. Kyle PM, Redman CWG. Comparative risk-benefit assessment of drugs used in the management of hypertension in pregnancy. Drug Safe 1992;7:223–234.

43. Wideswensson D, Montan S, Arulkumaran S, et al. Effect of methyldopa and isradipine on fetal heart rate pattern assessed by computerized cardiotocography in human pregnancy. Am J Obstet Gynecol 1993;169:1581–1585.

44. Serra-Serra V, Kyle PM, Chandran R, Redman CWG. The effect of nifedipine and methyldopa on maternal cerebral circulation. Br J Obstet Gynaecol 1997;104:532–537.

45. Gans ROB, Dekker GA. Preeclampsia: A state of sympathetic overactivity. N Engl J Med 1997; 336:1326.

46. Lund Johansen P. The effect of beta-blocker therapy on chronic hemodynamics. Prim Cardiol 1980;1:20–26.

47. Paran E, Holzberg G, Mazor M, et al. Beta-adrenergic blocking agents in the treatment of pregnancy-induced hypertension. Int J Clin Pharmacol Ther 1995;33:119–123.

48. Dubois D, Petitcolas J, Temperville B, et al. Beta blocker therapy in 125 cases of hypertension during pregnancy. Clin Exp Hypertens B 1983;2:41–59.

49. Mabie WC, Gonzalez AR, Sibai BM, Amon E. A comparative trial of labetalol and hydralazine in the acute management of severe hypertension complicating pregnancy. Obstet Gynecol 1987; 70:328–333.

50. Kaaja R, Hiilesmaa V, Holma K, Jarvenpaa AL. Maternal antihypertensive therapy with beta-blockers associated with poor outcome in very-low birthweight infants. Int J Gynecol Obstet 1992;38:195–199.

51. Dubois D, Petitcolas J, Temperville B, et al. Treatment of hypertension in pregnancy with beta-adrenoceptor antagonists. Br J Clin Pharmacol 1982;13:375S–378S.

52. Lardoux H, Gerard J, Elazquez G, Flouvat B. Which beta-blocker in pregnancy-induced hypertension? Lancet 1983;2:1194–1198.

53. Danti L, Valcamonico A, Soregaroli M, et al. Fetal and maternal Doppler modifications during therapy with antihypertensive drugs. J Matern Fetal Invest 1994;4:19–23.

54. Kaaja R, Hiilesmaa V, Holma K, Jarvenpaa AL. Maternal antihypertensive therapy with beta-blockers associated with poor outcome in very-low-birth-weight infants. Int J Gynecol Obstet 1992;38:195–199.

55. Lund Johansen P. Pharmacology of combined alpha-beta-blockade. Drugs 1984;28:35–50.

56. Hjertberg R, Faxelius G, Lagercrantz H. Neonatal adaptation in hypertensive pregnancy: A study of labetalol vs. hydralazine treatment. J Perinat Med 1993;21:69–75.

57. Lamming GD, Broughton Pipkin F, Symonds EM. Comparison of the alpha and beta blocking drug labetalol and methyldopa in the treatment of moderate and severe PIH. Clin Exp Hypertens [B] 1980;2:865–869.

58. Cruickshank DJ, Robertson AA, Campbell DM, MacGillivray I. Does labetalol influence the development of proteinuria in pregnancy hypertension? A randomized controlled study. Eur J Obstet Gynecol Reprod Biol 1992;45:47–51.

59. Greer IA, Walker JJ, Calder AA, Forbes CD. Inhibition of platelet aggregation in whole blood by adrenoceptor antagonists. Thromb Res 1985; 40:631–635.

60. Cruickshank DJ, Campbell D, Robertson AA, Mac-Gillivray I. Intra-uterine growth retardation and maternal labetalol treatment in a random allocation controlled study. J Obstet Gynaecol 1992; 12:223–227.

61. Walker JJ, Greer I, Calder AA. Treatment of acute pregnancy-related hypertension: Labetalol and hydralazine compared. Postgrad Med J 1983; 59:168–170.

62. Ayromlooi J, Tobias M, Berg P, Leff R. The effects of diazoxide upon fetal and maternal hemodynamics and fetal brain function and metabolism. Pediatr Pharmacol 1982;2:293–304.

63. Koch Weser J. Vasodilator drugs in the treament of hypertension. Arch Intern Med 1974;133:1017–1020.

64. Grunewald C, Carlstrom K, Lunell NO, et al. Dihydralazine in preeclampsia: Acute effects on atrial natriuretic peptide concentration and feto-maternal hemodynamics. J Matern Fetal Med 1993; 3:21–24.

65. Lipshitz J, Ahokas RA, Reynolds SL. The effect of hydralazine on placental perfusion in the spontaneously hypertensive rat. Am J Obstet Gynecol 1987;156:356–359.

66. Vink GJ, Moodley J. The effect of low-dose dihydrallazine on the fetus in the emergency treatment of hypertension in pregnancy. S Afr Med J 1982;62:475–477.

67. Visser W, Wallenburg HCS. A comparison between the hemodynamic effects of oral nifedipine and intravenous dihydralazine in patients with severe preeclampsia. J Hypertens 1995;13:791–795.

68. Visser W, Vanpampus MG, Treffers PE, Wallenburg HCS. Perinatal results of hemodynamic and conservative temporizing treatment in severe preeclampsia. Eur J Obstet Gynecol Reprod Biol 1994;53:175–181.

69. Voto LS, Lapidus AM, Catuzzi P, et al. Cadralazine for the treatment of preeclampsia: An open, non-comparative, dose-finding pilot study. Hypertension 1992;19:II132–II136.

70. Nissen JC. Treatment of hypertensive emergencies of pregnancy. Clin Pharm 1982;1:334–343.

71. Olivari MT, Bartorelli C, Polese A, et al. Treatment of hypertension with nifedipine, a calcium antagonistic agent. Circulation 1979;59:1056–1058.

72. Prevost RR, Akl SA, Whybrew WD, Sibai BM. Oral nifedipine pharmacokinetics in pregnancy-induced hypertension. Pharmacotherapy 1992; 12:174–177.

73. Walker JJ, Mathers A, Bjornsson S, et al. The effect of acute and chronic antihypertensive therapy on maternal and fetoplacental Doppler velocimetry. Eur J Obstet Gynecol Reprod Biol 1992;43:193–199.

74. Parisi VM, Salinas J, Stockmar EJ. Placental vascular responses to nicardipine in the hypertensive ewe. Am J Obstet Gynecol 1989;161:1039–1043.

75. Parisi VM, Salinas J, Stockmar EJ. Fetal vascular responses to maternal nicardipine administration in the hypertensive ewe. Am J Obstet Gynecol 1989;161:1035–1039.

76. Ahokas RA, Sibai BM, Mabie WC, Anderson GD. Nifedipine does not adversely affect uteroplacental blood flow in the hypertensive term-pregnant rat. Am J Obstet Gynecol 1988;159:1440–1445.

77. Tranquilli AL, Garzetti GG, Detommaso G, et al. Nifedipine treatment in preeclampsia reverts the increased erythrocyte aggregation to normal. Am J Obstet Gynecol 1992;167:942–945.

78. Maharaj B, Khedun SM, Moodley J, et al. A comparative study of intravenous isradipine and dihydralazine in the treatment of severe hypertension of pregnancy in black patients. Hypertens Pregn 1997;16:1–9.

79. Anthony J, Mantel G, Johanson R, Dommisse J. The hemodynamic and respiratory effects of intravenous nimodipine used in the treatment of eclampsia. Br J Obstet Gynaecol 1996;103:518–522.

80. Barron WM. The syndrome of preeclampsia. Gastroenterol Clin North Am 1992;21:851–872.

81. Lindheimer MD. Hypertension in pregnancy. Hypertension 1993;22:127–137.

82. Henriksen T. Hypertension in pregnancy: Use of antihypertensive drugs. Acta Obstet Gynecol Scand 1997;76:96–106.

83. Impey L. Severe hypotension and fetal distress following sublingual administration of nifedipine to a patient with severe pregnancy-induced hypertension at 33 weeks. Br J Obstet Gynaecol 1993;100:959–961.

84. Wacker J, Muller J, Grischke EM, et al. Antihypertensive therapy of pregnancy-induced-hypertension (PIH) with urapidil. Zentralbl Gynakol 1994;116:271–273.

85. Vargas G, Salmeron I, Sanchez AR, et al. Efficacy of isosorbide spray in preeclampsia (PE) treatment. Hypertension 1997;29:6.

86. Cody RJ, Tarazi RC, Bravo EL, Fouan FM. Haemodynamics of orally active converting enzyme inhibitor (SQ-14,225) in hypertensive patients. Clin Sci Mol Med 1978;55:453–457.

87. Todd PA, Goa KL. Enalapril: A reappraisal of its pharmacology and therapeutic use in hypertension. Drugs 1992;43:346–381.

88. Sibai BM, Abdella TN, Anderson GD, Dilts PV. Plasma volume findings in pregnant women with mild hypertension: Therapeutic considerations. Am J Obstet Gynecol 1983;145:539–543.

89. Aisenbrey GA, Corwin E, Catanzarite V. Effect of magnesium-sulfate on the vascular actions of nor-

epinephrine and angiotensin-II. Am J Perinatol 1992;9:477–480.

90. Pritchard JA. The use of the magnesium ion in the management of eclamptogenic toxaemias. Surg Gynecol Obstet 1955;100:131–135.

91. Pritchard JA, Cunningham FG, Pritchard SA. The Parkland Memorial Hospital protocol for treatment of eclampsia: Evaluation of 245 cases. Am J Obstet Gynecol 1984;148:951–963.

92. Zuspan FP. Problems encountered in the treatment of pregnancy-induced hypertension: A point of view. Am J Obstet Gynecol 1978;131:591–597.

93. Sibai BM, Graham JM, McCubbin JH. A comparison of intravenous and intramuscular magnesium sulfate regimens in preeclampsia. Am J Obstet Gynecol 1984;150:728–733.

94. AbiSaid D, Annegers JF, CombsCantrell D, et al. A case-control evaluation of treatment efficacy: The example of magnesium sulfate prophylaxis against eclampsia in patients with preeclampsia. J Clin Epidemiol 1997;50:419–423.

95. Walsh SW. Low-dose aspirin: Treatment for the imbalance of increased thromboxane and decreased prostacyclin in preeclampsia. Am J Perinatol 1989;6:124–132.

96. Lippert TH, Muck AO. Can prophylactic treatment of preeclampsia be performed with low-dose aspirin: Critical assessment of available studies. Geburtshilfe Frauenheilkd 1996;56:88–92.

97. The CLASP collaborators. CLASP: A randomized trial of low-dose aspirin for the prevention and treatment of preeclampsia among 9364 pregnant women. Lancet 1994;343:619–629.

98. Hauth JC, Goldenberg RL, Parker CR, et al. Low-dose aspirin: Lack of association with an increase in abruptio placentae or perinatal mortality. Obstet Gynecol 1995;85:1055–1058.

99. Uzan S, Merviel P, Beaufils M, et al. Aspirin during pregnancy: Indications and modalities from recent trials. Presse Med 1996;25:31–36.

100. Wallenburg HCS. Low-dose aspirin therapy in obstetrics. Curr Opin Obstet Gynecol 1995;7:135–139.

101. Wisdom SJ, Wilson R, McKillop JH, Walker JJ. Antioxidant systems in normal pregnancy and in pregnancy-induced hypertension. Am J Obstet Gynecol 1991;165:1701–1704.

102. Chen G, Wilson R, Cumming G, et al. Intracellular and extracellular antioxidant buffering levels in erythrocytes from pregnancy-induced hypertension. J Hum Hypertens 1994;8:37–42.

103. Stratta P, Canavese C, Porcu M, et al. Vitamin E supplementation in preeclampsia. Gynecol Obstet Invest 1994;37:246–249.

104. Gulmezoglu AM, Oosthuizen MMJ, Hofmeyr GJ. Placental malondialdehyde and glutathione levels in a controlled trial of antioxidant treatment in severe preeclampsia. Hypertens Pregn 1996; 15:287–295.

105. Gulmezoglu AM, Hofmeyr GJ, Oosthuisen MMJ. Antioxidants in the treatment of severe preeclampsia: An explanatory randomised controlled trial. Br J Obstet Gynaecol 1997;104:689–696.

105a. Chappell LC, Seed PT, Briley AL, et al. Effect of antioxidants on the occurrence of pre-eclampsia in women at increased risk: A randomized trial. Lancet 1999;354:810–816.

106. Lees C, Langford E, Brown AS, et al. The effects of s-nitrosoglutathione on platelet activation, hypertension, and uterine and fetal Doppler in severe preeclampsia. Obstet Gynecol 1996;88:14–19.

107. Ramanathan J, Sibai BM, Mabie WC, et al. The use of labetalol for attenuation of the hypertensive response to endotracheal intubation in preeclampsia. Am J Obstet Gynecol 1988;159:650–654.

108. McCombs J. Treatment of preeclampsia and eclampsia. Clin Pharm 1992;11:236–245.

109. Michael CA. The evaluation of labetalol in the treatment of hypertension complicating pregnancy. Br J Clin Pharmacol 1982;13:127S–131S.

110. Michael CA. Use of labetalol in the treatment of severe hypertension during pregnancy. Br J Clin Pharmacol 1979;8:211S–215S.

111. Barton JR, Hiett AK, Conover WB. The use of nifedipine during the postpartum period in patients with severe preeclampsia. Am J Obstet Gynecol 1990;162:788–792.

112. Walters BN, Redman CW. Treatment of severe pregnancy-associated hypertension with the calcium antagonist nifedipine. Br J Obstet Gynaecol 1984;91:330–336.

113. Friedman EA, Neff RK. Pregnancy outcome as related to hypertension, edema, and proteinuria. Perspect Nephrol Hypertens 1976;5:13–22.

114. Redman CW, Beilin LJ, Bonnar J. Treatment of hypertension in pregnancy with methyldopa: Blood pressure control and side effects. Br J Obstet Gynaecol 1977;84:419–426.

115. Rubin PC, Butters L, Clark DM, et al. Placebo-controlled trial of atenolol in treatment of pregnancy-associated hypertension. Lancet 1983; 1:431–434.

116. Lowe SA, Rubin PC. The pharmacological management of hypertension in pregnancy. J Hypertens 1992;10:201–207.

117. Easterling TR, Benedetti TJ, Carlson KC, et al. The effect of maternal hemodynamics on fetal growth in hypertensive pregnancies. Am J Obstet Gynecol 1991;165:902–906.

118. Greer IA, Walker JJ, Bjornsson S, Calder AA. Second line therapy with nifedipine in severe hypertension. Clin Exp Hypertens [B] 1989;8:277–292.

119. Plouin PF, Breart G, Maillard F, et al. Comparison of antihypertensive efficacy and perinatal safety of labetalol and methyldopa in the treatment of hypertension in pregnancy: A randomized controlled trial. Br J Obstet Gynaecol 1988;95:868–876.

120. Pickles CJ, Pipkin FB, Symonds EM. A randomized placebo controlled trial of labetalol in the treatment of mild to moderate pregnancy induced hypertension. Br J Obstet Gynaecol 1992;99:964–968.

121. Cruickshank DJ, Robertson AA, Campbell DM, MacGillivray I. Maternal obstetric outcome measures in a randomized controlled study of labetalol in the treatment of hypertension in pregnancy. Part B. Hypertension in pregnancy. Clin Exp Hypertens 1991;10:333–344.

122. Collins R, Duley L. Any antihypertensive therapy for pregnancy hypertension. *In* Enkin MW, Keirse MJNC, Renfrew MJ, Neilson JP (eds). Pregnancy and Childbirth Module. Available: Cochrane Database of Systematic Reviews Review No. 04426. Oxford: Update Software, 1995, Disk Issue 1: Cochrane Updates on Disk, 1995.

12

PREECLAMPSIA, ECLAMPSIA, and the CEREBRAL CIRCULATION: ABNORMALITIES in AUTOREGULATION and PERFUSION

Michael A. Belfort

Preeclampsia and eclampsia continue to be a major cause of maternal death. It is estimated that eclampsia causes 50,000 maternal deaths per year worldwide.[1] In the United States, preeclampsia and eclampsia are the second leading cause of maternal mortality[2, 3] and are associated with increased risk of abruptio placentae (placental abruption), disseminated intravascular coagulation (DIC), acute renal failure, and cerebral hemorrhage.[4] Data from the National Hospital Discharge Survey, conducted by the National Center for Health Statistics,[5, 6] indicate that the average incidence of preeclampsia in the United States is 26 cases per 1000 deliveries. The rate of severe preeclampsia (defined per American College of Obstetricians and Gynecologists guidelines)[7] increased from 2.9 cases per 1000 deliveries in 1984 to 5.2 cases per 1000 deliveries in 1986 and was seen without regard to racial group. Eclampsia occurred at an average annual rate of 0.56 per 1000 deliveries.

It is conservatively estimated that in the United States there are at least 90,000 to 100,000 women treated for preeclampsia per year.[6] Of these, approximately 18,000 to 20,000 patients have severe preeclampsia and 2000 to 2500 patients have eclampsia. Despite the use of prophylactic magnesium sulfate ($MgSO_4$) in preeclamptic women, patients still have seizures and some die. The percentage of patients who have a seizure while receiving prophylactic therapy for eclampsia (usually $MgSO_4$) is not well re-

ported but appears to be in the range of 0.3% to 4.3%.[8, 9, 9a]

ETIOLOGY OF ECLAMPSIA

The cause of seizures in eclampsia is unclear. Cerebral vasospasm, hypertensive encephalopathy and reversible posterior leukoencephalopathy,[10] and excitation of brain receptors all have been implicated.[11–14]

Cerebral vasospasm has been consistently described in eclampsia with a number of modalities, including angiography, computed tomography (CT),[15, 16] and transcranial Doppler (TCD) ultrasonography.[17–24] A factor in support of this finding is that blood flow velocity in the middle cerebral artery (MCA) is significantly higher in eclamptic women than in preeclamptic women.[20] The MCA is an important supplier of the cerebrum, where the seizure activity originates. One of the difficulties in interpreting this information is that most women studied have been examined after the event and after treatment with various drugs. Many of the agents used have potent vascular effects and may have caused cerebral vasodilatation. However, the persistence of severe vasospasm, even after such drug therapy, does suggest that the vasospasm was worse before therapy and that vasospasm is an important contributor to some eclamptic convulsions.

Of note is a case report by Hashimoto and associates,[25] who showed that MCA blood flow velocity increased only after the eclamptic seizures had resolved. They suggest that cerebral arterial vasospasm may be a consequence of eclampsia rather than the cause and that the true etiologic mechanism might lie in the arterioles, not the arteries. Until longitudinal studies in women who subsequently develop eclampsia are available, this theory will remain speculative.

Hypertensive encephalopathy has been suggested by some internists and neurologists as the cause of eclamptic seizures,[12, 21, 26–30] but this hypothesis has not been well accepted by the obstetric community. The typical findings in hypertensive encephalopathy include fibrinoid necrosis, fibrin thrombi, microinfarcts and microglial nodules, petechial hemorrhages, lacunar infarcts, and microhemorrhages,[31] and these have been present in some eclamptic women.[12, 26] In addition, experimental hypertensive encephalopathy can cause a "beaded" or "sausage string" appearance in the cerebral microvasculature, which represents areas of forced arteriolar dilatation separated by segments of normally reactive vessels.[32] This type of vascular architecture is typical of the segmental dilatation and spasm seen in the retinal and cerebral arteries of eclamptic women.[18]

Although it is generally thought that most women with severe preeclampsia have cerebral vasoconstriction and underperfusion, it is possible that some may demonstrate hypertensive encephalopathy with resultant cerebral overperfusion and focal edema.[33, 34] This might explain the failure of prophylactic medications and the persistent seizures seen in some eclamptic women.

Alterations in the cerebral circulation in preeclamptic and eclamptic women may occur despite minimal alterations in systemic blood pressure (BP).[35, 36] Some data suggest that the MCA, the vessel responsible for most of the parietal lobe blood flow, may not vasoconstrict in response to elevated BP.[36] Because most eclamptic seizures presumably result from a perturbation in the MCA distribution, the abnormal response in this vessel may indicate failure of local autoregulation.

A similar response, failure to protect an organ from excessive BP, has been reported by Kublickas and colleagues,[37] who showed decreased resistance in the renal artery in preeclampsia despite increasing perfusion pressure. Others have shown differential vascular abnormalities in the occipital lobes

in eclamptic women, a finding that is in concert with the frequently encountered visual disturbances and occasional reversible blindness seen in this disease.[17, 18] These data support the theory that in some preeclamptic patients, as a result of abnormal cerebral autoregulation, overperfusion of the brain may occur with resulting hypertensive encephalopathy.[38, 39] The BP at which the upper limit of cerebral autoregulation is exceeded is not known in pregnancy but is thought to be close to a diastolic pressure of 100 mmHg.[40]

Thus, eclampsia may well represent the end stage of at least two very different pathophysiologic pathways—one in which cerebral perfusion is low as a result of vasospasm (despite elevated systemic BP) and one in which cerebral perfusion is increased as a result of abnormal autoregulation and a failure of the normal protective reflexes.[41]

The systemic arterial pressure, the intracranial pressure, and the state of functioning of the autoregulatory reflexes play important roles in determining the cerebral perfusion at any specific time. If one accepts that vasospasm is the most likely cause of eclampsia based on current evidence, but that hypertensive encephalopathy can also cause seizures, it follows that therapy directed at counteracting one of these pathophysiologic processes may be ineffective at preventing seizures. In fact, certain kinds of therapy may potentially promote seizures under certain circumstances. Dihydralazine, for example, can severely disturb or even completely abolish cerebral autoregulation, resulting in increased flow and flow velocities[42] as well as increased intracranial pressure.[43] Use of this drug when it does not effectively control blood pressure but does abolish cerebral autoregulation may lead to hypertensive encephalopathy and an overperfusion syndrome. This process, however, has never been documented in an eclamptic patient and remains an educated speculation.

DOPPLER ULTRASOUND, CEREBRAL BLOOD VELOCITY, AND CEREBRAL BLOOD FLOW IN PREGNANCY

The normal cerebral blood flow changes of pregnancy are poorly documented compared with the physiologic alterations in other vascular beds during gestation. This is due, partly, to technical difficulties associated with in vivo studies of blood flow in the human brain. Angiography, the "gold standard" in the evaluation of the cerebral vasculature, is an invasive test and presents obvious ethical concerns for its use in normal pregnant women. Few data on the physiologic adaptations of the brain to pregnancy are available in the literature, and most texts concerning the changes of pregnancy do not address this issue at all. There are also ethical problems with using angiography and other methods involving radiation as well as magnetic resonance imaging (MRI) during pregnancy.

The advent of Doppler ultrasound, and in particular TCD ultrasound, has changed this. It is now possible to acquire Doppler-derived velocity information from most of the basal brain arteries (including almost all of the circle of Willis branches) with a noninvasive technique. Using these data, one can diagnose arterial malformations, functional abnormalities, and physiologic changes in brain blood velocity. One can detect direction and velocity of blood flow, and from this infer the presence of distal or proximal arterial constriction or dilatation. In addition, TCD ultrasound can be used to determine real-time changes over very short time intervals and to continuously monitor cerebral blood velocity during surgical procedures or experimental drug protocols. TCD ultrasound has been extensively used clinically by neurologists and neurosurgeons to detect and monitor cerebral vasospasm in patients with subarachnoid hemorrhage.[44-46]

Investigators are beginning to use TCD ultrasound to define pregnancy-induced and pregnancy-associated changes in the cerebral circulation. Williams and Wilson,[47] using a cross-sectional design, studied the MCA blood flow velocity in 154 normotensive pregnant women. They determined that the maximum systolic velocity remained constant during the first and second trimesters and then decreased from 29 to 36 weeks' gestation. The minimum diastolic velocity was not significantly altered throughout gestation. The mean blood flow velocity in the MCA decreased from a peak value at 21 to 24 weeks' gestation to a nadir at 33 to 36 weeks' gestation. The authors also pointed out that the decrease in systolic blood flow velocity did not correlate with the simulta-

neous decline in mean arterial pressure (MAP) during pregnancy, suggesting that this change is independent of MAP influence and most likely represents a specific physiologic cerebral adaptation. This information confirmed the long-held belief that, in a similar way to many other circulations, the cerebral circulation undergoes a decrease in resistance during pregnancy.

Irion and coworkers[48] supported these findings by observing a significant decrease in the systolic velocity, without change in the diastolic velocity, in the MCA at 26 weeks' gestation. Our group has data that support the work of these two groups by showing that there is a progressive decrease in the resistance index in the MCA during normal pregnancy with advancing gestation.[49]

MacKenzie and colleagues[50] established cross-sectional normative data on the systolic-diastolic (S/D) ratio, pulsatility index (PI), and resistance index (RI) for the ophthalmic and central retinal arteries in normal pregnant women from 20 to 41 weeks' gestation. These authors observed that the end-diastolic flow velocity, in both the ophthalmic and central retinal arteries, increased with advancing gestation, whereas the peak systolic velocity for both arteries was not altered as gestation advanced.

Belfort and associates[49, 51] also agreed that the PI of the central retinal artery negatively correlates with advancing gestational age by noting a decrease from 0.98 at 20 weeks' gestation to 0.85 at term. Using cross-sectional data, they also demonstrated a decrease in the RI of the ophthalmic and central retinal arteries during normal pregnancy as gestation advances.[49]

Belfort and coworkers[52] have defined the hemodynamic changes, specifically velocity, RIs, and cerebral perfusion pressure (CPP), in the MCA distribution of the brain during normal pregnancy. TCD ultrasound was used to determine the systolic, diastolic, and mean blood velocities in the MCAs in nonlaboring women studied longitudinally (at 4-week intervals) during normal gestation. The RI, PI, and CPP were calculated using the velocity and BP data. The mean value, along with the 5th and 95th percentiles, was defined; MCA velocities, RIs, and PIs decreased, whereas CPP increased during normal pregnancy (Figs. 12–1 to 12–3).

Figure 12–1 shows the mean velocity change, Figure 12–2 shows the RI change,

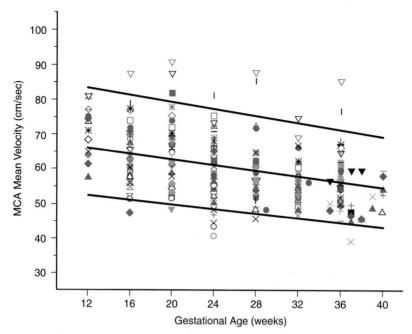

FIGURE 12–1. Middle cerebral artery (MCA) mean velocity data for normal pregnancy. The median line and the 5th and 95th percentiles are shown for gestational ages from 12 weeks to 40 weeks. (From Belfort MA, Tooke-Miller C, Allen JC, et al. Physiologic changes in velocity, resistance indices, and cerebral perfusion pressure in the middle cerebral artery distribution during normal pregnancy. Acta Obstet Gynecol Scand [in press]. © Munksgaard International Publishers, Ltd.).

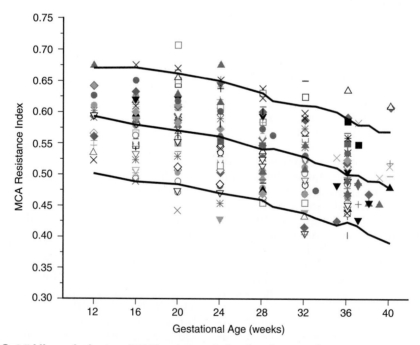

FIGURE 12–2. Middle cerebral artery (MCA) resistance index data for normal pregnancy. The median line and the 5th and 95th percentiles are shown for gestational ages from 12 weeks to 40 weeks. (From Belfort MA, Tooke-Miller C, Allen JC, et al. Physiologic changes in velocity, resistance indices, and cerebral perfusion pressure in the middle cerebral artery distribution during normal pregnancy. Acta Obstet Gynecol Scand [in press]. © Munksgaard International Publishers, Ltd.).

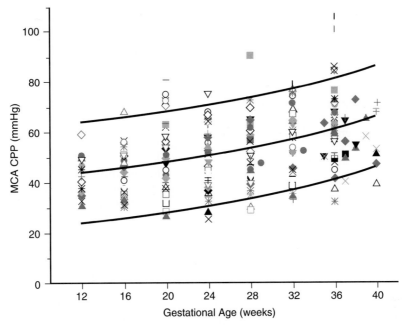

FIGURE 12–3. Middle cerebral artery (MCA) cerebral perfusion pressure (CPP) data for normal pregnancy. The mean line and the 5th and 95th percentiles are shown for gestational ages from 12 weeks to 40 weeks. (From Belfort MA, Tooke-Miller C, Allen JC, et al. Physiologic changes in velocity, resistance indices, and cerebral perfusion pressure in the middle cerebral artery distribution during normal pregnancy. Acta Obstet Gynecol Scand [in press]. © Munksgaard International Publishers, Ltd.).

and Figure 12–3 shows the CPP change during normal pregnancy. This study defined the normative ranges for MCA velocity, RIs, and CPP during normal human pregnancy using longitudinally collected data. The availability of a defined normal range should certainly help in the identification of abnormalities in cerebral hemodynamics during pregnancy and should be useful to both clinicians and researchers.

Doppler Ultrasound, Bias, and Confounders

Because of the dependence of Doppler-derived velocity measurements on the angle of insonation, various non–angle-dependent indices have been developed to assess downstream resistance and pulsatility. Of special interest to us has been the ability to combine various additional parameters (such as diastolic and mean BP) with velocity measurement to allow the development of more meaningful measures such as cerebral perfusion.[53] This aspect of the field is still in its infancy, and new indices are being developed as more sensitive and versatile ultrasound technology becomes available.

We more fully address this aspect of TCD ultrasound technology later.

Flow-Volume-Velocity Relationships

One of the most frequently mentioned problems with TCD ultrasound is the unclear relationship between cerebral blood flow volume and the flow velocities in the basal cerebral vessels, as assessed by TCD ultrasound. There are several important limitations to the use of TCD ultrasound in this respect, which stem mainly from the following facts:

1. The MCA diameter (3.82 ± 0.43 mm)[54] and the amount of tissue it supplies have significant interindividual variation.
2. The flow velocity within the main trunk of the MCA has a wide range of normality.
3. The angle of insonation and the attenuation of ultrasound beam are important in the calculation of the velocity.
4. Age-related changes are present.

Given all of these confounders, however, some data still show a good association between cerebral blood flow and cerebral blood velocity, as measured using Doppler ultrasound.[55–57] Furthermore, by using intraindividual comparisons under normocapnic and hypercapnic conditions, one can minimize these limitations.[58] In fact, the relative changes in cerebral blood flow velocity reflect the relative changes in regional cerebral blood flow.[59] Furthermore, Doppler measurements can accurately reflect changes in cerebral blood flow during dynamic testing of cerebral autoregulatory responses in humans.[56, 60, 61] The measurement of blood flow, however, is not a commonly performed procedure in pregnancy, and research in this field is only now beginning.

In terms of the reliability of the technique and reproducibility of the results, Aaslid and coworkers,[62] Lieb and colleagues,[63] and Harris and associates[64] have shown minimal interobserver variation for both transcranial and ocular blood velocity measurements. Intraobserver variation in our laboratory is less than 5% (4.5 ± 2.8%; mean ± standard deviation) for the central retinal artery RI, and similar for the ophthalmic artery RI (4.3 ± 3.0%).[64] These figures compare very well with those of others working in the same field.[65] Interobserver and intraobserver variability are periodically assessed in our laboratory. This assessment takes the form of two TCD ultrasound examinations performed in the same patient 5 minutes apart by each of the two individuals performing the studies in our laboratory. Ten different women are studied. The MCA velocity and BP are measured at each examination and the CPP is calculated. The two CPP results, generated at each examination by each examiner, are then compared for interobserver and intraobserver variability. The variations have always been less than 10%. This aspect of continued quality assurance is important in any vascular laboratory and maintains good habits.

A number of confounding influences can affect the interpretation of Doppler cerebral velocity data. These include any factors that may:

1. Increase the carbon dioxide (CO_2) or H^+ tension in the cerebral circulation.

2. Decrease or increase the hemoglobin concentration.

3. Independently alter the diameter of the vessel being studied at the point of insonation.

4. Introduce errors such as those possibly associated with cigarette smoking and changes in posture.

In pregnant women, gestational age is another important factor that must be considered; as the pregnancy progresses, significant hemodynamic changes occur.

Increased CO_2 tension leads to cerebral vasodilatation, as does acidosis. Patients undergoing cerebral Doppler studies, ideally, should be studied in a steady state, or end-tidal CO_2 tension should be measured in order to control for fluctuations. Even the minimal increases in tidal volume and respiratory rate associated with labor contractions may be important. Labor itself has been shown to be associated with decreases in mean MCA flow velocity.[66] Hemoconcentration and hemodilution are also important, and attention should be paid to the hematocrit level when blood loss or volume infusion may have altered the hemoglobin content of the blood during the study period.

The segmental nature of the vasospasm seen in some conditions, notably preeclampsia, is of concern as well because the same segment of artery can show completely different velocity profiles, depending on its state of contraction. Thus, if the region of vessel being insonated is likely to change, its diameter velocity readings may be inaccurate, particularly if an indication of downstream vascular condition is being extrapolated. In this regard, the M1 portion of the MCA is unlikely to change in diameter[44, 62, 67] because it is well supported by alveolar tissue in its bony canal. The angle of insonation is crucial because the velocity is related to the cosine of the angle of insonation (q). If q is less than 10 degrees, the error involved is almost negligible and acceptable for most purposes. Because of the anatomy of the bony canal through which the M1 portion of the MCA runs, the angle of insonation very rarely exceeds 10 degrees.[68] This ensures that, in almost all cases, once the optimal signal is obtained, the angle of insonation is less than 10 degrees.

The effect of maternal cigarette smoking on MCA blood flow velocities during normal pregnancy was described by Irion and coworkers.[48] They found that the systolic, diastolic, and mean velocities of the MCA, detected in both the left lateral decubitus and sitting positions, were significantly higher at 18 and 26 weeks' gestation in women who smoked cigarettes. They determined that the number of cigarettes smoked positively correlated with increased MCA velocities. One must take this factor into account when studying women known to smoke, and it is an important confounding factor in some earlier published studies. Similarly, one should also consider posture when studying pregnant women, especially preeclamptic pregnant women. A change from a lying to a sitting position may cause a significant increase in both systolic and diastolic velocities in the MCA in such patients.[69, 70]

Another important variable in pregnant women is gestational age. As pregnancy advances, the reduction in MCA velocity should be controlled for when women of different gestational ages are being compared.[71]

CEREBRAL PERFUSION PRESSURE

Under normal conditions, the arterioles in the cerebrovascular system are responsible for about 80% of the vascular resistance. Because arterioles have active smooth muscle tone, they do not behave simply like tubes of variable dimension. Smooth muscle tone in the arterioles reduces their diameter when systolic pressure is transmitted into them via the arteries. In addition, this tone also tends to close the arterioles when pressure falls during the pulse cycle.

Under conditions of low vascular resistance, the arterioles remain open throughout the pulse cycle and the active smooth muscle tone never causes them to close completely. However, even a slight increase in arteriolar tone will narrow the diameter of open arterioles and, in some cases, cause them to close completely when the pressure within them falls at the end of the pulse cycle.

The pressure at which an arteriole closes is its *critical closing pressure*.[72] Critical closing pressure explains why arterioles close as pressure falls during the pulse cycle and why fewer arterioles are open at the end of the pulse cycle than earlier, when pressure is at its systolic maximum. Thus, pressure at the end of a pulse cycle is less effective in perfusing the capillary bed than that early in the cycle. In the brain, CPP is reduced as arteriolar resistance rises abruptly as a result

of more and more arterioles reaching their critical closing pressure.

Another feature of arteriolar tone is its effect in delaying the flow of blood from arteries to capillaries.[73] When arteriolar tone is high, it reduces the rate of blood flow from arteries to capillaries. This maintains the arterial BP at a higher level for a longer portion of the pulse cycle than if the arteriolar tone was low and there was a rapid run-off of blood.

BP distends the arterial segments, and blood is effectively stored in the arteries while the pressure decays during the pulse cycle. The amount stored in each segment depends on the compliance of the artery and the pressure gradient between the lumen and the region outside the artery. The result of storing blood in the arteries and reducing the rate of flow through arterioles is to slow the deceleration of blood flow during the pulse cycle. The more compliant the arterial segment, the slower the deceleration during the pulse cycle. This feature of arteriolar tone interacting with arterial pressure and arterial compliance affects the shape of the velocity profile during the pulse cycle. When arteriolar tone is low, blood velocity rapidly rises to a maximum and falls quickly to a minimum. In contrast, when arteriolar tone is high, the blood flow velocity falls more slowly. The area under the pulsatile amplitude of the velocity waveform, and the height of the pulse velocity wave, may be used to estimate the proportion of blood flow stored in arterial segments during the peak of the pulse cycle and released when pressure falls during the cycle.

One of the major problems with today's Doppler indices is that they were initially developed for use in peripheral vascular examination of large-diameter arteries (e.g., femoral, dorsalis pedis, brachial).[74] Indices such as the PI and RI focus on the systolic component of the velocity profile. The traditional Doppler indices of hemodynamics (the RI and PI) provide limited data regarding arteriolar tone when applied to the cerebral circulation. Both the RI defined as $(velocity_{systolic} - velocity_{diastolic})/velocity_{systolic}$ and the PI defined as $(velocity_{systolic} - velocity_{diastolic})/velocity_{mean}$ are significantly influenced by the systolic velocity, which reflects large-caliber arterial constriction.[74] These indices were originally developed using older technology and larger-diameter arteries (e.g., femoral artery, aorta). The typical waveform shape from such arteries has a tall, peaked systolic component, a steep diastolic slope, and a low or nonexistent diastolic component.

The smaller-diameter arteries that are now easily visualized with modern equipment provide completely different waveforms from those seen in the larger-diameter, higher-velocity, and higher-resistance vessels. Using indices that focus on the systolic velocity tends to ignore aspects of waveform shape peculiar to lower resistance vascular beds. Specifically, the typical waveform seen in low-resistance, low-velocity, smaller-diameter arteries has a low systolic velocity, flatter diastolic downslope, and a proportionately higher diastolic velocity, than that seen in high-resistance, high-velocity arteries. Because of shape differences (Fig. 12–4), indices such as the RI that do not focus on the mean and diastolic velocities may be less representative and sensitive than those that do. Figure 12–4 shows the importance of waveform shape; although both waveforms have the same RI, there is obviously a difference in terms of the hemodynamics involved.

To take into account waveform shape, one must consider mean velocity and diastolic velocity to a greater extent. We therefore developed some new indices based on mean and diastolic velocity, and these have been very sensitive in showing changes in both cerebral and uterine circulations.[51, 75–77]

One of the indices that we developed was a Doppler method of assessing CPP. CPP has been studied, experimentally, with simulta-neous Doppler and pressure measurements and, in support of our contentions, Chan and associates[78] showed that CPP was more strongly associated with diastolic velocity than with systolic velocity. They also showed that as CPP decreased below a critical value of 70 mmHg, a progressive increase in TCD PI was observed (R = -0.942, $P < .0001$). At pressures above 70 mmHg, there was no correlation between PI and CPP. In most pregnant women, the CPP is usually above 70 mmHg in the third trimester. This fact further strengthens our contention that in order to infer changes in cerebral perfusion, the CPP is a much better index than the PI. The Chan study also demonstrated that the relationship between PI and CPP (CPP < 70 mmHg) held true in patients with both focal and diffuse pathologic processes and was the same whether changes in CPP resulted from alterations in intracranial pressure or BP.[78]

A further deficiency of the current cerebral Doppler assessment techniques is that they neglect to take into account the systemic arterial pressure, a vital component of CPP. Our method of estimating CPP considers simultaneously measured cerebral blood velocity and systemic arterial pressure and estimates CPP in the MCA.

In 1986, Aaslid and associates[79] validated a Doppler method of estimating CPP. They measured velocity in the MCA (Doppler ultrasound) and intraventricular pressure and radial arterial BP (direct strain gauge transducers) in 10 patients undergoing a supratentorial shunt procedure. They estimated CPP using the following ratio: (mean flow velocity)/(pulsatile amplitude of flow velocity) multiplied by the arterial BP. To increase the accuracy, Fourier analysis was used and only the amplitude of the first harmonic of the pulsatility in both flow velocity and arterial BP recordings was used. They expressed their calculations as

$$CPP = \frac{V_0}{V_1} \times ABP_1$$

where V_0 is the mean and V_1 is the amplitude of the first harmonic of the velocity waveform, and ABP_1 is the first harmonic of the arterial pressure wave. Their experimental results confirmed the validity of the method. The standard deviation between estimated CPP and measured CPP was 8.2

Resistance Index =

$$\frac{\text{Systolic velocity - Diastolic velocity}}{\text{Systolic velocity}}$$

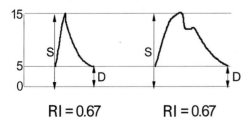

FIGURE 12–4. Two waveforms with completely different shapes can still have the same resistance index (RI) value—an indication of the lack of sensitivity of this parameter. S, systolic velocity; D, diastolic velocity.

mmHg at a CPP of 40 mmHg, and the mean deviation was only 1 mmHg.

We have adapted the method of Aaslid and associates[79] by altering the formula to reflect the area under the pulsatile amplitude of the flow velocity and arterial BP waveforms rather than the first harmonic. Our equation,[51, 52] using areas under pulsatile amplitudes, is as follows:

$$CPP = \frac{Velocity_{mean}}{Velocity_{mean} - Velocity_{diastolic}} \times (BP_{mean} - BP_{diastolic})$$

Validation of Doppler-Based Formula for Noninvasive Estimation of Cerebral Perfusion Pressure

Validation of our formula has been an important goal for our team in order to use the formula clinically and to establish the credibility of the technique. Because it is ethically and logistically impossible to validate the formula using normal pregnant women as controls, we have been forced to use data from patients with cerebral pathology. There are obviously problems with extrapolating information derived from patients with intracranial disease, but under the circumstances this model offers the best attempt to validate our formula.

We have now validated our formula, and initial results have been promising.[80] We studied 20 patients with an epidural in situ with TCD of the maternal MCA to measure systolic, diastolic, and mean velocities. A pressure transducer was connected to the epidural catheter, and pressure was recorded. A Dinamap monitor was used to measure BP. Of the 20 laboring women studied, all had normal pregnancies. The mean age was 28 ± 7 years, and the mean gestational age was 39 ± 2 weeks. The mean BP was 77 ± 12 mmHg. The directly measured and the Doppler-estimated CPPs were compared using Bland-Altman plots and regression analysis. The Bland-Altman[81] plot showed a mean difference of 2.2 mmHg at a mean CPP of 65 ± 12 mmHg, with a standard deviation of 4.8 mmHg. The regression analysis showed an R = 0.92 , an R^2 = 0.86, and a P < .0001 (Fig. 12–5). Although this technique is promising, further validation work is required before it should be used as a clinical tool.

Cerebral Blood Velocity and Mean Arterial Pressure

One of the most interesting and remarkable studies in this field has been that of Kyle and coworkers,[35] who assessed the maternal cerebral circulation with TCD ultrasound during an intravenous angiotensin II infusion in 110 normotensive women at 28 weeks' gestation. They noted a significant rise in BP and a fall in heart rate as a result of the angiotensin II infusion. There was a simultaneous decrease in the systolic velocity and PI in the MCA associated with an increase in the diastolic and mean velocities. All values returned to baseline levels 10 minutes after infusion.

FIGURE 12–5. A regression plot of the invasively measured cerebral perfusion pressure (CPP) data (CPP Direct) versus the noninvasively measured CPP data (CPP Doppler).

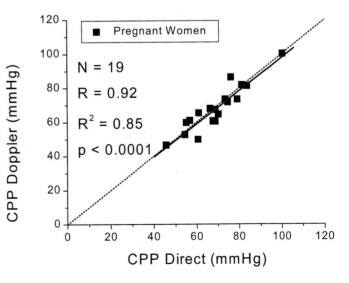

The authors suggested that the alterations in blood flow velocity were related to the rise in BP rather than to a direct effect of angiotensin II on the cerebral circulation. The study did show that increasing cerebral perfusion in a normal pregnant woman causes cerebral vasodilatation and decreased cerebral resistance. This is possibly related to release of vasodilator substances from the normal endothelium. This finding is supported by our data[82] showing a negative correlation between MAP and cerebral resistance within the normal autoregulatory range. Presumably, within the usual range of BP and autoregulation, there is a threshold over which the cerebral vasculature begins to constrict in order to protect itself from overperfusion. Obviously, this point was not reached in the study by Kyle and coworkers.[35] A similar study in preeclamptic women may well show that angiotensin II has a different effect on the cerebral circulation in this group. To date this study has not been performed.

Cerebral Blood Velocity and Central Hemodynamic Indices

It has long been known that the orbital vessels reflect major physiologic and pathologic changes in other vascular beds. Funduscopy was, at one time, one of the few important indicators of cerebral edema and disordered cerebral blood flow caused by a variety of conditions.

In the 1990s, it was shown that blood flow velocity and RI from the ophthalmic and central retinal arteries were related to the oxygen delivery index, oxygen consumption index, cardiac index, and systemic vascular RI in critically ill pregnant or early postpartum women requiring invasive monitoring.[83] The ophthalmic artery RI showed a positive correlation with oxygen consumption index, oxygen delivery index, and cardiac index. Only the ophthalmic artery diastolic velocity correlated with the oxygen consumption index, oxygen delivery index, and the cardiac index. No other correlation between the other central retinal or ophthalmic Doppler indices and respiratory or hemodynamic parameters was noted.

The study suggests that orbital Doppler sonography may have value in the noninvasive evaluation of systemic hemodynamic or respiratory parameters in critically ill parturient women. Van Bel and colleagues[84] reported that the systolic velocity in the vertebral artery of dogs shows a strong relationship to the myocardial contractile state. Because of this, the authors suggested that indices combining peak systolic velocity with other velocity measurements should not be used in noninvasive assessment of cerebral vascular resistance. Our CPP equation specifically excludes systolic velocity for this reason.

Cerebral Perfusion Pressure in Normal Pregnancy and in the Puerperium

The development and testing of our formula for the CPP have been discussed. The need for more sensitive indices is apparent because the RI and PI are insensitive to many waveform changes. This raises the question of how reliable these indices are in accurately representing changes in vasoconstriction. In fact, in special circumstances, such as subarachnoid hemorrhage, a decreasing RI may actually represent worsening vasospasm and increasing intracranial pressure instead of decreasing vasospasm.[85] This was one of the main reasons we pursued the development of CPP as a more representative parameter for measuring and comparing cerebral hemodynamics in pregnancy and preeclampsia.

Figure 12–3 shows normative data and 95th percentiles for MCA CPP from our studies of 65 pregnant women. Figure 12–6 shows the normative data for the anterior, middle, and posterior cerebral arteries in the same women. These data demonstrate that normal pregnancy is associated with a significant increase in CPP in all three vessels that takes at least 3 months to revert to prepregnancy levels. These rather large changes are important to consider in analyses of cerebral hemodynamics in pregnant women.

SEIZURES IN PREECLAMPTIC-ECLAMPTIC WOMEN

The etiology of the seizures in preeclampsia is the subject of heated debate. Cerebral vasospasm, hypertensive encephalopathy, and excitation of brain receptors have all been implicated.[18, 86–88] The study of cerebral blood flow velocity in preeclampsia using

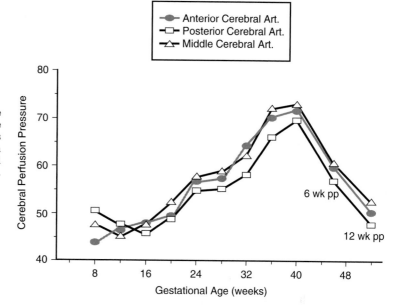

FIGURE 12–6. Changes in the mean cerebral perfusion pressure (CPP) in the three major arteries of the brain tend to follow each other during normal gestation and during the postpartum period. Art., artery; pp, post partum.

TCD ultrasound and orbital ultrasound has improved our understanding of this condition as well as the cerebral effects of medications (MgSO$_4$, nimodipine) used in the management of patients with preeclampsia.

Cerebral vasospasm has been demonstrated in both preeclamptic and eclamptic women,[17, 18, 87–90] and this vasoconstriction is probably an important part of the pathophysiology of the disease. For many years, debate has centered on the contribution of hypertensive encephalopathy to eclampsia, with many neurologists supporting a central role for this mechanism. Obstetric lore has dictated that eclampsia is an ischemic event resulting from severe vasospasm. Data from our studies have shed light on the pathophysiology of eclampsia and suggest that both hypertensive encephalopathy and ischemia may be involved, either sequentially or simultaneously. Unfortunately, most available data have been collected after the fact, that is, after the patient has manifested symptoms of the disease process and has received some form of therapy. Thus, whether cerebral vasoconstriction precedes seizure activity in eclamptic women is unclear.

Severe cerebral vasospasm in patients with both preeclampsia and eclampsia responds to MgSO$_4$ and calcium channel blocker therapy with vasodilatation and cessation (or prevention) of seizures. From this response, it has been assumed that severe ischemia precedes seizures, and most treatment strategies have been developed with this in mind. Our group, however, has shown that seizure activity in one patient was actually preceded by apparent overperfusion, strengthening the argument that in at least some cases, eclampsia is a result of hypertensive encephalopathy (Fig. 12–7).

Zunker and associates[89] have shown pathologically elevated MCA flow velocities (up to twice the normal value) in preeclamptic and eclamptic women. Many of these patients had extremely elevated velocities despite a MAP below 150 mmHg. These investigators suggested that their findings were a result of forced vasodilatation, probably resulting from passive overdistention of cerebral arterioles and vasogenic edema rather than vasospasm.

Williams and MacLean[70] studied the MCA blood flow velocity in 10 preeclamptic women using TCD ultrasound. They concluded that preeclamptic women experienced a 30% rise in systolic, diastolic, and mean blood flow velocities upon changing from the left lateral decubitus position to the sitting position. This finding is in contrast to the lack of a postural effect on cerebral blood flow velocities noted in a normal gestation. In the preeclamptic group, they also found no concomitant change in BP as a result of the change in posture. This finding supported the clinical evidence that has long suggested that preeclampsia is a condi-

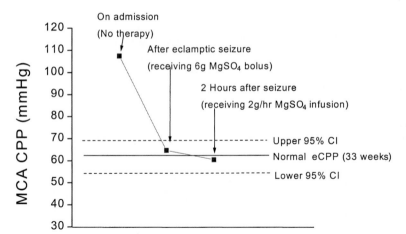

FIGURE 12–7. Middle cerebral artery (MCA) cerebral perfusion pressure (CPP) data for a patient who was studied before and after an eclamptic convulsion. These data indicate that cerebral hyperperfusion may be important in the pathophysiology of eclampsia. CI, confidence interval; eCPP, estimated cerebral perfusion pressure.

tion of increased vascular reactivity that is sensitive to, and sometimes stimulated by, postural changes.

Naidu and colleagues[90] showed in the largest study of its type that the pathophysiologic mechanism of eclamptic seizures appears to be related to primary cerebral vasospasm with resultant ischemia and cerebral edema involving mainly the watershed areas and parieto-occipital lobes of the brain. Using imaging and ultrasonographic techniques, they studied 65 women with eclampsia within 48 hours after delivery. Unenhanced cerebral CT scans were performed in all the women and single photon emission computed tomography (SPECT) scans were performed in 63 women using technetium 99m–hexamethyl propylenamine oxime (^{99m}Tc-HMPAO) as a tracer of regional cerebral blood flow. MCA blood flow velocity waveforms were measured using 2-MHz pulsed Doppler ultrasonography via the transtemporal approach. SPECT scanning revealed perfusion deficits in the watershed areas in all women, 75% of whom had concomitant deficits in the parieto-occipital areas of the brain. Hypodensities (cerebral edema) were reported in 38 CT scans (58.5%), with parieto-occipital involvement in 97.4% of cases. Increased flow velocity measurements in the middle and posterior cerebral arteries were recorded in 36 (85.7%) women undergoing TCD ultrasound.

These data contradict those of Morriss and associates,[91] who studied 28 women with eclampsia and severe preeclampsia using phase-contrast MRI. These authors found no evidence of vasospasm, despite seeing brain lesions in all women with preeclampsia.

They questioned the role of vasospasm and cerebral hypoperfusion in preeclampsia. This study has been criticized because the number of patients was small and imaging was performed on most of those studied hours after the seizure and hours after initiation of vasodilator therapy ($MgSO_4$).

Cerebral vasospasm as a component of the pathophysiology in eclamptic women has been consistently described with TCD ultrasound.[19, 20, 92, 93] This is illustrated by elevated MCA blood flow velocities and high RIs and PIs in some patients. Blood flow velocity in the MCA is significantly higher in eclamptic women than in preeclamptic women.[92] An even further increase in cerebral blood flow velocity was found in the postconvulsive phase in eclamptic women.

One of the difficulties in interpreting this information is that most women studied have been examined after the event and after treatment with various drugs. Many of the agents used have potent vascular effects and may have caused cerebral vasodilatation. However, the presence of severe vasospasm after such drug therapy does suggest that the vasospasm was worse before therapy and that vasospasm is an important contributor to some eclamptic convulsions.

Alterations in the cerebral circulation occur in preeclamptic and eclamptic women despite minimal alterations in BP.[53, 92] This may help to explain patients who have seizures despite low BP or, even more commonly, no sudden change in BP preceding the event. Significantly elevated MCA blood flow velocities in both preeclamptic and eclamptic women have been noted without concomitant BP elevations.[92] This phenomenon may be the result of disordered cerebral autoregulation in preeclampsia and invokes the theory that the disease is capable of regionally affecting vascular smooth muscle function. There are data that support this theory of regional malfunction.

We have shown that there is no significant correlation between the MAP and MCA RI in preeclamptic women.[53] In the same preeclamptic patients, however, there was a correlation between the MAP and the RIs in the central retinal and ophthalmic arteries. These data are interesting because it appears that the MCA, the vessel responsible for the majority of the parietal lobe blood flow, may behave differently than other regional small arteries in preeclampsia. Because most eclamptic seizures occur in the MCA distribution, the abnormal response in this vessel may indicate failure of local autoregulation. A similar response—failure to protect an organ from excessive BP—has been reported by Kublickas and coworkers,[37] who showed decreased resistance in the renal artery in preeclampsia despite increasing perfusion pressure. Our data also suggest that there is a differential response between the large-caliber and small-caliber cerebral vessels in normotensive and preeclamptic parturients and that these vessels behave differently in relation to MAP in preeclampsia.

We have reported on the CPP in the MCA in both mild and severe preeclamptic women.[94] The study findings suggest that in preeclampsia the brain can be (1) normally perfused, (2) underperfused, or (3) overperfused. In general, so-called mild preeclampsia is associated with normal CPP although in rare instances the CPP has been low (Fig. 12–8).[95] In contrast, severe preeclampsia is associated with normal and higher CPP. Most patients in both groups have "normal" CPP, depending on individual response to the disease. Figure 12–8 shows that 100% of patients with severe preeclampsia had normal or high CPP (44/44), whereas in women with mild preeclampsia 50/54 (93%) had normal or low CPP, and 4/54 (7%) had high CPP. The figure also shows that 57% of the women with severe preeclampsia and 85% with mild preeclampsia have normal CPP ($P = .004$).

In terms of explaining seizure activity based on CPP, data are scarce. Speculative models have been developed, but none is proven. In one model, initial vasospasm is followed by cerebral ischemia and reduced CPP. BP is elevated in response to this, with an increase in CPP to within the normal range (mild preeclampsia). If vasospasm persists, MAP increases to improve perfusion. If this fails, ischemia occurs. Usually, however, the increased MAP normalizes the CPP and autoregulatory influences maintain CPP within the normal range. If the MAP increase overwhelms the ability of the vasculature to regulate the CPP, overperfusion and hypertensive encephalopathy result. Extrapolation of this model suggests that the mechanism of eclampsia in women with "mild preeclampsia," or low BP prior to the

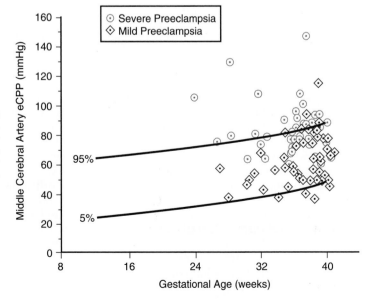

FIGURE 12–8. Data from women with mild and severe preeclampsia plotted against the normative 5th and 95th percentiles. Most patients have normal cerebral perfusion pressure (CPP) values, but low and high CPP may be seen in patients with preeclampsia.

seizure, is cerebral ischemia. This concept is supported by Hansen and associates[96] and Demarin and colleagues,[97] who showed that women with mild preeclampsia had lower MCA velocities than women with severe preeclampsia.

In contrast, the mechanism for eclampsia in women with "severe preeclampsia" may more likely be due to an overperfusion syndrome (i.e., hypertensive encephalopathy). This is a concept worthy of further research and one that may affect the way we manage these patients, such as choosing the appropriate medications on the basis of CPP measurements rather than empiricism. For example, a woman with severe preeclampsia and an elevated CPP may be better served by having her BP lowered with an agent having minimal cerebral vasodilatory action (e.g., labetalol) in order to minimize the risk of worsening the overperfusion. A patient with very low CPP may be better treated with an agent that vasodilates the cerebral vasculature as well as reduces BP (e.g., nimodipine). Although the concept of low CPP is attractive, further investigation is required because very few of our patients had low CPP.

The question of the interrelationship between cerebral capillary critical closing pressure (i.e., "resistance" in the cerebral capillaries) and CPP needs to be investigated. There may well be an important relationship between the two that controls the amount of blood perfusing the brain. In some situations, even a high CPP may be insufficient to adequately perfuse the brain (i.e., when critical closing pressure is very high), resulting in an ischemic seizure. In other situations, a "normal" CPP may cause overperfusion (i.e., when critical closing pressure is very low). We are actively researching this interrelationship.

It is difficult to discern whether elevated velocity indicates ischemia or hyperemia because high MCA velocities can occur in both situations.[98] This is one reason why we believe that using the CPP to evaluate the cerebral perfusion status may be preferable to simply using a velocity estimation.

Posterior Cerebral Circulation

One of the current deficiencies in cerebrovascular research in preeclampsia is the lack of knowledge regarding the posterior circulation. The posterior circulation is known to be susceptible to the lesions of hypertensive encephalopathy.[99] CT and MRI scans in eclamptic women frequently demonstrate edema in the region of the posterior circulation and occipital lobes.[98, 99] However, few data exist for Doppler studies in these patients. There is good circumstantial evidence to suggest that sympathetic vascular innervation may be at fault, given the known regional heterogeneity of this system. The sympathetic innervation of intracranial arteries is known to protect the brain from marked increases in BP.[100, 101] In addition, the internal carotid system is much better supplied with sympathetic innervation than the vertebrobasilar system.[102] Acute hypertension may thus stimulate the sympathetic nerves and lead to more efficient protection of the anterior circulation than the posterior circulation. This may explain the more commonly seen edema in the occipital lobes of preeclamptic and eclamptic women and may indicate breakthrough of autoregulation in the vertebrobasilar and posterior cerebral artery distributions.[103] In this regard, it has been reported that preeclamptic women have abnormalities in the sympathetic nervous system.[103, 104]

Orbital Doppler Findings

Orbital Doppler sonography has been used to demonstrate the link between vasospasm in the central retinal artery in a patient with preeclampsia and visual symptoms.[105] Treatment with $MgSO_4$ in this same patient resulted in increased blood flow velocity and decreased resistance, accompanied by resolution of visual symptoms. This finding suggested that the visual disturbances in preeclampsia may be attributed to central retinal artery vasospasm and ischemia rather than occipital lobe edema[106] or cerebral vein thrombosis.[107] Again, this is evidence for a regional vascular response to the disease.

Additional investigation of the ophthalmic circulation has revealed significantly elevated systolic, diastolic, and mean velocities in preeclamptic women compared with normotensive women[108]; women with mild preeclampsia also have a paradoxically low ophthalmic artery PI compared with normotensive women. This situation is reversed and becomes elevated in patients with severe preeclampsia.

We have proposed a model to explain these unexpected differences. The ophthalmic artery has anastomoses with branches of the external carotid artery and thus connects with the peripheral circulation. In mild preeclampsia, resistance may be decreased in the ophthalmic artery as a compensation for cerebral ischemia resulting from MCA vasospasm. Subsequently, as the disease process progresses, worsening dysfunction in the ophthalmic artery and its anastomosis may cause vasoconstriction and an increase in resistance.

CEREBRAL AUTOREGULATION, CEREBRAL PERFUSION, AND CHOICE OF ANTISEIZURE AGENT

The increase or decrease in CPP noted with the use of certain drugs in preeclamptic women is probably not excessive in most circumstances. However, in patients who are critically balanced in terms of cerebral perfusion, changes of even minimal magnitude may be important.

Some data suggest that cerebral[36] and renal[37] autoregulation is disordered in preeclampsia and that autoregulation in the MCA in particular may be affected. The main support for this hypothesis comes from a paper published by our group.[36] In this study, 24 normal pregnant women; 18 preeclamptic women in whom data had been simultaneously collected from the MCA, the ophthalmic artery, and the central retinal artery; and 79 preeclamptic women (42 with headache and 37 without headache) in whom data from the MCA only was available were studied. The three groups were similar in terms of their demographic characteristics. The preeclamptic patients had significantly higher BP and significantly more proteinuria than the normal pregnant women ($P < .05$). There were no differences in the mean RI values for the three vessels between the two groups of patients in each analysis.

Preeclamptic women demonstrated a different relationship between BP and RI in the ophthalmic artery and central retinal artery than did normal pregnant women. However, in the MCA, preeclampsia did not appear to affect the RI response to increasing MAP in women with headache. In preeclamptic women without headache the relationship seen in the ophthalmic artery and central renal artery was preserved in the MCA. These findings may be explained as showing a failure in the autoregulatory capacity of the MCA in preeclampsia, and this failure may be accompanied by the physical symptom of headache. The MCA is the primary blood supply of the parietal lobes, and pressure-passive overperfusion in this region may well account for eclamptic convulsions.

Knowledge of the underlying CPP status is obviously of value in a scientifically considered therapeutic approach. By measuring the CPP and comparing it with normative data, the clinician can choose the eclampsia prophylactic drug best suited to the CPP of the patient. When it is not possible to measure CPP, it is advisable that $MgSO_4$ (with or without labetalol) be used in women in whom cerebral overperfusion may be an issue (chronic hypertensives and in women with superimposed preeclampsia), whereas a drug such as nimodipine (a calcium antagonist with preferential cerebral vasodilator properties) may be a good alternative in women with suspected severe cerebral vasospasm associated with minimal elevation in systemic BP.

Eclampsia and Cerebrovascular Alterations

Using our model of estimated CPP, we analyzed data from one of our patients with unremitting eclamptic convulsions.[19] We compared these data with data in the literature derived from three patients who suffered a single convulsion that was controlled by BP management.[20] This analysis suggested a difference between the two types of patients that is in keeping with our hypothesis.

In our single patient with unremitting eclampsia (demonstrating CT changes consistent with severe cerebral ischemia), Doppler analysis of the MCA showed a very high PI (1.55), high systolic velocity (173 cm/sec), and low CPP (CPP = 42 mmHg). This profile represented a state of combined arterial and arteriolar constriction—consistent with severe cerebral vasospasm and ischemia.

In contrast, the patients of Williams and Wilson[20] had low pulsatility (PI = 0.57), high systolic velocity (142 cm/sec), and elevated CPP (86 mmHg). This profile, with arteriolar constriction to protect the capillary circulation, is more consistent with hypertensive encephalopathy than cerebral ischemia, with higher pressures in the capillaries perfusing the MCA distribution than that seen in our patient. These data are further circumstantial evidence to support our hypothesis that eclamptic convulsions can result from at least two different causes.

Chronic Hypertension and Superimposed Preeclampsia

The state of the CPP in patients with chronic hypertension and the change in CPP wrought by superimposed preeclampsia are unknown. It appears that superimposed preeclampsia may be associated with CPP.[109] We have some preliminary (unpublished) data regarding 15 women with chronic hypertension and 15 women with superimposed preeclampsia. All of the women were studied before labor and before any treatment or volume expansion. The two groups were similar in most demographic criteria, although patients with superimposed preeclampsia had significantly more proteinuria. MAP was similar for the two groups, and there were no significant differences in systolic or diastolic pressure. The RI and PI were not significantly different. The absolute CPP was significantly higher in the patients with superimposed preeclampsia.

On the basis of these findings, we believe that the development of superimposed preeclampsia significantly increases the CPP in women with chronic hypertension and that this is not directly related to an increase in BP. This CPP increase may be useful in distinguishing superimposed preeclampsia from chronic hypertension. It may also explain the increased risk for eclampsia seen in these patients. Our data also suggest that CPP is not directly related to BP and that preeclampsia has an independent effect on CPP.

The study's findings indicate that women with chronic hypertension may have elevated or normal CPP, whereas women with chronic hypertension and superimposed preeclampsia are more likely to have elevated CPP similar to that seen in severe preeclampsia. Thus, the presence of superimposed preeclampsia in a woman who has previously had chronic hypertension may

indicate the supervention of cerebral overperfusion, with the attendant risk of eclamptic seizures resulting from hypertensive encephalopathy rather than cerebral ischemia. These data suggest that BP control in such patients should be with agents that lower BP without having a significant vasodilatory effect on the cerebral arteries (i.e., a β-blocker). Because these women are at risk for hypertensive encephalopathy, increasing the CPP may precipitate convulsions. These findings may explain the high eclampsia rate in patients with superimposed preeclampsia who were treated with nimodipine.[8]

Preeclampsia, Headache, and Abnormal Cerebral Perfusion

Headache has long been recognized as an important harbinger of eclampsia, and in more than 80% of cases of eclampsia the patient reported an antecedent headache.[107] The character of these headaches has not been defined; in many instances, they are diffuse and poorly characterized. This is partly because of an inadequate understanding of the pathophysiology of headache in preeclampsia.

In nonpregnant individuals, nitroglycerin-induced headache (believed to be caused by cerebral vasodilatation) is associated with a significant reduction in MCA velocity without any change in BP.[110] These and other data show that Doppler ultrasonography is playing an important role in the research of the pathophysiology of headache. Evidence is now emerging that begins to link headache and abnormal CPP.[111, 112]

Preeclamptic patients with headache are more likely to have abnormal CPP than those of similar gestational age without headache. Figure 12–9 shows the results of a study that we performed.[94, 95] Preeclamptic women with headache were more likely to have an abnormal CPP value than those without headache. Women with headache had abnormal CPP (20/42 [48%]) more commonly than women without headache (8/37 [22%]). In Figure 12–9, 18 patients with headache and 7 without headache had values above the 95th percentile ($P = .04$, odds ratio = 3.21 [1.04 – 10.22]), and only two patients with headache and one without headache had CPP values below the 5th percentile. The findings support the notion that

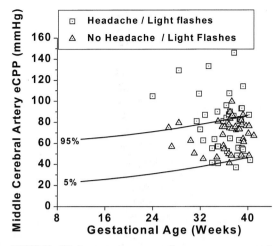

FIGURE 12–9. Data from preeclamptic women with and without headache and flashes of light. Women with headache are more likely to have elevated and abnormal cerebral perfusion pressure (CPP) than those without headache, suggesting that elevated CPP may be associated with headache in preeclampsia. eCPP, estimated cerebral perfusion pressure.

preeclamptic women with headache who have an abnormal CPP are more likely to have a high CPP than a low CPP (43% versus 5%).

Ohno and associates[113] have shown that preeclamptic women with visual disturbances have higher MCA velocities than preeclamptic women without visual disturbances. We suggest that in preeclamptic patients headache is strongly associated with abnormal cerebral perfusion. Although some preeclamptic women without headache have abnormal CPP, those with headache have significantly greater deviation from the norm.[94, 95] Of interest is that both elevated MCA CPP and decreased MCA CPP were associated with headache. Presumably, both underperfused ischemic brain (low CPP) and overperfused encephalopathic brain (high CPP) can stimulate an epileptiform discharge and cause an eclamptic seizure. This further supports the theory that both ischemia and hypertensive encephalopathy may be involved in the pathophysiology of eclamptic seizures and suggests that headache is a symptom with at least two pathophysiologic pathways in preeclampsia. Patients with headache are also more likely to have abnormal cerebral autoregulation, as we have shown.[95] Preeclamptic women with headache had an abnormal MCA RI response to increasing MAP, as opposed to those without headache, when the

RI appropriately increased to counter high CPP.[95]

The abnormal CPP theory remains to be confirmed with rigorous studies, but evidence is mounting to support it. Figure 12–7 shows the CPP from a preeclamptic woman who presented with intermittent headache at 33 weeks' gestation. CPP was measured and was noted to be elevated—suggestive of imminent hypertensive encephalopathy and the potential for cerebral overperfusion. In view of her immature gestational age and moderately elevated BP, the patient was observed overnight and hematologic and biochemical profiles were started. The following morning, the patient vomited and almost immediately had an eclamptic convulsion. This is the first case that we are aware of in which abnormal CPP was measured before an eclamptic convulsion. It is not unreasonable to suggest that the increased BP caused by the vomiting precipitated an acute hypertensive encephalopathy and eclampsia. The underlying propensity to overperfusion already existed and the protective autoregulation may well have failed, allowing sudden overperfusion. Any cause of acute BP increase (pain, emotion, physical exertion, coughing, drugs, or sudden increases in BP) may well have had the same effect.

Although never shown to occur before a seizure, cerebral ischemia may have the same outcome. We and others have demonstrated severe cerebral underperfusion and vasospasm in women who have had, or who are currently having, eclamptic seizures. There is obviously a danger involved in extrapolating findings after the fact, because the eclamptic seizure itself may have caused the release of vasoconstrictor substances that resulted in vasospasm. Unfortunately, until longitudinal data are available from women before and after eclamptic seizures, this point will remain speculative.

In 1998, Williams and coworkers[114] showed that, in postpartum women who had had preeclampsia, CPP remained elevated for at least 1 week. They hypothesized that this elevation may put these patients at risk for postpartum seizures. A longitudinal study to test this hypothesis remains to be done.

Both cerebral hemispheres must be examined independently, and assessment should not be based on an average CPP. This is because it is possible to see very different perfusion status in the two hemispheres;

that is, it is not uncommon to see normal CPP in one hemisphere and very abnormal perfusion pressure in the other. Averaging the two results would diminish the significance of the abnormal finding and may obscure the immediacy of the problem.

Magnesium Sulfate: Effect on Cerebral and Orbital Vessels in Preeclampsia

The use of $MgSO_4$ for the treatment of preeclampsia has been well supported[1, 115] even though we know little of its mechanism of action. The cerebral vasodilatory response to $MgSO_4$ infusion was used to indirectly confirm the presence of cerebral vasoconstriction or vasospasm in preeclampsia.[116–120] Whether this response is the result of calcium antagonism or the endothelial release of prostacyclin or nitric oxide is debatable.[121]

TCD ultrasound evaluation of the MCA during an infusion of $MgSO_4$ demonstrated a significant decrease in the PI compared with pretreatment Doppler measurements.[114, 115] MCA mean velocity increases significantly after treatment with $MgSO_4$.[82, 122] Reduction in the MCA PI during $MgSO_4$ therapy suggests that vasospasm in small-caliber vessels distal to the MCA is alleviated. The effect of $MgSO_4$ on the smaller caliber vessels distal to the MCA[118–120] (central retinal artery and posterior ciliary artery) has been evaluated during $MgSO_4$ infusion. Both the central retinal and posterior ciliary artery PIs and RIs were significantly reduced as a result of the infusion. In addition, increases in both the peak systolic velocity and the end-diastolic velocity in the central retinal artery have been demonstrated during an infusion of $MgSO_4$ in a preeclamptic patient who was experiencing scotomata.[105] $MgSO_4$ appears to exert its major effect on the central retinal vasculature, resulting in a 125% increase in the end-diastolic velocity; there is much less of an increase in the systolic velocity (42%). These data are consistent with the theory that the visual disturbance associated with preeclampsia results from central retinal artery vasospasm with resultant retinal ischemia.

$MgSO_4$ has clearly been associated with increased blood flow velocity and decreased resistance in both large-caliber and small-caliber cerebral vessels in women with preeclampsia. These findings suggest that one of its protective mechanisms is the alleviation of vasospasm in cerebral vessels. Of importance, however, is the fact that the vasodilatory effect of $MgSO_4$ appears to be temporary, as demonstrated by Naidu and colleagues,[90] who used MRI, SPECT, and Doppler studies.

$MgSO_4$ also has a hypotensive action consequent on its peripheral vasodilatory activity. These two effects, cerebral vasodilation and reduction of BP, may be important in different ways in the two proposed mechanisms for eclampsia. Cerebral vasodilation alleviates cerebral ischemia and increases CPP. Hypotension reduces CPP and prevents hypertensive encephalopathy.

Nimodipine: Effect on Cerebral and Orbital Vessels in Preeclampsia

Nimodipine, a 1,4-dihydropyridine calcium antagonist, has selective cerebral vasodilator properties without the same degree of antihypertensive effect seen with other dihydropyridines (e.g., nifedipine).[121] The use of sublingually and intravenously administered nimodipine has been associated with resolution of eclamptic seizures.[88, 121]

Belfort and colleagues[88] described the effects of nimodipine on the central retinal artery in an eclamptic patient. Using orbital color flow Doppler ultrasonography, they noted a reduction in the central retinal artery PI from 1.04 to 0.53 (49%) within 40 minutes of nimodipine administration. This was associated with a cessation of seizure activity in the patient who had previously had recalcitrant convulsions despite adequate control of BP. This case is thought to represent that group of eclamptic women who have persistent cerebral ischemia on the basis of unresolved vasospasm. In such patients, further reduction in BP may contribute to continued seizures as a result of worsened ischemia. Cerebral vasodilation with increased perfusion pressure, rather than decreased cerebral perfusion, is needed, and nimodipine appears to be well suited to this purpose.

Belfort and associates[123] further investigated the effects of nimodipine in patients with severe preeclampsia using transcranial and orbital Doppler sonography. One hour after nimodipine administration, the ophthalmic artery PI and the central retinal artery systolic velocity and PI were significantly decreased. This did not happen in the MCA, suggesting that nimodipine may be more effective in reducing vasospasm in smaller-caliber vessels than in the larger vessels (MCA).

MILD PREECLAMPSIA AND CEREBRAL HEMODYNAMICS AFTER TREATMENT

There is a paucity of data addressing the optimal CPP for women with preeclampsia. We believe that therapy should be aimed at maintaining CPP within the normal range. Given that in some cases mild preeclampsia is associated with low CPP,[82, 122] we studied the effects of nimodipine versus $MgSO_4$ on CPP in such a group of women.[53] We showed that the change in CPP was significantly different between the two groups (0 to 30 minutes). The change in CPP after nimodipine (median percentage change from baseline [25% to 75%]) was significantly more positive than after the $MgSO_4$.

Nimodipine appears to cause an increase in CPP, compared with $MgSO_4$, and may be more suitable than $MgSO_4$ when CPP is very low. Although our experiment showed an apparent advantage in certain patients, $MgSO_4$ has been used for many years without evidence of compromise in mild preeclampsia.

Obviously, there is more to cerebral perfusion than simply CPP. Nimodipine may have an advantage over $MgSO_4$ in one specific situation—when the vasospasm is so severe that $MgSO_4$ may not be as effective a cerebral vasodilator as nimodipine. In such a case, giving a patient an agent that reduces MAP proportionately more than it relieves cerebral vasospasm may result in worsened CPP and subsequent seizures. This may explain the rare failures that we see with $MgSO_4$ as a prophylactic and therapeutic agent.

POSTPARTUM CEREBRAL CHANGES ASSOCIATED WITH PREECLAMPSIA

Preeclamptic and normotensive patients have been evaluated with TCD ultrasound in the immediate and extended postpartum periods.[124–127] Williams and McLean[124] investigated 46 preeclamptic women in the antepartum period and again at 24 and 48 hours post partum. They determined that these patients had more elevated systolic, diastolic, and mean velocities in the MCA 24 hours after delivery than before delivery. They also demonstrated a further increase in all velocities at 48 hours post partum. The same investigators also found that preeclamptic women, when compared with normotensive women, had elevated cerebral blood flow velocities in the antepartum period and at 24 and 48 hours post partum. These data suggest that the cerebral vasculature of some preeclamptic women is in a vasoconstricted state before delivery as well as immediately post partum (i.e., up to 48 hours after delivery) compared with normotensive women.

Transcranial and orbital Doppler sonography have been used to evaluate preeclamptic women during the postpartum period in an effort to evaluate the duration of the changes wrought by the disease process.[126] Compared with normotensive women, preeclamptic women had significantly lower RIs in the larger diameter arteries at 6 weeks post partum. Also, the diastolic and mean velocities in the ophthalmic artery and the systolic velocity in the central retinal artery were significantly increased in preeclamptic women at 6 weeks post partum.

In a select group of preeclamptic women, the evaluation was also performed at 12 weeks post partum. We showed that the ophthalmic artery mean velocity and the central retinal artery systolic and diastolic velocities were elevated in previously preeclamptic women.[128]

From these data, it may be concluded that the cerebral vasculature in previously preeclamptic women continues to exhibit changes as late as 12 weeks post partum. This suggests that preeclamptic women have persistent vasoconstriction in the arterioles distal to the central renal artery, as well as compensatory vasodilatation in the ophthalmic artery, beyond the time period traditionally regarded as the puerperium.

TCD ultrasound has the potential to revolutionize our knowledge of cerebral blood velocity, pressure, and flow in pregnant women. The data presented in this chapter are exciting and hold the promise of further findings in the future, some of which may well result in management changes.

References

1. Which anticonvulsant for women with eclampsia? Evidence from the Collaborative Eclampsia Trial [published erratum in Lancet 1995;346:258]. Lancet 1995;345:1455–1463.
2. Kaunitz AM, Hughes JM, Grimes DA, et al. Causes of maternal mortality in the United States. Obstet Gynecol 1985;65:605–612.
3. Rochat RW, Koonin LM, Atrash HK, Jewett JF. Maternal mortality in the United States: Report from the Maternal Mortality Collaborative. Obstet Gynecol 1988;72:91–97.
4. Abdella TN, Sibai BM, Hays JM Jr, Anderson GD. Relationship of hypertensive disease to abruptio placentae. Obstet Gynecol 1984;63:365–370.
5. Saftlas AF, Olson DR, Franks AL, et al. Epidemiology of preeclampsia and eclampsia in the United States, 1979–1986. Am J Obstet Gynecol 1990; 163:460–465.
6. Graves EJ. Utilization of short-stay hospitals, United States, 1986, annual summary. Washington, DC: National Center for Health Statistics, 1988; U.S. Department of Health and Human Services Pub No. 88-1757(Public Health Service). Vital and Health Statistics Series 13, No. 96.
7. ACOG Technical Bulletin. Hypertension in pregnancy. No. 219, January 1996 (replaces No. 91, February 1986). Committee on Technical Bulletins of the American College of Obstetricians and Gynecologists.
8. Belfort MA, Anthony J, Saade G. Interim report of the nimodipine vs. magnesium sulfate for seizure prophylaxis in severe preeclampsia study: An international, randomized, controlled trial. Am J Obstet Gynecol 1998;178:10.
9. Burrows RF, Burrows EA. The feasibility of a control population for a randomized control trial of seizure prophylaxis in the hypertensive disorders of pregnancy. Am J Obstet Gynecol 1995;173:929–935.
9a. Hall DR, Odendaal HJ, Smith M. Is the prophylactic administration of magnesium sulfate in women with preeclampsia indicated prior to labor? Br J Gynaecol 2000;107:903–908.
10. Hinchey J, Chaves C, Appignani B, et al. A reversible posterior leukoencephalopathy syndrome. N Engl J Med 1996;334:494–500.
11. Horn EH, Filshie M, Kerslake RW, Jaspan T. Widespread cerebral ischaemia treated with nimodipine in a patient with eclampsia. BMJ 1990; 301:794.
12. Richards A, Graham D, Bullock R. Clinicopathological study of neurological complications due to hypertensive disorders of pregnancy. J Neurol Neurosurg Psychiatry 1988;51:416–421.
13. Cotton DB, Janusz CA, Berman RF. Anticonvulsant effects of magnesium sulfate on hippocampal seizures: Therapeutic implications in preeclampsia-eclampsia. Am J Obstet Gynecol 1992;166: 1127–1134; discussion 1134–1136.
14. Hallak M, Berman RF, Irtenkauf SM, et al. Peripheral magnesium sulfate enters the brain and increases the threshold for hippocampal seizures in rats. Am J Obstet Gynecol 1992;167:1605–1610.
15. Beausang-Linder M, Bill A. Cerebral circulation in acute arterial hypertension: Protective effects of sympathetic nervous activity. Acta Physiol Scand 1981;111:193–199.
16. Digre KB, Varner MW, Osborn AG, Crawford S. Cranial magnetic resonance imaging in severe preeclampsia vs eclampsia. Arch Neurol 1993; 50:399–406.
17. Will AD, Lewis KL, Hinshaw DB Jr, et al. Cerebral vasoconstriction in toxemia. Neurology 1987; 37:1555–1557.
18. Trommer BL, Homer D, Mikhael MA. Cerebral vasospasm and eclampsia. Stroke 1988;19:326–329.
19. Van den Veyver IB, Belfort MA, Rowe TF, Moise KJ. Cerebral vasospasm in eclampsia: Transcranial Doppler ultrasound findings. J Matern Fetal Med 1994;3:9–13.
20. Williams KP, Wilson S. Maternal cerebral blood flow changes associated with eclampsia. Am J Perinatol 1995;12:189–191.
21. Vandenplas O, Dive A, Dooms G, Mahieu P. Magnetic resonance evaluation of severe neurological disorders in eclampsia. Neuroradiology 1990; 32:47–49.
22. Duncan R, Hadley D, Bone I, et al. Blindness in eclampsia: CT and MR imaging. J Neurol Neurosurg Psychiatry 1989;52:899–902.
23. Ito T, Sakai T, Inagawa S, et al. MR angiography of cerebral vasospasm in preeclampsia. AJNR Am J Neuroradiol 1995;16:1344–1346.
24. Lewis LK, Hinshaw DB Jr, Will AD, et al. CT and angiographic correlation of severe neurological disease in toxemia of pregnancy. Neuroradiology 1988;30:59–64.
25. Hashimoto H, Kuriyama Y, Naritomi H, Sawada T. Serial assessments of middle cerebral artery flow velocity with transcranial Doppler sonography in the recovery stage of eclampsia: A case report. Angiology 1997;48:355–358.
26. Govan ADT. The pathogenesis of eclamptic lesions. J Pathol Microbiol 1961;24:561–575.
27. Sanders TG, Clayman DA, Sanchez-Ramos L, et al. Brain in eclampsia: MR imaging with clinical correlation. Radiology 1991;180:475–478.
28. Crawford S, Varner MW, Digre KB, et al. Cranial magnetic resonance imaging in eclampsia. Obstet Gynecol 1987;70:474–477.
29. Donaldson JO. Magnesium sulfate and eclampsia [letter]. Arch Neurol 1989;46:945–946.
30. Donaldson JO. Eclamptic hypertensive encephalopathy. Semin Neurol 1988;8:230–233.
31. Chester EM, Agamanolis DP, Banker BQ, Victor M. Hypertensive encephalopathy: A clinicopathologic study of 20 cases. Neurology 1978;28:928–939.
32. Kontos HA, Wei EP, Dietrich WD, et al. Mechanism of cerebral arteriolar abnormalities after acute hypertension. Am J Physiol 1981;240:H511–H527.
33. Hatashita S, Hoff JT, Ishii S. Focal brain edema associated with acute arterial hypertension. J Neurosurg 1986;64:643–649.
34. Gotoh O, Asano T, Koide T, Takakura K. Ischemic brain edema following occlusion of the middle cerebral artery in the rat: I. The time courses of the brain water, sodium and potassium contents and blood-brain barrier permeability to ^{125}I-albumin. Stroke 1985;16:101–109.
35. Kyle PM, de Swiet M, Buckley D, et al. Noninvasive assessment of the maternal cerebral circulation by transcranial Doppler ultrasound during angiotensin II infusion. Br J Obstet Gynaecol 1993;100:85–91.

36. Belfort MA, Saade GR, Grunewald C, et al. Effects of blood pressure on orbital and middle cerebral artery resistances in healthy pregnant women and women with preeclampsia. Am J Obstet Gynecol 1999;180:601–607.

37. Kublickas M, Grunewald C, Nisell H, et al. Interpretation of pulsatility index in studies on renal circulation of normal and preeclamptic pregnancies. Eur J Ultrasound 1994;1:137–142.

38. Schwartz RB, Jones KM, Kalina P, et al. Hypertensive encephalopathy: Findings on CT, MR imaging, and SPECT imaging in 14 cases. AJR Am J Roentgenol 1992;159:379–383.

39. Vliegen JH, Muskens E, Keunen RW, et al. Abnormal cerebral hemodynamics in pregnancy-related hypertensive encephalopathy. Eur J Obstet Gynecol Reprod Biol 1993;49:198–200.

40. Symon L, Held K, Dorsch NW. A study of regional autoregulation in the cerebral circulation to increased perfusion pressure in normocapnia and hypercapnia. Stroke 1973;4:139–147.

41. Nag S, Robertson DM, Dinsdale HB. Cerebral cortical changes in acute experimental hypertension: An ultrastructural study. Lab Invest 1977;36:150–161.

42. Rowe GG, Maxwell GM, Crumpton CW. The cerebral haemodynamic response to administration of hydralazine. Circulation 1962;25:970–972.

43. Overgaard J, Skinhoj E. A paradoxical cerebral hemodynamic effect of hydralazine. Stroke 1975;6:402–410.

44. Arnolds BJ, von Reutern GM. Transcranial Doppler sonography. Examination technique and normal reference values. Ultrasound Med Biol 1986;12:115–123.

45. Aaslid R, Huber P, Nornes H. A transcranial Doppler method in the evaluation of cerebrovascular spasm. Neuroradiology 1986;28:11–16.

46. Aaslid R, Huber P, Nornes H. Evaluation of cerebrovascular spasm with transcranial Doppler ultrasound. J Neurosurg 1984;60:37–41.

47. Williams K, Wilson S. Maternal middle cerebral artery blood flow velocity variation with gestational age. Obstet Gynecol 1994;84:445–448.

48. Irion O, Moutquin JM, Williams K, Forest JC. Reference values and influence of smoking on maternal middle cerebral artery blood flow [abstract]. Am J Obstet Gynecol 1996;174:367.

49. Belfort MA, Yared M, Saade G, et al. Cerebrovascular resistance decrease in normal pregnancy: Normative data for middle cerebral, central retinal and ophthalmic arteries and comparison with preeclamptic pregnancy [abstract]. Am J Obstet Gynecol 1995;172:382.

50. MacKenzie F, De Vermette R, Nimrod C, et al. Doppler sonographic studies on the ophthalmic and central retinal arteries in the gravid woman. J Ultrasound Med 1995;14:643–647.

51. West MS, Belfort MA, Herd JA, et al. Normative longitudinal data for three new Doppler cerebral hemodynamic indices during pregnancy. J Soc Gynecol Invest 1997;4:200A.

52. Belfort MA, Tooke-Miller C, Allen JC, et al. Physiologic changes in velocity, resistance indices, and cerebral perfusion pressure in the middle cerebral artery distribution during normal pregnancy. Acta Obstet Gynecol Scand (in press).

53. Belfort MA, Saade GR, Yared M, et al. Change in estimated cerebral perfusion pressure after treatment with nimodipine or magnesium sulfate in patients with preeclampsia. Am J Obstet Gynecol 1999;181:402–407.

54. Gabrielsen TO, Greitz T. Normal size of the internal carotid, middle cerebral and anterior cerebral arteries. Acta Radiol [Diagn] (Stockh) 1970;10:1–10.

55. Kochs E, Hoffman WE, Werner C, et al. Cerebral blood flow velocity in relation to cerebral blood flow, cerebral metabolic rate for oxygen, and electroencephalogram analysis during isoflurane anesthesia in dogs. Anesth Analg 1993;76:1222–1226.

56. Larsen FS, Olsen KS, Hansen BA, et al. Transcranial Doppler is valid for determination of the lower limit of cerebral blood flow autoregulation. Stroke 1994;25:1985–1988.

57. Dahl A, Russell D, Nyberg-Hansen R, et al. Cerebral vasoreactivity in unilateral carotid artery disease: A comparison of blood flow velocity and regional cerebral blood flow measurements. Stroke 1944;25:621–626.

58. Ringelstein EB, Sievers C, Ecker S, et al. Noninvasive assessment of CO_2-induced cerebral vasomotor response in normal individuals and patients with internal carotid artery occlusions. Stroke 1988;19:963–969.

59. Kirkham FJ, Padayachee TS, Parsons S, et al. Transcranial measurement of blood velocities in the basal cerebral arteries using pulsed Doppler ultrasound: Velocity as an index of flow. Ultrasound Med Biol 1986;12:15–21.

60. Newell DW, Aaslid R, Lam A, et al. Comparison of flow and velocity during dynamic autoregulation testing in humans. Stroke 1994;25:793–797.

61. Tiecks FP, Lam AM, Aaslid R, Newell DW. Comparison of static and dynamic cerebral autoregulation measurements. Stroke 1995;26:1014–1019.

62. Aaslid R, Markwalder TM, Nornes H. Noninvasive transcranial Doppler ultrasound recording of flow velocity in basal cerebral arteries. J Neurosurg 1982;57:769–774.

63. Lieb WE, Cohen SM, Merton DA, et al. Color Doppler imaging of the eye and orbit: Technique and normal vascular anatomy. Arch Ophthalmol 1991;109:527–531.

64. Harris A, Spaeth GL, Sergott RC, et al. Retrobulbar arterial hemodynamic effects of betaxolol and timolol in normal-tension glaucoma. Am J Ophthalmol 1995;120:168–175.

65. Erickson SJ, Hendrix LE, Massaro BM, et al. Color Doppler flow imaging of the normal and abnormal orbit. Radiology 1989;173:511–516.

66. Williams KP, Galerneau F, Wilson S. Effect of labor on maternal cerebral blood flow velocity. Am J Obstet Gynecol 1998;178:59–61.

67. Kontos HA, Wei EP, Navari RM, et al. Responses of cerebral arteries and arterioles to acute hypotension and hypertension. Am J Physiol 1978;234:H371–H383.

68. Gibo H, Carver CC, Rhoton AL Jr, et al. Microsurgical anatomy of the middle cerebral artery. J Neurosurg 1981;54:151–169.

69. Williams K, MacLean C. Transcranial assessment of maternal cerebral blood flow velocity in normal vs. pre-eclamptic women (variation with maternal posture). A preliminary study. J Perinat Med 1994;22:291–294.

70. Williams K, MacLean C. Transcranial assessment of maternal cerebral blood flow velocity in normal

vs. hypertensive states: Variations with maternal posture. J Reprod Med 1994;39:685–688.

71. Serra-Serra V, Kyle PM, Chandran R, Redman CW. Maternal middle cerebral artery velocimetry in normal pregnancy and postpartum. Br J Obstet Gynaecol 1997;104:904–909.

72. Dewey RC, Pieper HP, Hunt WE. Experimental cerebral hemodynamics: Vasomotor tone, critical closing pressure, and vascular bed resistance. J Neurosurg 1974;41:597–606.

73. Sainz A, Cabau J, Roberts VC. Deceleration vs. acceleration: A haemodynamic parameter in the assessment of vascular reactivity: A preliminary study. Med Eng Phys 1995;17:91–95.

74. Gosling RG, King DH. Ultrasonographic angiography. *In* Hascus AW, Adamson L (eds). Arteries and Veins. Edinburgh: Churchill Livingstone, 1975, p 61.

75. Belfort MA, West MS, Giannina G, et al. Physiologic changes in cerebral perfusion pressure in the 3 main arterial distributions of the brain during normal pregnancy and in the postpartum period [abstract]. J Soc Gynecol Invest 1997;4:146A.

76. Belfort MA, West MS, Giannina G, et al. Cerebral perfusion pressure is significantly lower in mild preeclampsia than in severe preeclampsia: Pathophysiologic implications for eclampsia. J Soc Gynecol Invest 1997;4:142A.

77. Giannina G, Hanley M, Belfort MA, et al. Introduction of the steady flow index in uterine artery Doppler velocimetry in pregnancy. J Soc Gynecol Invest 1997;4:270A.

78. Chan KH, Miller JD, Dearden NM, et al. The effect of changes in cerebral perfusion pressure upon middle cerebral artery blood flow velocity and jugular bulb venous oxygen saturation after severe brain injury. J Neurosurg 1992;77:55–61.

79. Aaslid R, Lundar T, Lindegaard KF, Nornes H. Estimation of cerebral perfusion pressure from arterial blood pressure and transcranial Doppler recordings. *In* Miller JD, Teasdale GM, Rowen JO, et al (eds). Intracranial Pressure. Vol 6. Berlin: Springer-Verlag, 1986, p 226–229.

80. Belfort MA, Tooke-Miller C, Varner MW, et al. Evaluation of a non-invasive transcranial Doppler and blood pressure based method for the evaluation of cerebral perfusion pressure in pregnant women. J Hypertens Pregn (in press).

81. Bland JM, Altman DG. Statistical methods for assessing agreement between two methods of clinical measurement. Lancet 1986;1:307–310.

82. Belfort MA, Grunewald C, Saade GR, et al. Preeclampsia may cause both overperfusion and underperfusion of the brain: A cerebral perfusion based model [letter]. Acta Obstet Gynecol Scand 2000 (in press).

83. Belfort MA, Saade GR. Oxygen delivery and consumption in critically ill pregnant patients: Association with ophthalmic artery diastolic velocity. Am J Obstet Gynecol 1994;171:211–217.

84. Van Bel F, Steendijk P, Teitel DF, et al. Cerebral blood flow velocity: The influence of myocardial contractility on the velocity waveform of brain supplying arteries. Ultrasound Med Biol 1992; 18:441–449.

85. Klingelhofer J, Dander D, Holzgraefe M, et al. Cerebral vasospasm evaluated by transcranial Doppler ultrasonography at different intracranial pressures. J Neurosurg 1991;75:752–758.

86. Donaldson JO. Does magnesium sulfate treat eclamptic convulsions? Clin Neuropharmacol 1986;9:37–45.

87. Castren O, Saarikoski S, Siimes A. Vascular reactivity in normal pregnancy and in pregnancies complicated by hypertension. Int J Obstet Gynecol 1973;11:236–246.

88. Belfort MA, Carpenter RJ Jr, Kirshon B, et al. The use of nimodipine in a patient with eclampsia: Color flow Doppler demonstration of retinal artery relaxation. Am J Obstet Gynecol 1993;169:204–206.

89. Zunker P, Ley-Pozo J, Louwen F, et al. Cerebral hemodynamics in pre-eclampsia/eclampsia syndrome. Ultrasound Obstet Gynecol 1995;6:411–415.

90. Naidu K, Moodley J, Corr P, Hoffmann M. Single photon emission and cerebral computerised tomographic scan and transcranial Doppler sonographic findings in eclampsia. Br J Obstet Gynaecol 1997;104:1165–1172.

91. Morriss MC, Twickler DM, Hatab MR, et al. Cerebral blood flow and cranial magnetic resonance imaging in eclampsia and severe preeclampsia. Obstet Gynecol 1997;89:561–568.

92. Williams K, McLean C. Maternal cerebral vasospasm in eclampsia assessed by transcranial Doppler. Am J Perinatol 1993;10:243–244.

93. Qureshi AI, Frankel MR, Ottenlips JR, Stern BJ. Cerebral hemodynamics in preeclampsia and eclampsia. Arch Neurol 1996;53:1226–1231.

94. Belfort MA, Saade GR, Grunewald C, et al. Association of cerebral perfusion pressure with headache in women with pre-eclampsia. Br J Obstet Gynaecol 1999;106:814–821.

95. Belfort MA, Saade GR, Grunewald C, et al. Association of cerebral perfusion pressure with headache in women with pre-eclampsia [letter]. Br J Obstet Gynaecol 2000 (in press).

96. Hansen WF, Burnham SJ, Svendsen TO, et al. Transcranial Doppler findings of cerebral vasospasm in preeclampsia. J Matern Fetal Med 1996;5:194–200.

97. Demarin V, Rundek T, Hodek B. Maternal cerebral circulation in normal and abnormal pregnancies. Acta Obstet Gynecol Scand 1997;76:619–624.

98. Romner B, Bellner J, Kongstad P, Sjoholm H. Elevated transcranial Doppler flow velocities after severe head injury: Cerebral vasospasm or hyperemia? J Neurosurg 1996;85:90–97.

99. Aguglia U, Tinuper P, Farnarier G, Quattrone A. Electroencephalographic and anatomo-clinical evidences of posterior cerebral damage in hypertensive encephalopathy. Clin Electroencephalogr 1984;15:53–60.

100. Edvinsson L, Owman C, Sjoberg NO. Autonomic nerves, mast cells, and amine receptors in human brain vessels: A histochemical and pharmacological study. Brain Res 1976;115:377–393.

101. Edvinsson L, Owman C, Siesjo B. Physiological role of cerebrovascular sympathetic nerves in the autoregulation of cerebral blood flow. Brain Res 1976;117:519–523.

102. Manfredi M, Beltramello A, Bongiovanni LG, et al. Eclamptic encephalopathy: Imaging and pathogenetic considerations. Acta Neurol Scand 1997;96:277–282.

103. Greenwood JP, Stoker JB, Walker JJ, Mary DA. Sympathetic nerve discharge in normal pregnancy

and pregnancy-induced hypertension [published erratum in J Hypertens 1998;16:1219]. J Hypertens 1998;16:617–624.

104. Schobel HP, Fischer T, Heuszer K, et al. Preeclampsia—a state of sympathetic overactivity. N Engl J Med 1996;335:1480–1485.

105. Belfort MA, Saade GR. Retinal vasospasm associated with visual disturbance in preeclampsia: Color flow Doppler findings. Am J Obstet Gynecol 1993;169:523–525.

106. Plazzi G, Tinuper P, Cerullo A, et al. Occipital lobe epilepsy: A chronic condition related to transient occipital lobe involvement in eclampsia. Epilepsia 1994;35:644–647.

107. Monteiro ML, Hoyt WF, Imes RK. Puerperal cerebral blindness: Transient bilateral occipital involvement from presumed cerebral venous thrombosis. Arch Neurol 1984;41:1300–1301.

108. Hata T, Senoh D, Hata K, Kitao M. Ophthalmic artery velocimetry in preeclampsia. Gynecol Obstet Invest 1995;40:32–35.

109. Belfort MA, Grunewald C, Nisell H, et al. Pregnant women with chronic hypertension and superimposed preeclampsia have a cerebral overperfusion state similar to that seen in severe preeclampsia [abstract]. J Soc Gyncol Invest 1999;6:68A.

110. Tegeler CH, Davidai G, Gengo FM, et al. Middle cerebral artery velocity correlates with nitroglycerin-induced headache onset. J Neuroimaging 1996;6:81–86.

111. Basoglu T, Ozbenli T, Bernay I, et al. Demonstration of frontal hypoperfusion in benign exertional headache by technetium-99m-HMPAO SPECT. J Nucl Med 1996;37:1172–1174.

112. Jorgensen LG. Transcranial Doppler ultrasound for cerebral perfusion. Acta Physiol Scand Suppl 1995;625:1–44.

113. Ohno Y, Kawai M, Wakahara Y, et al. Transcranial assessment of maternal cerebral blood flow velocity in patients with pre-eclampsia. Acta Obstet Gynecol Scand 1997;76:928–932.

114. Williams KP, Galerneau F, Wilson S. Changes in cerebral perfusion pressure in puerperal women with preeclampsia. Obstet Gynecol 1998;92:1016–1019.

115. Pritchard JA, Pritchard SA. Standardized treatment of 154 consecutive cases of eclampsia. Am J Obstet Gynecol 1975;123:543–552.

116. Belfort MA, Moise KJ Jr. Effect of magnesium sulfate on maternal brain blood flow in preeclampsia: A randomized, placebo-controlled study. Am J Obstet Gynecol 1992;167:661–666.

117. Belfort MA, Saade GR, Moise KJ Jr. The effect of magnesium sulfate on maternal and fetal blood flow in pregnancy-induced hypertension. Acta Obstet Gynecol Scand 1993;72:526–530.

118. Belfort MA. Doppler assessment of retinal blood flow velocity during parenteral magnesium treatment in patients with preeclampsia. Magnes Res 1993;6:239–246.

119. Belfort MA. The effect of magnesium sulphate on blood flow velocity in the maternal retina in mild pre-eclampsia: A preliminary colour flow Doppler study. Br J Obstet Gynaecol 1992;99:641–645.

120. Belfort MA, Saade GR, Moise KJ Jr. The effect of magnesium sulfate on maternal retinal blood flow in preeclampsia: A randomized placebo-controlled study. Am J Obstet Gynecol 1992;167:1548–1553.

121. Anthony J, Johanson RB, Duley L. Role of magnesium sulfate in seizure prevention in patients with eclampsia and pre-eclampsia. Drug Saf 1996;15:188–199.

122. Belfort MA, Grunewald C, Saade GR, et al. Preeclampsia may cause both overperfusion and underperfusion of the brain: A cerebral perfusion based model. Acta Obstet Gynecol Scand 1999;78:586–591.

123. Belfort MA, Saade GR, Moise KJ Jr, et al. Nimodipine in the management of preeclampsia: Maternal and fetal effects. Am J Obstet Gynecol 1994;171:417–424.

124. Williams KP, McLean C. Peripartum changes in maternal cerebral blood flow velocity in normotensive and preeclamptic patients. Obstet Gynecol 1993;82:334–337.

125. Belfort MA, Saade GR, Cruz A, et al. Postpartum preeclamptic patients have decreased resistance in their larger diameter cerebral arteries than normal postpartum [abstract]. Circulation 1995;92:1421.

126. Bogousslavsky J, Despland PA, Regli F, Dubuis PY. Postpartum cerebral angiopathy: Reversible vasoconstriction assessed by transcranial Doppler ultrasounds. Eur Neurol 1989;29:102–105.

127. Raps EC, Galetta SL, Broderick M, Atlas SW. Delayed peripartum vasculopathy: Cerebral eclampsia revisited. Ann Neurol 1993;33:222–225.

128. Giannina G, Belfort MA, Cruz AL, Herd JA. Persistent cerebrovascular changes in postpartum preeclamptic women: A Doppler evaluation. Am J Obstet Gynecol 1997;177:1213–1218.

13 RANDOMIZED TRIALS for PREVENTION and TREATMENT of ECLAMPTIC CONVULSIONS

Andrea Witlin and Baha M. Sibai

Approximately 5% to 7% of all pregnancies are complicated by preeclampsia. The incidence of eclamptic seizures (eclamptic convulsions) in women with preeclampsia is less than 1%. In the United States, magnesium sulfate (MgSO$_4$) is used for seizure prophylaxis in women with preeclampsia and for therapy of eclamptic convulsions. Alternatives to MgSO$_4$ as a prophylactic agent in women with severe preeclampsia have been suggested, including phenytoin,[1] diazepam,[2] nimodipine,[3] and aggressive antihypertensive therapy.[4] Nonetheless, these alternative therapies have not provided equivalent results to those of MgSO$_4$ therapy. Even though MgSO$_4$ has been used for more than 70 years, its mode of action has yet to be elicited.

HISTORICAL PERSPECTIVE

MgSO$_4$ use was first reported in the early 1900s for control of tetanic convulsions.[5] Shortly thereafter, Lazard reported on the use of MgSO$_4$ for control of eclamptic convulsions with an associated fivefold (30% versus 5.8%) reduction of maternal mortality.[6] MgSO$_4$ therapy was heralded as an improvement to the previously used eliminative measures for therapy of eclampsia—enemas, castor oil, and phlebotomy.[6] MgSO$_4$ therapy was thus adopted for treatment of eclamptic convulsions on the basis of observational studies and anecdotal experience. As a natural extension to its use for therapy of eclamptic seizures, MgSO$_4$ was then adapted for prophylaxis of seizures in women with severe preeclampsia.

The modern obstetric use of MgSO$_4$ therapy for preeclampsia and eclampsia has been credited to Pritchard, who popularized the intramuscular (IM) route of administration of MgSO$_4$ (a 10-g IM load followed by 5 g IM every 4 h).[7] The continuous intravenous infusion was recommended by Zuspan (a 4-g intravenous [IV] load followed by 1 g/h)[8] and subsequently modified by Sibai (a 6-g IV load followed by 2 g/h).[9, 10] According to Pritchard,[7] appropriate serum levels of magnesium for treatment of eclamptic convulsions were 3.5 to 7 mEq/L or, correspondingly, 4.2 to 8.4 mg/dL (magnesium level mg/dL = 1.2 × magnesium level mEq/L).[7] However, no study has ever correlated explicit serum levels of magnesium with abolishment of seizure activity in a fashion analogous to the use of minimal inhibitory concentration and selection of antimicrobial agents. The concept of appropriate magnesium levels is based on Pritchard's clinical experience that most eclamptic seizures were successfully treated when the aforementioned magnesium levels were attained.[7]

RANDOMIZED TRIALS

There are five randomized trials comparing MgSO$_4$ with either phenytoin or placebo for inpatients with hypertensive disorders of pregnancy. Only one of these trials[1] had an adequate sample size to evaluate the effects of seizure prophylaxis in these women; the remaining trials primarily evaluated side effects of MgSO$_4$ therapy (Table 13–1).[1, 11–14]

221

TABLE 13-1. RANDOMIZED TRIALS OF MAGNESIUM SULFATE (MgSO₄) VERSUS PHENYTOIN OR PLACEBO FOR HYPERTENSIVE DISORDERS IN PREGNANCY

| AUTHOR | CONTROL GROUP | CONVULSIONS | |
		MgSO₄	Control
Appleton et al[11]	Phenytoin	0/24	0/23
Friedman et al[12]	Phenytoin	0/60	0/43
Atkinson et al[13]	Phenytoin	0/28	0/26
Lucas et al[1]	Phenytoin	0/1049	10/1089
Witlin et al[14]	Placebo	0/67	0/68
All authors		0/1228*	10/1249 (0.8%)*

*$P < .001$.

The largest randomized trial was reported by Lucas and associates.[1] More than 2000 women with various hypertensive disorders of pregnancy were assigned to either an IM magnesium regimen or a phenytoin regimen administered during labor and post partum. The authors found no seizures among 1049 patients receiving MgSO₄ and 10 cases of eclampsia (1%) among 1089 patients receiving phenytoin. MgSO₄ was considered superior to phenytoin for seizure prophylaxis in such patients. However, there are no placebo-controlled trials with adequate sample size to address the efficacy of MgSO₄ for this purpose. Therefore, the design and completion of such a trial are urgently needed.

Witlin and colleagues[14] studied 135 women with mild preeclampsia at or later than 37 weeks' gestation in a randomized, placebo-controlled trial of MgSO₄ for seizure prophylaxis. The authors noted that 10% of women progressed to a clinical diagnosis of

severe preeclampsia despite use of MgSO₄ prophylaxis. This incidence of progression to severe preeclampsia was similar in the placebo control group. The mean magnesium level in the magnesium-treated women was 4.7 ± 1.0 mg/dL.[14] For women in the placebo cohort progressing to severe preeclampsia, it was suggested that there was sufficient time to safely initiate MgSO₄ therapy for treatment of severe preeclampsia. This assumed "safety net" must be further evaluated in a larger trial.

There are four randomized trials comparing the use of antihypertensive drugs alone versus antihypertensive drugs plus parenteral MgSO₄ (Table 13–2).[4, 15–17] Two of these trials had inadequate sample size for this purpose,[4, 15] whereas the other two had adequate sample size.

The trial by Belfort and coworkers[16] compared the use of MgSO₄ with nimodipine (a calcium channel blocker with cerebral vasodilatory effects). The authors found lower incidence of eclampsia in the MgSO₄ group (1.5% versus 3.6%), but the difference was not statistically significant. The trial by Coetzee and colleagues[17] was double-blind, comparing IV MgSO₄ with IV saline in 685 patients with severe preeclampsia. The authors found a significant reduction in development of eclampsia in the group receiving magnesium (see Table 13–2). Therefore, it is apparent that MgSO₄ prophylaxis should be used in all patients with severe preeclampsia during labor and post partum.

Moodley and Moodley[4] are among several authors advocating the use of aggressive antihypertensive therapy in women with severe preeclampsia as an alternative to sei-

TABLE 13-2. RANDOMIZED TRIALS OF MAGNESIUM SULFATE (MgSO₄) THERAPY VERSUS NO ANTICONVULSANT THERAPY FOR SEVERE PREECLAMPSIA

| AUTHOR | ANTIHYPERTENSIVE THERAPY | TREATMENT OF CONVULSIONS | | RR (95% CI) |
		MgSO₄ No. (%)	Control No. (%)	
Moodley and Moodley[4]	Dihydralazine, nifedipine	1/112 (0.9)	0/116 (0)	N/A
Chen et al[15]	Hydralazine, methyldopa, nifedipine	0/34	0/34	N/A
Belfort et al[16]	Nimodipine, hydralazine	5/324 (1.5)	11/303 (3.6)	0.43 (0.15–1.21)
Coetzee et al[17]	Hydralazine, labetalol	1/345 (0.3)	11/340 (3.2)*	0.09 (0.01–0.69)
All studies		7/815 (0.86)	22/793 (2.8)	0.31 (0.13–0.72)

*Placebo-controlled.

CI, confidence interval; N/A, not applicable; RR, relative risk.

zure prophylaxis. They explored this hypothesis in a randomized controlled trial using the rapid-acting antihypertensive agents dihydralazine and nifedipine. Although the conclusions are limited by the small sample size, the authors suggested that aggressive use of antihypertensive medication alone might be sufficient therapy for severe preeclampsia.[4] In the future, this recommendation may be enhanced by selection of agents with combined antihypertensive, cerebrovasodilator, and decreased platelet aggregation action.

MgSO$_4$ does not prevent recurrent seizures in all eclamptic patients. There are six observational studies describing the rate of subsequent seizures in eclamptic women receiving MgSO$_4$ (Table 13–3).[18–22] The overall rate of recurrent seizures among these studies is 10%. This failure rate of MgSO$_4$ was also used as a reason to conduct randomized trials comparing it with other traditional anticonvulsants.

In the 1990s, several randomized trials were reported comparing the efficacy of MgSO$_4$ with other anticonvulsants in eclamptic women (Table 13–4).[2, 23–26] Four of these trials[23–26] had limited sample size, and only one multicenter trial had adequate sample size for this purpose.

The Collaborative Eclampsia Trial[2] was conducted in several centers in South Africa and South America. The trial included 1680 women with eclampsia who were assigned to MgSO$_4$, phenytoin, or diazepam therapy in two different randomization schemes. The trial demonstrated that MgSO$_4$ was superior to both phenytoin and diazepam for the treatment of *recurrent* seizures in eclamptic women (see Table 13–4). In addition, MgSO$_4$ reduced the risk of maternal death by one fourth over those treated with diazepam, relative risk (RR) 0.7 (95% confidence interval [CI] 0.4–1.4) and reduced the risk of maternal death by half over those treated with phenytoin, RR 0.5 (95% CI 0.2–2.0). Furthermore, there was a decreased incidence of pneumonia, less need for mechanical ventilation, and fewer admissions to the intensive care unit (ICU) in women receiving magnesium therapy.

Data by Bhalla and associates[25] also indicated that MgSO$_4$ was superior to lytic cocktail in eclamptic women.

TABLE 13–3. OBSERVATIONAL STUDIES ON SUBSEQUENT CONVULSIONS IN WOMEN WITH ECLAMPSIA RECEIVING MAGNESIUM SULFATE

AUTHOR	NO. OF PATIENTS WITH ECLAMPSIA	RECURRENT CONVULSIONS No.	(%)
Pritchard and Pritchard (1975)[18]	85	3	(3.5)
Gedekoh et al (1981)[19]	52	1	(1.9)
Pritchard et al (1984)[20]	83	10	(12.0)
Dunn et al (1986)[21]	13	5	(38.5)
Sibai and Ramanathan (1991)[22]	315	41	(13.0)
Dommisse (1990)[23]	100	3	(3.0)
All studies	648	63	(9.7)

TABLE 13–4. RANDOMIZED TRIALS COMPARING MAGNESIUM SULFATE (MgSO$_4$) THERAPY WITH OTHER ANTICONVULSANT AGENTS FOR ECLAMPSIA

AUTHOR	ANTIHYPERTENSIVE THERAPY	RECURRENT SEIZURES MgSO$_4$ No. (%)	Other No. (%)	RR (95% CI)
Dommisse[23]	Dihydralazine	0/11 (0)	4/11 (36.7)*	
Crowther[24]	Dihydralazine	5/24 (20.8)	7/27 (26)†	0.8 (0.29–2.2)
Bhalla et al[25]	Nifedipine	1/45 (2.2)	11/45 (24.4)‡	0.09 (0.01–0.68)
Friedman et al[26]	Nifedipine, labetalol	0/11 (0)	2/13 (15.4)*	
Collaborative Trial[2]	NR	60/453 (13.2)	126/452 (27.9)†	0.48 (0.36–0.63)
	NR	22/388 (5.7)	66/387 (17.1)*	0.33 (0.21–0.53)
All studies		88/922 (9.4)	216/935 (23.1)	0.41 (0.32–0.51)

*Phenytoin.
†Diazepam.
‡Lytic cocktail.
CI, confidence interval; NR, not reported; RR, relative risk.

Crowther[24] identified a trend toward lower maternal morbidity (recurrent convulsions, cardiopulmonary problems, disseminated intravascular coagulation, and acute renal failure) in the magnesium-treated cohort, RR 0.6 (95% CI 0.3–1.2). In addition, there was a trend toward improved neonatal outcome in the magnesium-treated group with regard to a 5-minute Apgar score below 7, need for intubation and positive pressure ventilation, and neonatal intensive care unit (NICU) admission.

The aforementioned randomized trials had also adequate information to compare the rate of maternal death between those receiving MgSO$_4$ and those receiving other agents (Table 13–5).[2, 23–26] The overall results demonstrated that MgSO$_4$ therapy was associated with significantly lower maternal mortality in eclampsia than that observed with other anticonvulsant agents (3.8% versus 5.1%; $P < .05$).

RETROSPECTIVE STUDIES

A few retrospective studies[27–30, 30a] have evaluated the frequency of eclampsia in women not receiving seizure prophylaxis (Table 13–6). The incidence of eclampsia ranges from one in 555 for women with hypertension[30] to one in 78 in women with severe preeclampsia.[29] The heterogeneity of these conditions (ranging from nonproteinuric hypertension[30] to severe preeclampsia[29]) warrants cautious interpretation of the data. Walker[30] limited evaluation to women with hypertension (without preeclampsia) only, Chua and Redman[29] limited investigation to women

with severe preeclampsia only, and the conclusions of Olah and coworkers[31] are limited by small sample size (n = 56). The two largest studies are reviewed next in greater detail.

Odendaal and Hall[28] from South Africa prospectively studied 1001 women with severe preeclampsia treated with MgSO$_4$ for seizure prophylaxis based on the clinical presentation suggestive of "impending eclampsia." Of this group, 510 women received MgSO$_4$ therapy and 491 women were monitored without benefit of MgSO$_4$ therapy. A total of five women developed eclampsia, two before delivery (both receiving MgSO$_4$ therapy) and three after delivery (none receiving MgSO$_4$ therapy). Two of the three postpartum seizures occurred more than 48 hours after delivery. It is not known whether the magnesium-treated cohort represented a group of "higher-risk" women who were appropriately treated with MgSO$_4$ or whether "impending eclampsia" could not be reliably anticipated.

Burrows and Burrows[27] performed an 8-year retrospective, single-institution, cross-sectional study of 1559 hypertensive pregnant women (more than half with severe disease) managed without seizure prophylaxis. Seizures occurred in 4.3% of those with preeclampsia and in 2.1% of those with chronic hypertension and superimposed preeclampsia. The likelihood of seizures was 17.4 times greater in women with preeclampsia (95% CI 5.2–60.2) and 8.1 times greater for women with chronic hypertension and superimposed preeclampsia (95% CI 1.3–49.4) compared with women with gestational hypertension or chronic hy-

TABLE 13–5. MATERNAL DEATHS IN TRIALS COMPARING MAGNESIUM SULFATE (MgSO$_4$) THERAPY WITH OTHER ANTICONVULSANT AGENTS FOR ECLAMPSIA

| | | MATERNAL DEATHS | | |
| | | MgSO$_4$ | Other | |
AUTHOR	COMPARISON GROUP	No. (%)	No. (%)	RR (95% CI)
Dommisse[23]	Phenytoin	0/11	0/11	
Crowther[24]	Diazepam	1/24 (4.2)	0/27	
Bhalla et al[25]	Lytic cocktail	0/45	2/45 (4.4)	
Friedman et al[26]	Phenytoin	0/11	0/13	
Collaborative Trial[2]	Phenytoin	10/388 (2.6)	20/387 (5.2)	0.50 (0.24–1.00)
	Diazepam	17/453 (3.8)	23/452 (5.1)	0.74 (0.40–1.36)
All studies		28/932 (3.0)	45/935 (4.8)	0.62 (0.39–0.99)

CI, confidence interval; RR, relative risk.

TABLE 13–6. OBSERVATIONAL STUDIES ON ECLAMPSIA IN WOMEN WITH PREECLAMPSIA NOT RECEIVING PROPHYLACTIC THERAPY

AUTHOR	CLASSIFICATION OF DISEASE	NO. OF PATIENTS	ECLAMPSIA	
			No.	(%)
Chua and Redman (1987–1990)[29]	Severe preeclampsia	78	1	(1.3)
Nelson (1951–1953)[30a]	Gestational hypertension	527	2	(0.38)
Nelson (1951–1953)[30a]	Preeclampsia*	216	6	(2.8)
Walker (1981–1989)[30]	Hypertensive disorders	3885	7	(0.18)
Burrows and Burrows (1986–1993)[27]	Gestational hypertension	745	1	(0.13)
	Preeclampsia*	457	9†	(1.9)
Odendaal and Hall (1983–1993)[28]	Severe preeclampsia	491	3	(0.6)

*Includes mild and severe preeclampsia.
†Includes convulsion only during and after delivery.

pertension. This incidence of seizures seems in sharp contrast to that noted previously in women with severe preeclampsia (see Table 13–3). It appears that the authors have either reported upon a cohort of patients at exceedingly high risk for seizure or that their results confirm the utility of $MgSO_4$ seizure prophylaxis in a population of women with severe preeclampsia (level II-2 evidence).[32]

In summary, a review of randomized trials indicates $MgSO_4$ to be the ideal agent to use for prophylaxis in women with severe preeclampsia and for the treatment of eclamptic convulsions. Information is limited regarding the need for $MgSO_4$ as prophylaxis in women with mild hypertension or mild preeclampsia.

CONCLUSION

$MgSO_4$ therapy for prophylaxis of eclamptic seizures exemplifies current obstetric care in the United States for women with preeclampsia and eclampsia, respectively. As reviewed earlier, $MgSO_4$ therapy for eclampsia appears to be well supported by level I evidence.[32] There appears to be strong support (level I, II-1, II-2 evidence)[32] for seizure prophylaxis with $MgSO_4$ and antihypertensive and cerebrovasodilator agents for women with severe preeclampsia when the data of Coetzee and colleagues[17] and Belfort and coworkers[16] are examined collectively. However, there is limited evidence to support routine seizure prophylaxis in women with mild gestational hypertension or preeclampsia.[1]

Although $MgSO_4$ for seizure prophylaxis is deemed advantageous, its potential for diminishing the morbidity associated with eclampsia is limited. Up to 40% of all eclamptic seizures occur before birth (before hospitalization) prior to women receiving recent medical attention.[33, 34] In addition, up to 49.2% of seizures occur at a gestational age less than 36 weeks, when the greatest fetal morbidity and mortality occurs.[33, 34] An additional 16% of eclamptic seizures occur more than 48 hours post partum.[35]

Therefore, $MgSO_4$ therapy for seizure prophylaxis can be expected to have a potential effect on reduction of seizures that occur only during delivery and within 12 to 24 hours after delivery. This represents only about 45% to 50% of all eclamptic seizures. Moreover, intensive maternal and fetal surveillance accompanies intrapartum therapy and thus decreases potential untoward effects from seizures.

The obstetric use of $MgSO_4$ in the early part of the 20th century appears to have been a serendipitous discovery that we are only now beginning to comprehend. In the 1990s, it was used to ameliorate endothelial cell dysfunction and to decrease platelet adhesiveness, presumed to be partially responsible for the pathophysiology of preeclampsia.[36, 37] Through further understanding of the pathophysiology of preeclampsia and role of $MgSO_4$ therapy, we may be able to improve on our current therapy.

Until the efficacy of $MgSO_4$ is properly evaluated in a research trial with sufficient statistical power, its judicious use should be retained in the management strategy of women with hypertensive disorders of pregnancy. *Continued close intrapartum and postpartum surveillance is crucial for optimal maternal and perinatal outcome.*

Irrespective of MgSO$_4$ therapy, progression from mild to severe disease cannot be predicted without close maternal surveillance. Although the duration of postpartum MgSO$_4$ seizure prophylaxis has never been studied in a clinical trial, the current opinion is that MgSO$_4$ therapy should be continued for up to 12 to 24 hours post partum, depending on the severity of the disease. A presumptive diagnosis of eclampsia not responsive to MgSO$_4$ therapy should raise the suspicion of an underlying central nervous system lesion, and neuroimaging studies should be performed promptly.[38]

References

1. Lucas MJ, Leveno KJ, Cunningham FG. A comparison of magnesium sulfate with phenytoin for the prevention of eclampsia. N Engl J Med 1995; 333:201–205.
2. Which anticonvulsant for women with eclampsia? Evidence from the Collaborative Eclampsia Trial. Lancet 1995;345:1455–1463.
3. Belfort MA, Saade GR, Moise KJ, et al. Nimodipine in the management of preeclampsia: Maternal and fetal effects. Am J Obstet Gynecol 1994;171:417–424.
4. Moodley J, Moodley VV. Prophylactic anticonvulsant therapy in hypertensive crises of pregnancy: The need for a large randomized trial. Hypertens Pregn 1994;13:245–252.
5. Alton BH, Lincoln GC. The control of eclampsia convulsions by intraspinal injections of magnesium sulphate. Am J Obstet Gynecol 1925;9:167–177.
6. Lazard EM. A preliminary report on the intravenous use of magnesium sulphate in puerperal eclampsia. Am J Obstet Gynecol 1925;9:178–188.
7. Pritchard JA. The use of the magnesium ion in the management of eclamptogenic toxemias. Surg Gynecol Obstet 1955;100:131–140.
8. Zuspan FP. Treatment of severe preeclampsia and eclampsia. Clin Obstet Gynecol 1966;9:954–972.
9. Sibai BM, Lipshitz J, Anderson GD, Dilts PV. Reassessment of intravenous MgSO$_4$ therapy in preeclampsia-eclampsia. Obstet Gynecol 1981;57:199–202.
10. Sibai BM. Magnesium sulfate is the ideal anticonvulsant in preeclampsia-eclampsia. Am J Obstet Gynecol 1990;162:1141–1145.
11. Appleton MP, Kuehl TJ, Raebel MA, et al. Magnesium sulfate versus phenytoin for seizure prophylaxis in pregnancy-induced hypertension. Am J Obstet Gynecol 1991;165:907–913.
12. Friedman SA, Lim KH, Baker CA, Repke JT. Phenytoin versus magnesium sulfate in preeclampsia: A pilot study. Am J Perinatol 1993;10:233–238.
13. Atkinson MW, Guinn D, Owen J, Hauth JC. Does magnesium sulfate affect the length of labor induction in women with pregnancy-associated hypertension? Am J Obstet Gynecol 1995;173:1219–1222.
14. Witlin AG, Friedman SA, Sibai BM. The effect of magnesium sulfate therapy on the duration of labor

15. Chen F, Chang S, Chu K. Expectant management in severe preeclampsia: Does magnesium sulfate prevent the development of eclampsia? Acta Obstet Gynecol Scand 1995;74:181–185.
16. Belfort M, Anthony J, Saade G, and the Nimodipine Study Group. Interim report of the nimodipine vs. magnesium sulfate for seizure prophylaxis in severe preeclampsia study: An international, randomized, controlled trial. Am J Obstet Gynecol 1998;178:S3.
17. Coetzee EJ, Dommisse J, Anthony J. A randomized controlled trial of intravenous magnesium sulphate versus placebo in the management of women with severe pre-eclampsia. Br J Obstet Gynaecol 1998;105:300–303.
18. Pritchard JA, Pritchard SA. Standardized treatment of 154 consecutive cases of eclampsia. Am J Obstet Gynecol 1975;123:543–552.
19. Gedekoh RH, Hayashi TT, MacDonald HMM. Eclampsia at Magee-Women's Hospital 1970 to 1980. Am J Obstet Gynecol 1981;140:860–866.
20. Pritchard JA, Cunningham FG, Pritchard SA. The Parkland Memorial Hospital protocol for treatment of eclampsia: Evaluation of 245 cases. Am J Obstet Gynecol 1984;148:951–963.
21. Dunn R, Lee W, Cotton DB. Evaluation of computerized axial tomography of eclamptic women with seizures refractory to magnesium sulfate therapy. Am J Obstet Gynecol 1986;155:267–268.
22. Sibai BM, Ramanathan J. The case for magnesium sulfate in preeclampsia-eclampsia. Int J Obstet Anesth 1992;1:167–175.
23. Dommisse J. Phenytoin sodium and magnesium sulphate in the management of eclampsia. Br J Obstet Gynaecol 1990;97:104–109.
24. Crowther C. Magnesium sulphate versus diazepam in the management of eclampsia: A randomized controlled trial. Br J Obstet Gynaecol 1990;97:110–117.
25. Bhalla AK, Dhall GI, Dhall K. A safer and more effective treatment regimen for eclampsia. Aust N Z J Obstet Gynecol 1994;34:144–148.
26. Friedman SA, Schiff E, Kao L, Sibai BM. Phenytoin versus magnesium sulfate in patients with eclampsia: Preliminary results from a randomized. Abstract 452. Poster presented at 15th Annual Meeting of the Society of Perinatal Obstetricians, Atlanta, January 23–28, 1995. Am J Obstet Gynecol 1995;175(1 pt 2):384.
27. Burrows RF, Burrows EA. The feasibility of a control population for a randomized control trial of seizure prophylaxis in the hypertensive disorders of pregnancy. Am J Obstet Gynecol 1995;173:929–935.
28. Odendaal HJ, Hall DR. Is magnesium sulfate prophylaxis really necessary in patients with severe preeclampsia? J Mat Fet Inv 1996;6:14–18.
29. Chua S, Redman CWG. Are prophylactic anticonvulsants required in severe pre-eclampsia? Lancet 1991;337:250–251.
30. Walker JJ. Hypertensive drugs in pregnancy. Hypertens Pregn 1991;18:845–872.
30a. Nelson TR. A clinical study of preeclampsia: II. Obstet Gynaecol Br Empire 1955;62:58–66.
31. Olah KS, Redman CWG, Gee H. Management of severe, early pre-eclampsia: Is conservative man-

agement justified? Eur J Obstet Gynecol Reprod Biol 1993;51:175–180.

32. Fisher M (ed). Guide to Clinical Preventive Services: An Assessment of the Effectiveness of 169 Interventions: Report of the U.S. Preventive Services Task Force. Baltimore: Williams & Wilkins, 1989, pp 388–389.

33. Douglas KA, Redman CWG. Eclampsia in the United Kingdom. BMJ 1994;309:1395–1400.

34. Sibai BM. Eclampsia. VI. Maternal-perinatal outcome in 254 consecutive cases. Am J Obstet Gynecol 1990;163:1049–1055.

35. Lubarsky SL, Barton JR, Friedman SA, et al. Late postpartum eclampsia revisited. Obstet Gynecol 1994;83:502–505.

36. Ravn HB, Vissinger H, Kristensen SD, et al. Magnesium inhibits platelet activity: An infusion study in healthy volunteers. Thromb Haemost 1996; 75:939–944.

37. Gawaz M, Ott I, Reininger AJ, Neumann FJ. Effects of magnesium on platelet aggregation and adhesion. Thromb Haemost 1994;72:912–918.

38. Witlin AG, Friedman SA, Egerman RE, et al. Cerebrovascular disorders complicating pregnancy: Beyond eclampsia. Am J Obstet Gynecol 1997; 176:1139–1148.

14 PRECONCEPTION COUNSELING for WOMEN with a HISTORY of HYPERTENSIVE DISORDERS

Robert S. Egerman and Baha M. Sibai

Periodically, obstetricians face questions from women (or from their family members) regarding expectations of future pregnancy outcomes after a hypertensive disorder has complicated an antecedent pregnancy. This chapter reviews the salient features of counseling women with a history of chronic hypertension or a history of preeclampsia and its variants. This format intends to give the clinician a concise, accessible source of information for appropriate patient counseling.

CHRONIC HYPERTENSION AND PREGNANCY

Mild Hypertension

Chronic hypertension complicates 1% to 3% of pregnancies. As in the nonpregnant state, most cases of diagnosed chronic hypertension are *primary*, or essential, hypertension. (An attempt should be made to confirm the absence of *secondary* causes, particularly in a young woman.) Additionally, patients with an underlying anatomic renal abnormality causing urinary reflux and scarring are further predisposed to preeclampsia.[1]

Regarding pregnancy outcome in patients with mild chronic hypertension, as defined by diastolic blood pressure 90 to 110 mmHg, Sibai and colleagues monitored 211 patients in whom antihypertensive medication was discontinued (Table 14–1).[2] By the second trimester, half of the patients experienced a decrease in mean arterial pressure (MAP),

one third experienced no change, and the remainder experienced an increase.[2] A severe exacerbation in the degree of hypertension was seen during the third trimester in 4% of those patients whose blood pressure initially decreased, in 16% of those women whose blood pressure remained unchanged, and in 32% of those whose blood pressure worsened. This study demonstrated that most gravid women with mild hypertension do not need medication, inasmuch as only 13% of women in this series required treatment later in the pregnancy.

Superimposed preeclampsia occurred in 10% of pregnancies. The likelihood of development of preeclampsia in a patient with mild chronic hypertension did not differ from that of the general obstetric population. Of the group without superimposed preeclampsia, no differences were seen between the hypertensive group and the control group regarding small-for-gestational-age (SGA) infants (defined as below the 10th percentile), prematurity, or abruptio placen-

TABLE 14–1. COURSE OF MILD CHRONIC HYPERTENSION IN PREGNANCY

	WORSE (%)	NO CHANGE (%)	BETTER (%)
Blood pressure course in mild chronic hypertension	17	34	49
Development of severe hypertension in subgroup above	32	16	4

229

tae. With antenatal testing, perinatal mortality approached that of the general population in Sibai's series.[2]

In contrast, from a study by McCowan and associates[3] (in which SGA was defined as below the 5th percentile) in 155 women whose pregnancies were complicated by pure chronic hypertension without superimposed preeclampsia, more than twice as many hypertensive women delivered SGA infants (10.9%) compared with control subjects (4.1%). McCowan's group used a lower blood pressure threshold for initiating antihypertensive therapy; 30% of women with chronic hypertension without superimposed preeclampsia were treated with various agents. Perinatal loss and prematurity were not affected by chronic hypertension.[3]

Barton and colleagues[4] studied the effect of maternal age as a confounding factor regarding perinatal outcomes in pregnancies complicated by mild chronic hypertension. No significant differences were apparent in the 20- to 30-year-old group compared with patients 35 years of age and older in terms of gestational age at delivery or birth weight. The authors reported an increase in stillborn infants among the older gravidas, 5/379 versus 0/379, $P = .063$. Furthermore, the presence of proteinuria, defined as greater than 1+ on urine dipstick, was associated with earlier gestational age and lower birth weights at delivery.

Sibai and coworkers[5] reviewed perinatal risk factors in women with chronic hypertension enrolled in a multicenter trial of aspirin for the prevention of preeclampsia. Preeclampsia developed in 25% of 763 gravidas. The presence of proteinuria in early pregnancy did not affect the frequency of preeclampsia; however, proteinuria was associated with delivery at less than 35 weeks' gestation (36% versus 16%), as well as SGA (23% versus 10%). Women who had had hypertension for 4 or more years and those who had experienced preeclampsia during an antecedent pregnancy had a greater likelihood of preeclampsia than subjects without these risk factors (31% versus 22% and 32% versus 23%, respectively).

Furthermore, from the same study, the overall frequency of abruptio placentae was 1.5% among women with chronic hypertension. This frequency was not affected by maternal age, duration of chronic hypertension, level of diastolic blood pressure, or presence of proteinuria at baseline examination. In patients in whom superimposed preeclampsia developed, the frequency of abruptio placentae increased to 3% compared with 1% in those without this process ($P = .04$).

In conclusion, patients with mild chronic hypertension in whom superimposed preeclampsia does not develop and who are given appropriate maternal and fetal surveillance typically have favorable pregnancy outcomes. Development of severe hypertension or superimposed preeclampsia portends greater complications for the mother as well as the fetus.

Severe Hypertension

Treatment of severe chronic hypertension is necessary to prevent cardiovascular, cerebrovascular, renal, and retinal end-organ injury. With diastolic blood pressure at or above 110 mmHg, pregnant women are at increased risk for development of superimposed preeclampsia and preterm delivery.

Sibai and Anderson[6] reported that in 44 women with severe hypertension during the first trimester, the uncorrected perinatal mortality was as high as 25%. This occurred despite treatment to keep systolic pressures below 160 mmHg and diastolic pressures below 110 mmHg. The majority of infants were delivered before 37 weeks' gestation. Furthermore, in that series 19/44 (43%) experienced transient renal deterioration and 23/44 (52%) experienced superimposed preeclampsia. When pregnancies affected by preeclampsia were compared with pregnancies not affected, perinatal outcomes—including mean gestational age at delivery (28.6 versus 36.5 weeks), birth weight (827 versus 2632 g), growth restriction (78% versus 5%), and perinatal mortality (48% versus 0%)—were worse in the group with preeclampsia.

An increase in abruptio placentae is noted in pregnancies complicated by hypertensive disease. This increase ranges between 0.5% and 10% and leads to significant perinatal morbidity. It is interesting that medical treatment of the chronic hypertension does not alter the frequency of abruptio placentae, superimposed preeclampsia, or preterm delivery.[7]

LARGE BODY MASS INDEX

The association between obesity and pregnancy-induced hypertension is apparent.[8]

Additionally, excessive weight is a risk factor for numerous other cardiovascular and metabolic disturbances.

In an analysis of 4314 healthy nulliparous women participating in the Calcium for Preeclampsia Prevention study (CPEP), higher body mass indices (BMIs) correlated with the development of preeclampsia (Table 14–2).[9] The odds ratio was adjusted for confounding factors, including systolic and diastolic blood pressure, ethnicity, smoking, and maternal age. Furthermore, a weight gain of 2 pounds per week or greater was associated with an increased risk of preeclampsia regardless of whether the weight gain began in the second or third trimester.

DIABETES AND PREGNANCY

As anticipated, pregestational diabetes is a significant risk factor for preeclampsia. Hanson and Persson found a fourfold increase in the frequency of preeclampsia among Swedish women with type 1 diabetes compared with the background population. Additionally, the poorer the glycemic control (as reflected by glycosylated hemoglobin values), the greater the frequency of preeclampsia.[10]

In a study from Denmark involving women with type 1 diabetes, the presence of microalbuminuria (urinary excretion, 30–300 mg/24 h) was associated with a greater risk of preeclampsia (60%) than in patients with normal albumin excretion (4%).[11] This study also demonstrated that the longer the duration of diabetes, the greater the risk for preeclampsia.

For patients without a history of pregestational diabetes, higher values on the 1-hour glucose screen indicate an increased risk for preeclampsia.[12] Interestingly, these investigators found that after adjustment for BMI, race, and hypertensive disorder, patients with gestational diabetes did not show a statistically significant increase in risk for preeclampsia. It was concluded that insulin resistance may play a role in the pathogenesis of preeclampsia.

PREECLAMPSIA

Overview of Risk

Recurrence of preeclampsia depends on a number of risk factors, including (1) development of underlying medical processes, (2) body habitus, (3) smoking, (4) psychosocial strain, and (5) current partner.[13] Trupin and associates[14] studied a cohort in California of several thousand women. The overall frequency of preeclampsia among nulliparous patients, multiparous patients with a new partner, and multiparous patients with the same partner was 3.2%, 3%, and 1.9%, respectively.

In a study from a large Norwegian database, Lie and coworkers[15] found the overall risk of preeclampsia in their population to be 3% during the first pregnancy and 1.7% during the second pregnancy if the woman had the same partner and 1.9% if the partner for the subsequent pregnancy was different. As expected, if a woman has had a history of preeclampsia, she is at higher risk for preeclampsia during future pregnancies.

Lie and coworkers reported that the relative risk of preeclampsia in the second pregnancy was increased to 11.8 (confidence interval [CI] 11.1–12.6) if the mother had a history of preeclampsia during the antecedent pregnancy and if her partner was the same; the risk increased to 8.2 (CI 5.9–11.3) if the mother's partner was different. Also, if the father in a previous preeclamptic pregnancy changed partners, the new partner had a heightened risk of preeclampsia as well, with a relative risk of 1.8 (CI 1.2–2.6). The genetics of preeclampsia remain elusive and complex.

A second-trimester blood pressure measurement is an important tool for risk assessment for preeclampsia. In a large cohort from the National Institute of Child Health and Development Network of Maternal-Fetal Medicine Units, increased mean arterial blood pressure correlated with a greater risk for preeclampsia in women with diabetes, hypertension, multiple gestations, or a history of preeclampsia.[16]

TABLE 14–2. BODY MASS INDICES FOR PREECLAMPSIA

BMI (kg/m²)	ADJUSTED ODDS RATIO	95% CONFIDENCE INTERVAL
26 to <35	2.21	1.30–3.75
>35	3.38	1.79–5.81

BMI, body mass index.

Finally, in determining risk factors for preeclampsia in healthy nulliparous women, Sibai and associates[17] prospectively monitored 2947 subjects. Preeclampsia developed in 5.3% of patients. Four characteristics were identified as predictors of preeclampsia:

- Systolic blood pressure
- Obesity
- Previous abortions or miscarriages
- Smoking

Both smoking and previous pregnancy losses (<20 weeks' gestation) provided some protection in this population.

Mild and Severe Disease

In a large series from Sibai and coworkers,[18] 406 women with a history of preeclampsia-eclampsia were monitored through subsequent pregnancies and compared with 409 normotensive subjects. In the normotensive group, the frequency of mild preeclampsia, severe preeclampsia, and eclampsia during the second pregnancy was 2.4%, 4.6%, and 0.6%, respectively. These percentages were similar for subsequent pregnancies. The preeclampsia-eclampsia group, in contrast, experienced recurrences of mild preeclampsia, severe preeclampsia, and eclampsia at frequencies of 19.5%, 25.9%, and 1.4%, respectively, during the second pregnancy, and of 6.8%, 12.2%, and 1.7%, respectively, for subsequent pregnancies.

The long-term risks of preeclampsia were noted from this series. Chronic hypertension developed in 24% of the women from the preeclamptic group who experienced hypertension during the second pregnancy and developed in only 6% in women who remained normotensive during the second pregnancy. Onset of preeclampsia before 31 weeks' gestation portends a greater likelihood of future hypertension.

Regarding recurrence of complications from severe preeclampsia, renal failure and hepatic rupture are discussed next. Recurrent pulmonary edema has been reported, but the risk for recurrence is unknown.[19]

Early Severe Preeclampsia

The frequency of severe preeclampsia recurrence depends on the trimester in which disease occurred during the index pregnancy. In a study of 125 women who presented with severe preeclampsia during the second trimester, 108 patients had 169 additional pregnancies.[20] Recurrence of preeclampsia occurred in 110/169 (65%) of pregnancies. Of those pregnancies complicated by preeclampsia, approximately one third occurred at or before 27 weeks' gestation, another third at 28 to 36 weeks' gestation, and the final third at 37 to 40 weeks' gestation. The patients with recurrent second-trimester preeclampsia were those in whom chronic hypertension was more likely either to already exist or to develop than their counterparts who experienced preeclampsia later in pregnancy.

HELLP Syndrome

Sibai and colleagues[21] studied 341 cases of HELLP (hemolysis, elevated liver enzymes, low platelets) syndrome post partum; 14% had preexisting chronic hypertension; the remainder were normotensive. Monitored for at least 2 years, 139 normotensive and 13 hypertensive women became pregnant. Of the normotensive patients, monitored through 192 subsequent pregnancies, 65% remained normotensive during the pregnancy, 25% experienced preeclampsia, and 10% experienced gestational hypertension. HELLP syndrome recurred in only 4% in the subsequent pregnancy. Preterm delivery occurred in 21%. In the patients with preexisting hypertension, 20 subsequent pregnancies were monitored, with 69% experiencing preeclampsia with a recurrence of HELLP syndrome in 8% and preterm delivery in 80%.

In another series by Sullivan and associates,[22] 64 patients with a history of class 1 or 2 HELLP syndrome (platelet count < 100,000/mL) were studied through 81 subsequent pregnancies. Chronic hypertension complicated 9% of these subsequent pregnancies. HELLP syndrome recurred in 18% of patients. From this study, the greater the severity of HELLP syndrome in the index pregnancy, the more severe the recurrence.

Acute renal failure develops in 7.4% of patients with HELLP syndrome.[23] In Sibai and Ramadan's series of 32 patients, six had preexisting chronic hypertension and 26 became preeclamptic.[23] The majority of patients experienced acute tubular necrosis. Three deaths occurred in the "pure preeclampsia" group and one in the chronic hypertension group. Of the surviving 23 patients with HELLP syndrome from the "pure preeclampsia" group, all had normal renal function at follow-up at 4 years; of the five survivors with preexisting hypertension, two had persistent failure requiring chronic dialysis, one was left with impaired renal function, and two had normal, functioning kidneys. Therefore, chronic hypertension when coupled with HELLP syndrome may contribute to significant renal dysfunction. Additionally, during pregnancy the antiphospholipid antibody syndrome can resemble HELLP syndrome and cause renal failure.[24] Recurrence rate in this setting is addressed later in the chapter.

Few data exist regarding recurrence of liver hemorrhage; however, recurrence has been reported with preeclampsia and careful monitoring is warranted.[25]

Eclampsia

Chesley and coworkers[26] monitored 270 women who survived an eclamptic pregnancy between 1931 and 1951. Chronic hypertension occurred with higher than anticipated frequency in multiparous, but not nulliparous, patients following an eclamptic pregnancy. The increased remote mortality found in the multiparous group was attributed to hypertension.

More recently, pregnancy outcome after eclampsia (Table 14–3) was studied by Sibai and colleagues[27] in 23 multiparous and 159 nulliparous patients, with 25 and 254 subsequent pregnancies, respectively. Twenty-two per cent of subsequent pregnancies were complicated by preeclampsia, 1.9% by eclampsia, 2.5% by abruptio placentae, and 2.7% by perinatal death. In the nulliparous group, 75% remained normotensive; of the remainder, 13% experienced mild preeclampsia and 9% experienced severe preeclampsia. Eclampsia recurred in 2.1%. Of the multiparous patients, preeclampsia recurred in 22%; in 75% of these cases the preeclampsia was mild, and there were no recurrences of eclampsia in this group.

The gestational age at which eclampsia occurred in the index pregnancy of nulliparae has an effect on subsequent pregnancy. From the same series, nulliparous patients who had eclampsia at or before 30 weeks' gestation had a 44% chance of recurrence of preeclampsia and 1.8% chance for eclampsia. Had the index eclamptic event occurred between 31 and 36 weeks' gestation or between 37 and 41 weeks' gestation, the risk of recurrent preeclampsia fell to 34% and 10%, respectively. It is notable that the risk of recurrent eclampsia was not altered by

---

TABLE 14–3. PREGNANCIES FOLLOWING ECLAMPSIA IN WOMEN WITHOUT PREEXISTING CHRONIC HYPERTENSION

OUTCOME	NULLIPAROUS WOMEN (n = 159)		MULTIPAROUS WOMEN (n = 23)		TOTAL (n = 182)	
	No.	(%)	No.	(%)	No.	(%)
No. of pregnancies	334		32		366*	
Normotensive pregnancies	254	76	25	78	279	76.2
Preeclampsia-eclampsia	80	24	7	22	87	23.8
Mild	43	12.9	5	15.6	48	13.1
Severe	30	9.0	2	6.3	32	8.8
Eclampsia	7	2.1	0		7	1.9
Preterm (<37 weeks' gestation)	48	14.4	2	6.3	50	13.7
IUGR (<10th percentile)	20	5.9	2	6.3	22	6.0
Abruptio placentae	9	2.7	0		9	2.5
Perinatal deaths	10	3.0	0		10	2.7

IUGR, intrauterine growth restriction.
*There were 370 births (four sets of twins), all in nulliparous women.
From Sibai BM, Sarinoglu C, Mercer BM. Eclampsia: VII. Pregnancy outcome after eclampsia and long-term prognosis. Am J Obstet Gynecol 1992;166:1757–1763.

TABLE 14–4. OUTCOME IN SUBSEQUENT PREGNANCIES IN NULLIPARAE ACCORDING TO GESTATIONAL AGE AT ONSET OF ECLAMPSIA IN INDEX PREGNANCY

| | WEEKS' GESTATION | | | | | | | |
| | ≤30 wk | | 31–36 wk | | 37–41 wk | | | |
	No.	%	No.	%	No.	%	SIGNIFICANCE	ODDS RATIO*
No. of women	26		55		78			
No. of pregnancies	54†		116†		164‡			
Preeclampsia-eclampsia	24	44.4	39	33.6	17	10.4	<0.0001	6.9:1
Mild	9	16.7	25	21.6	9	5.5	<0.01	3.4:1
Severe	14	25	12	10.3	4	2.5	<0.0001	14:1
Eclampsia	1	1.8	2	1.7	4	2.4	N.S.	
Preterm (<37 weeks' gestation)	19	35.2	18	15.5	11	6.7	<0.0001	7.5:1
IUGR	10	18.5	6	5.2	4	2.5	<0.0001	8.4:1
Abruptio placentae	4	7.4	4	3.4	1	0.6	<0.004	13:1
Perinatal deaths	3	5.5	4	3.4	3	1.8	0.15	3.1:1

IUGR, intrauterine growth restriction (<10th percentile); N.S., not significant.
*Comparison of ≤30 versus 37–41 weeks' gestation.
†One set of twins in each group.
‡Two sets of twins = 166 births.
From Sibai BM, Sarinoglu C, Mercer BM. Eclampsia: VII. Pregnancy outcome after eclampsia and long-term prognosis. Am J Obstet Gynecol 1992;166:1757–1763.

the gestational age of the index pregnancy (Table 14–4).

Lopez-Llera[28] reported 24 patients with recurrent eclampsia. From this series, maternal and fetal outcomes were worse among the pregnancies complicated by recurrent eclampsia. Furthermore, having had normal pregnancies after the first episode of eclampsia does not eliminate the risk of recurrent eclampsia.

GESTATIONAL HYPERTENSION

Gestational hypertension is a category of ambiguity. Generally, if hypertension develops after 20 weeks' gestation, the diagnosis is preeclampsia. Occasionally, given no other evidence of preeclampsia, the patient may be exhibiting gestational hypertension. Many of these patients have underlying chronic hypertension or the early development of preeclampsia. If the diagnosis remains gestational hypertension, the outcome of the pregnancy is good without pharmacotherapy.[29]

THROMBOPHILIA

Interest has emerged regarding the association between thrombophilia and pregnancy loss, preeclampsia, and abruptio placentae.

Initially, the focus was directed toward the antiphospholipid antibodies: lupus anticoagulant and anticardiolipin antibodies.

In a series of 43 women with a history of severe preeclampsia prior to 34 weeks' gestation, Branch and associates[30] reported a 16% frequency of antiphospholipid antibodies. No antiphospholipid antibodies were detected in 100 control subjects.

Several reports are disparate regarding this association; however, a meta-analysis by Zhang and associates[8] concluded that women with an antiphospholipid antibody were twice as likely as antibody-negative women to experience pregnancy-induced hypertension. Anticardiolipin antibody was interpreted as positive in this analysis if there were 15 or more units.

Dekker and colleagues[31] studied 101 patients in Amsterdam with severe preeclampsia with onset before 34 weeks' gestation; 39% of patients had chronic hypertension. For the entire group with early-onset preeclampsia, frequencies of protein S deficiency, protein C deficiency, antithrombin III deficiency, and lupus anticoagulant were 24.7%, 1.2%, 1.2%, and 0%, respectively. Activated protein C resistance was present in 16% of subjects, hyperhomocysteinemia in 17.7%, and a positive anticardiolipin antibody (≥15 units) in 15.8%. Unlike the women with chronic hypertension, the normotensive women tended to have higher rates of hemostatic and metabolic abnormalities.

In a larger study from the Amsterdam group, 345 patients with severe preeclampsia were compared with 67 women with uncomplicated pregnancies.[32] The frequency of activated protein C resistance was 11.3% among preeclamptic women compared with 1.5% among the controls. Only half of the preeclamptic subjects had the factor V Leiden mutation. Hyperhomocysteinemia was more common in the study group, as were anticardiolipin antibodies; however, statistical significance was not reached when the criterion for anticardiolipin positivity was 20 units or greater. Higher rates of hemostatic abnormalities were evident in the preeclamptic women who required delivery before 28 weeks' gestation.

Kupferminc and coworkers[33] studied the frequency of genetic thrombophilia in 110 Israeli women with obstetric complications, including severe preeclampsia, fetal growth restriction, abruptio placentae, and stillbirth and compared them with 110 women with uncomplicated pregnancies. Of the study group, 31% had severe preeclampsia. Patients with the factor V Leiden mutation (heterozygous or homozygous) had a relative risk of severe preeclampsia of 5.3 (CI 1.8–15.6). Homozygosity for the methylenetetrahydrofolate reductase mutation and heterozygosity for the prothrombin 20210 mutation carried a relative risk of 2.9 (CI 1.0–8.5) and 2.2 (CI 0.4–13.9), respectively.

Contrarily, De Groot and associates[34] compared the frequency of hereditary coagulation abnormalities in 163 subjects with preeclampsia with a control group. In their series from the Netherlands, similar prevalences were seen among the hypertensive and control subjects for the presence of factor V Leiden, prothrombin 20210A allele, protein C, protein S, and antithrombin III deficiencies. It is uncertain why an unexpectedly high frequency of factor V Leiden (9.2%) was found among the control subjects in this series.

Livingston and colleagues[35] compared the frequency of maternal and fetal gene of factor V Leiden, methylenetetrahydrofolate reductase, and prothrombin 20210 mutation in severe preeclamptic and normotensive pregnancies. Neither maternal nor fetal genetic polymorphisms were associated with the development of preeclampsia, HELLP syndrome, eclampsia, growth restriction, or

abruptio placentae. The findings were similar in African American and Caucasian subsets.

Future studies will likely clarify the inherent risks to a pregnancy from an inherited thrombophilia as well as the appropriate laboratory evaluation for women with a history of severe preeclampsia or other obstetric complications.

References

1. Bukowski TP, Betrus GG, Aquilina JW, Perlmutter AD. Urinary tract infections and pregnancy in women who underwent antireflux surgery in childhood. J Urol 1998;159:1286–1289.
2. Sibai BM, Abdella TN, Anderson GD. Pregnancy outcome in 211 patients with mild chronic hypertension. Obstet Gynecol 1983;61:571–576.
3. McCowan LME, Buist RG, North RA, Gamble G. Perinatal morbidity in chronic hypertension. Br J Obstet Gynaecol 1996;103:123–129.
4. Barton JR, Bergauer NK, Jacques DI, et al. Does advanced maternal age affect pregnancy outcome in women with mild hypertension remote from term? Am J Obstet Gynaecol 1997;176:1236–1243.
5. Sibai BM, Lindheimer M, Hauth J, et al. Risk factors for preeclampsia, abruptio placentae and adverse neonatal outcomes among women with chronic hypertension. N Engl J Med 1998;339:667–671.
6. Sibai BM, Anderson GD. Pregnancy outcome of intensive therapy in severe hypertension in first trimester. Obstet Gynecol 1986;67:517–522.
7. Sibai BM, Mabie WC, Shamsa F, et al. A comparison of no medication versus methyldopa or labetalol in chronic hypertension during pregnancy. Am J Obstet Gynecol 1990;162:960–967.
8. Zhang J, Zeisler J, Hatch MC, Berkowitz G. Epidemiology of pregnancy-induced hypertension. Epidemiol Rev 1997;19:218–232.
9. Sibai BM, Ewell M, Levine RJ, et al. Risk factors associated with preeclampsia in healthy nulliparous women. The Calcium for Preeclampsia Prevention (CPEP) Study Group. Am J Obstet Gynecol 1997;177:1003–1010.
10. Hanson U, Persson B. Epidemiology of pregnancy-induced hypertension and preeclampsia in type 1 (insulin-dependent) diabetic pregnancies in Sweden. Acta Obstet Gynecol Scand 1998;77:620–624.
11. Ekbom P and the Copenhagen Pre-eclampsia in Diabetic Pregnancy Study Group. Pre-pregnancy microalbuminuria predicts pre-eclampsia in insulin-dependent diabetes mellitus. Lancet 1999; 353:377.
12. Joffe GM, Esterlitz JR, Levine RJ, et al. The relationship between abnormal glucose tolerance and hypertensive disorders of pregnancy in healthy nulliparous women. Am J Obstet Gynecol 1998; 179:1032–1037.
13. Dekker GA. Risk factors for preeclampsia. Clin Obstet Gynecol 1999;42:422–435.
14. Trupin LS, Simon LP, Kenazi B. Change in paternity: A risk factor for preeclampsia in multiparas. Epidemiology 1996;7:240–244.
15. Lie RT, Rasmussen S, Brunborg H, et al. Fetal and

maternal contributions to risk of pre-eclampsia: Population based study. BMJ 1998;316:1343–1347.

16. Caritis S, Sibai B, Hauth J, et al. Predictors of preeclampsia in women at high risk. Am J Obstet Gynecol 1998;179:946–951.

17. Sibai BM, Gordon T, Thom E, et al. Risk factors for preeclampsia in healthy nulliparous women: A prospective multicenter study. Am J Obstet Gynecol 1995;172(2 pt 1):642–648.

18. Sibai BM, El-Nazer A, Gonzalez-Ruiz A. Severe preeclampsia-eclampsia in young primigravid women: Subsequent pregnancy outcome and remote prognosis. Am J Obstet Gynecol 1986; 155:1011–1016.

19. Gottlieb JE, Darby MJ, Gee MH, Fish JE. Recurrent noncardiac pulmonary edema accompanying pregnancy-induced hypertension. Chest 1991;100: 1730–1732.

20. Sibai BM, Mercer B, Sarinoglu C. Preeclampsia in the second trimester: Recurrence risk of long-term prognosis. Am J Obstet Gynecol 1991;165(5 pt 1):1408–1412.

21. Sibai BM, Ramadan MK, Chari RS, Friedman SA. Pregnancies complicated by HELLP syndrome (hemolysis, elevated liver enzymes, and low platelets): Subsequent pregnancy outcome and long-term prognosis. Am J Obstet Gynecol 1995;172(1 pt 1):125–129.

22. Sullivan CA, Magann EF, Perry KG Jr, et al. The recurrence risk of the syndrome of hemolysis, elevated liver enzymes, and low platelets (HELLP) in subsequent gestations. Am J Obstet Gynecol 1994;171:940–943.

23. Sibai BM, Ramadan MK. Acute renal failure in pregnancies complicated by hemolysis, elevated liver enzymes, and low platelets. Am J Obstet Gynecol 1993;168:1682–1690.

24. Kon SP, Kwan JT, Raftery MJ. Reversible renal failure due to the antiphospholipid antibody syndrome, pre-eclampsia and renal thrombotic microangiopathy. Clin Nephrol 1995;44:271–273.

25. Greenstein D, Henderson JM, Boyer TD. Liver hemorrhage: Recurrent episodes during pregnancy complicated by preeclampsia. Gastroenterology 1994;106:1668–1671.

26. Chesley LC, Annitto JE, Cosgrove RA. The remote prognosis of eclamptic women: Sixth periodic report. Am J Obstet Gynecol 1976;124:446–459.

27. Sibai BM, Sarinoglu C, Mercer BM. Eclampsia: VII. Pregnancy outcome after eclampsia and long-term prognosis. Am J Obstet Gynecol 1992;166:1757–1763.

28. Lopez-Llera M. Recurrent eclampsia: Clinical data, morbidity and pathogenic considerations. Eur J Obstet Gynecol Reprod Biol 1993;50:39–45.

29. Sibai BM. Drug therapy: Treatment of hypertension in pregnant women. N Engl J Med 1996;335:257–265.

30. Branch DW, Andres R, Digre KB, et al. The association of antiphospholipid antibodies with severe preeclampsia. Obstet Gynecol 1989;73:541–545.

31. Dekker GA, de Vries JIP, Doelitzsch PM, et al. Underlying disorders associated with severe early-onset preeclampsia. Am J Obstet Gynecol 1995; 173:1042–1048.

32. van Pampus MG, Dekker GA, Wolf H, et al. High prevalence of hemostatic abnormalities in women with a history of severe preeclampsia. Am J Obstet Gynecol 1999;180:1146–1150.

33. Kupferminc MJ, Eldor A, Steinman N, et al. Increased frequency of genetic thrombophilia in women with complications of pregnancy. N Engl J Med 1999;340:9–13.

34. De Groot CJM, Bloemenkamp KWM, Duvekot EJ, et al. Preeclampsia and genetic risk factors for thrombosis: A case-control study. Am J Obstet Gynecol 1999;181:975–980.

35. Livingston JC, Barton JR, Park V, et al. Maternal and fetal genetic thrombophilias are not associated with severe preeclampsia. Am J Obstet Gynecol 2000 (submitted).

15

ACUTE and LONG-TERM MANAGEMENT of HYPERTENSION in NONPREGNANT WOMEN

Phyllis August and Suzanne Oparil

There is no clear-cut dividing line between normal and high blood pressure. Sir George Pickering eloquently emphasized that the relationship between arterial pressure and adverse outcome is quantitative: the higher the blood pressure, the worse the prognosis.[1] However, the realities of clinical practice necessitate an operational definition, which Kaplan has suggested as "that level of blood pressure at which the benefits of action exceed the risks and costs of inaction."[2] Hypertension is thus defined by the Joint National Committee for the Detection and Treatment of Hypertension as a systolic blood pressure of 140 mmHg or greater, a diastolic blood pressure of 90 mmHg or greater, or both.[3]

EPIDEMIOLOGY

Hypertension is a common disorder, with as many as 50 million Americans affected.[4] The prevalence of hypertension increases with age, is greater in African Americans, and is greater in members of lower socioeconomic groups.[5] Hypertension is the most common reason for visits to a physician, accounting for at least 27 million visits per year. Overall, mean arterial pressure is higher in both normotensive and hypertensive men than in women.[6] In all ethnic groups, men tend to have higher mean systolic and diastolic blood pressures than women (by 6–7 mmHg and 3–5 mmHg, respectively), and through middle age the prevalence of hypertension is higher among men than among women (Fig. 15–1).

The National Health and Nutrition Examination Survey (NHANES) found that hypertension is more prevalent among women than among men after age 59 years. Furthermore, the Community Hypertension Evaluation Clinic (CHEC) Program, which screened 1 million Americans between 1973 and 1975, found that mean diastolic pressure was higher in men than in women at all ages, whereas mean systolic pressure was higher in men than in women until age 50 years for blacks and until age 65 years for whites and was higher in women thereafter.[7]

RISKS OF HYPERTENSION

Hypertension is associated with an increase in risk of most forms of cardiovascular disease, particularly in the coronary, cerebrovascular, renal, and peripheral vascular beds. The Framingham Heart Study clearly documented that the risks of coronary heart disease, stroke, and deaths from all causes were two to four times higher in women with definite or treated hypertension compared with their normotensive counterparts; the magnitude of the increase in risk with hypertension was similar in men. However, the rate of death was twice as high in men compared with women. Women with hypertension survive longer than men, which may explain the greater prevalence of hypertension in older women.

Hypertension causes vascular damage by a variety of mechanisms. The classic vascular lesions are:

1. Hyperplastic or proliferative arteriolosclerosis.
2. Hyaline arteriolosclerosis with thickening and hyalinization of the intima and media, resulting in narrowing of vascular lumen.

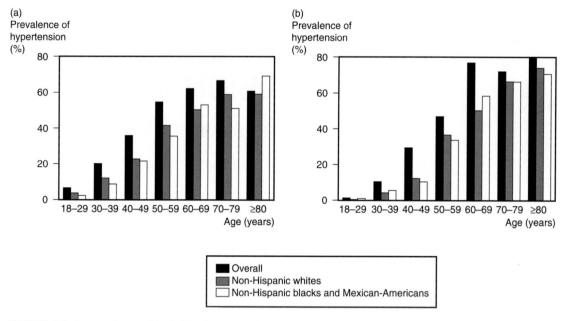

FIGURE 15–1. Prevalence of high blood pressure by age and race/ethnicity for men (a) and women (b) in the United States population aged 18 years or older. (Modified from Burt VI, Whelton P, Rocella EJ, et al. Prevalence of hypertension in the U.S. adult population: Results of the Third National Health and Nutrition Examination Survey, 1988–1991. Hypertension 1995;25:305–313.)

3. Small aneurysms in cerebral penetrating arterioles.

4. Nodular arteriosclerosis or atherosclerosis resulting in plaque formation and thrombi.

5. Exacerbation of congenital defects in blood vessel architecture.

These pathologic processes result in specific dysfunction of the heart, brain, and kidney and circulation.

The relationship of hypertension to stroke is most clearly demonstrated. The most prevalent type of stroke is atheroembolic brain infarction, resulting from atherosclerosis and thrombosis. This type of stroke is three times more common in persons with definite hypertension than in normotensive individuals,[8] and the incidence is similar in women and men. Systolic hypertension is more important than diastolic hypertension in increasing risk for stroke. The benefits of lowering blood pressure have been most dramatically demonstrated with respect to stroke. Reducing elevated blood pressure reduces overall stroke incidence by at least 40%, a phenomenon that has been observed in many clinical trials.

Hypertension is associated with left ventricular hypertrophy (LVH) and congestive heart failure, and the risk of these complications increases with increasing blood pressure.[9] The prevalence of LVH is 10 times higher in individuals with blood pressures of greater than 160/95 mmHg than in normotensive persons. Overall mortality is significantly increased when LVH is present. Antihypertensive therapy can reduce the risk of cardiac failure substantially in hypertensive individuals.

The incidence of coronary heart disease is increased significantly in hypertensive individuals, and the effect is continuous, with higher rates associated with higher blood pressure. The development of atherosclerosis is determined by other modifiable risk factors in addition to blood pressure, including smoking, hypercholesterolemia, and diabetes. This is perhaps why treatment of hypertension has a less dramatic effect on preventing coronary artery disease than on stroke (Fig. 15–2).[10]

Malignant hypertension is an uncommon sequela of poorly controlled, severe hypertension characterized by fibrinoid necrosis of the arterioles of the kidney and the eye, leading to deterioration in renal function and papilledema. This form of accelerated hypertension, which previously was responsible for many cases of end-stage renal dis-

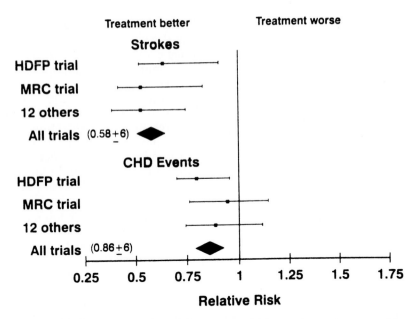

FIGURE 15–2. Estimated relative risk (with confidence intervals) for strokes and coronary heart disease (CHD) events in clinical trials of antihypertensive therapy. HDFP, Hypertension Detection and Follow-up Program; MRC, Medical Research Council. (From Collins R, Peto R, MacMahon S, et al. Blood pressure, stroke and coronary heart disease. Part 2: Short term reductions in blood pressure: Overview of randomized drug trials in their epidemiological context. Lancet 1990;335:827–838.)

ease, is rarely seen in patients receiving adequate antihypertensive treatment.

The degree to which mild to moderate essential hypertension leads to renal dysfunction has been debated. Although pathologic changes in the renal blood vessels are frequently demonstrable in renal tissue from individuals with hypertension, clinically significant renal failure does not develop in most patients with essential hypertension. This is not the case in African Americans, in whom essential hypertension is still a major risk factor for end-stage renal disease. In patients with renal disease resulting from diabetic nephropathy or other forms of glomerulonephritis, hypertension clearly contributes to progressive loss of renal function, and lowering blood pressure has beneficial effects on slowing the progression of disease.[11]

RATIONALE FOR TREATMENT

Many large clinical trials have demonstrated the benefits of lowering blood pressure with respect to prevention of cardiovascular morbidity and mortality. The benefits are most dramatic for severe hypertension and less so for milder disease. Benefits of therapy have

been documented in elderly individuals as well as those with isolated systolic hypertension.[12, 13] Although several large clinical trials demonstrating the benefits of treating hypertension either did not include women or included insufficient numbers to be statistically significant, several points are worth emphasizing.[14]

The Hypertension Detection and Follow-up Program demonstrated a reduction in stroke in all women receiving stepped-care therapy, with the greatest benefits seen in African American women and in older women. Because of the relatively low incidence of death, the Hypertension Detection and Follow-up Program and the Medical Research Council Trial did not demonstrate a decrease in mortality in women in the active or stepped-care treatment groups.

At present, the evidence is insufficient to warrant less aggressive treatment of hypertension in women; African-American women require particularly aggressive treatment. This view is supported by a meta-analysis of the effects of antihypertensive treatment on cardiovascular outcomes in women and men.[15] Antihypertensive treatment clearly reduced the incidence of strokes in women. A reduction in coronary events was not as apparent in women, although the investigators attributed this to the difference in untreated risk in men and women.

DIAGNOSTIC CATEGORIES

Hypertension is classified as either *essential* (primary), or *secondary*. Secondary hypertension (discussed later) is most commonly due to renal disease, renovascular disease, adrenal disease, thyroid dysfunction, or Cushing's syndrome.

Essential Hypertension

When no identifiable cause of hypertension is apparent, a diagnosis of essential hypertension is made. About 95% of hypertensive individuals fall into this category. Abundant evidence suggests that essential hypertension is a heterogeneous disorder, with different pathogenetic features playing a greater or lesser role in individual cases. A detailed discussion of the pathogenesis of essential hypertension is beyond the scope of this chapter; however, several important biochemical, hormonal, metabolic, and genetic abnormalities are summarized here.

Genetic Influence

Although there are now several well-documented monogenic forms of hypertension, such as Liddle's syndrome, glucocorticoid remediable aldosteronism, and apparent mineralocortocoid excess,[16] the consensus is that essential or primary hypertension is a polygenic disorder, which does not follow the classic mendelian rules of inheritance. Thus, the likelihood of identifying one or a few genes that have a major impact on the development of hypertension is small. Nevertheless, it is also likely that within the umbrella of individuals characterized as having essential hypertension, additional forms of monogenic hypertension will be discovered.

Polymorphisms in several genes, including the angiotensinogen gene,[17] α-adducin,[18] and the glucocorticoid receptor,[16] have been linked to the development of hypertension in humans. Although heredity plays a role in pathogenesis, several environmental factors, including obesity, diet, and perhaps stress, contribute to the expression of elevated blood pressure.

Renal Mechanisms

There is abundant evidence that renal mechanisms, either directly or indirectly, play an important role in subpopulations of hypertensive individuals. A variety of renal abnormalities have been proposed, including (1) renal ischemia leading to chronic nonsuppressible renin secretion,[19] (2) decreased renal mass leading to a reduction in nephron number,[20] and (3) decreased glomerular filtration rate (GFR) and reduced sodium excretory capacity.[21] Evidence to support these hypotheses is abundant and is based on epidemiologic, experimental, and clinical studies. A role for renal sodium retention in the pathogenesis of hypertension is supported by the efficacy of diuretic therapy in a majority of hypertensive individuals. Similarly, a role for nonsuppressible renin secretion is supported by the efficacy of agents that interrupt the renin-angiotensin system.

Hormonal Role

The most outstanding examples of a role for hormones in the pathogenesis of hypertension are secondary hypertension due to hyperaldosteronism, Cushing's disease, and renovascular hypertension. The renin-angiotensin system is also important in primary or essential hypertension (see preceding paragraph). This is particularly relevant in individuals with normal or high plasma renin activity in whom renin secretion may be increased by renal ischemia or who have abnormalities in the ability to modulate renin secretion appropriately to changes in sodium intake.[22]

A significant number of hypertensive individuals (~30%) have low or suppressed plasma renin activity, an expected response to volume overload; indeed, low-renin hypertension is often associated with increased sensitivity to salt restriction or diuretic therapy. The mechanism of sodium-volume excess leading to low-renin hypertension is not known. Clearly, renal factors may be important, but it has recently been proposed that some cases of low-renin hypertension may reflect abnormal cortisol or mineralocorticoid metabolism or abnormalities in sodium channel structure akin to the defect observed in *Liddle's syndrome*, a rare form of genetic hypertension characterized by low renin and aldosterone levels.

Sympathetic Nervous System

The role of the sympathetic nervous system in the pathogenesis of primary hypertension is supported by a large body of indirect experimental and clinical observations, including increased heart rate and plasma levels of catecholamines in response to a variety of stimuli in hypertensive individuals and in animals.[23] Dysregulation of baroreceptor sensitivity, leading to decreased inhibition of central mechanisms and increased sympathetic outflow, may also be involved.[24] Furthermore, there are well-established interactions between the sympathetic nervous system and the renin-angiotensin system that may play a role in the pathogenesis of hypertension.[23] Sympathetic nervous system activity and function are difficult to measure accurately in humans, making progress in this area somewhat slower than in other areas of hypertension research.

Vascular Structure and Function

It is beyond the scope of this chapter to review the expanding field of vascular biology and the role of abnormalities of vascular structure and function in the genesis and the maintenance of hypertension. However, several important areas of investigation worth mentioning include (1) vascular hypertrophy and remodeling of blood vessels, (2) alterations in ion transport, (3) signal transduction in vascular smooth muscle and endothelial cells, and (4) functional alterations of endothelial cells, leading to impaired ability to generate vasodilator (e.g., nitric oxide and prostacyclin) and vasoconstrictor substances. Additionally, interactions between nitric oxide, prostacyclin, platelets, and lipids lead to alterations in vascular function that are important in regulating the development of atherosclerotic lesions.

Metabolic Disturbances

The common occurrence of obesity, type 2 diabetes, and hypertension in the same individuals as well as the observation that a significant percentage of nonobese individuals with hypertension have insulin resistance and hyperinsulinemia has led to the concept that insulin resistance is important in the genesis of primary hypertension.[25] Hyperinsulinemia and resistance to the insulin-mediated peripheral utilization of glucose have been reported in hypertensive subjects and may predate the development of overt hypertension. Proposed mechanisms for the hypertensive effects of hyper-

insulinemia include (1) increased renal sodium retention, (2) salt sensitivity, (3) sympathetic nervous system activation, (4) impaired vasodilation, and (5) alterations in transmembrane electrolyte transport.[2]

Dietary Factors

The role of sodium in the pathogenesis of at least some, if not most, cases of primary hypertension has been established.[26] Other dietary components may also contribute to blood pressure elevation. Several studies document the inverse relationship between dietary calcium intake and blood pressure,[27] and increased dietary calcium in the form of both supplements and food sources has lowered blood pressure in experimental models and in human clinical trials.[28, 29] The mechanism by which calcium deficiency contributes to hypertension is unclear but is likely to involve alterations in calcium regulatory hormones (e.g., parathyroid hormone, vitamin D) that have vascular effects, perhaps by their ability to alter levels of intracellular free calcium in vascular smooth muscle.

Some data link hypertension and its vascular complications to a low potassium intake.[30] The importance of dietary potassium as well as calcium is underscored by the Dietary Approaches to Stop Hypertension Study, in which a high-potassium, high-calcium diet led to a significant reduction in blood pressure compared with a control group.[29]

Environment and Behavior

Several environmental factors influence blood pressure, and modification of these factors is an important aspect of treatment. Obesity and excess alcohol intake contribute to hypertension; weight loss, increased physical activity, and decreased alcohol intake are all effective strategies for lowering blood pressure. The roles of specific behavioral patterns, and of emotional stress on the genesis of hypertension have been more difficult to demonstrate. This remains an area of ongoing investigation.

Diagnosis

Appropriate management of hypertension involves (1) establishing the correct diagnosis (essential or secondary), (2) assessing the presence of other cardiovascular risk factors, (3) determining the extent of target organ damage or dysfunction, and, finally, (4) instituting proper therapy. The current classification schema for hypertension in adults is shown in Table 15–1.

The diagnosis of hypertension should not be made on the basis of a single blood pressure measurement. Initial elevated readings should be confirmed on at least two subsequent visits over the course of one to several weeks, depending on the severity of hypertension. Proper technique is essential and includes proper position, appropriate cuff size, and generally at least two readings. Patients should be seated with their arms bared, supported at heart level. The bladder of the cuff should encircle at least 80% of the arm. Equipment should be calibrated, particularly automatic devices. Systolic and diastolic blood pressure should be recorded, with disappearance of sound (phase V) used as the diastolic pressure.

Office blood pressures may not accurately reflect a patient's usual blood pressure (in as many as 25% of patients). These individuals have hypertension only in the doctor's office and are thus said to have "white coat hypertension." If this is suspected, ambulatory blood pressure monitoring may be helpful in documenting normotension outside of the clinic. Other circumstances in which ambulatory blood pressure monitoring may be useful are in the evaluation of resistant hypertension and the evaluation of adverse drug reactions.[31] Home blood pressure monitoring may also be useful for individuals with discrepancies between office and outside blood pressures.

Secondary hypertension should be considered in all new diagnoses of hypertension. Historical features suggestive of secondary hypertension include hypertension at a young age (<25 years of age) or hypertension that first appears at an older age (>60 years of age). Patients with resistant or severe hypertension are more likely to have secondary hypertension, as are those with malignant hypertension. Physical findings suggestive of secondary hypertension include:

- Abdominal bruits (renovascular hypertension)
- Delayed or absent femoral arterial pulses and decreased blood pressure in the lower extremities compared with the upper extremities (coarctation of the aorta)
- Truncal obesity and striae (Cushing's syndrome)
- Tachycardia, orthostatic hypotension, and sweating (pheochromocytoma)

Important aspects of the medical history of a hypertensive patient include:

- Family history of hypertension and other cardiovascular diseases
- Cardiovascular disease symptoms such as chest pain and shortness of breath
- Duration of hypertension
- History of smoking and exercise
- Dietary evaluation, including sodium intake, alcohol, calcium, fruits and vegetables, and fats
- Responses to medications, including side effects
- Use of over-the-counter and illicit drugs (decongestants, nonsteroidal anti-inflammatory drugs, cocaine)

Physical examination should include:

- At least two blood pressure measurements
- Measurement of height and weight
- Funduscopic examination
- Examination for carotid bruits
- Examination of the heart for size, murmurs, and arrhythmias
- Examination of the abdomen for bruits and aortic pulsation

TABLE 15–1. CLASSIFICATION OF BLOOD PRESSURE FOR ADULTS AGE 18 AND OLDER

CATEGORY	SYSTOLIC (mmHg)		DIASTOLIC (mmHg)
Normal	<130	and	<85
High normal	130–139	or	85–89
Hypertension			
Stage 1 (mild)	140–159	or	90–99
Stage 2 (moderate)	160–179	or	100–109
Stage 3 (severe)	≥180	or	≥110

From The Sixth Report of the Joint National Committee on Prevention, Detection, Evaluation, and Treatment of High Blood Pressure. Arch Intern Med 1997;157:2413–2446.

- Examination of the extremities for bruits, decreased pulses, and other signs of peripheral vascular disease (e.g., loss of secondary skin structures)

Routine laboratory examination of the hypertensive patient should include:

- Complete blood count
- Blood glucose
- Electrolytes
- Creatinine
- Uric acid
- Calcium
- Lipid profile
- Urinalysis
- Electrocardiogram

The need for additional laboratory examinations is determined by the presence of suggestive historical, physical, or laboratory features in individual cases. In some patients, additional investigations are necessary to rule out secondary hypertension; in others, the presence of newly diagnosed cardiovas-

cular risk factors, such as diabetes or cardiovascular disease, warrants additional testing. In our practice, in addition to routine laboratory testing, all patients with newly diagnosed hypertension undergo renin-sodium profiling. Plasma renin activity from peripheral venous blood is measured, and ideally the patient brings in a 24-hour urine collection to assess sodium intake. Although this test has been controversial, when measured accurately, the plasma renin activity, indexed with a 24-hour urine sodium excretion, provides helpful information regarding secondary hypertension and is useful in guiding antihypertensive therapy (Fig. 15–3). Very low plasma renin activity suggests primary aldosteronism; a high renin activity value is consistent with renovascular hypertension. Baseline renin levels are also useful in helping one decide whether to use anti–renin system drugs (in patients with medium or high renin levels) such as β-blockers, angiotensin-converting enzyme (ACE) inhibitors or angiotensin II receptor antago-

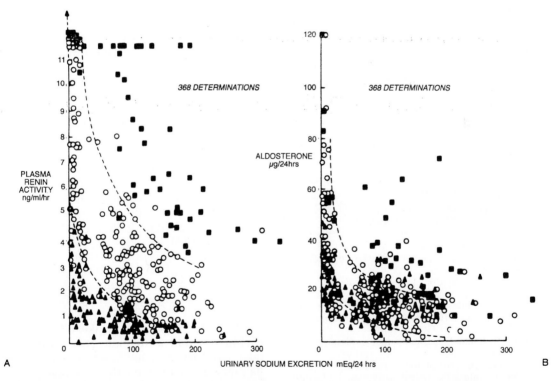

FIGURE 15–3. Relation of the noon ambulatory plasma renin activity *(A)* and of the corresponding daily urinary aldosterone excretion *(B)* to the concurrent daily rate of urinary sodium excretion. The *dashed lines* define the normal range derived from the study of normotensive people. ▲, low-renin essential hypertension; ○, normal-renin essential hypertension; ■, high-renin essential hypertension. Three major subgroups are defined by the appropriateness or normality of the plasma renin activity in relation to the rate of sodium excretion, which is used as an index of dietary intake and of sodium balance. (From Brunner HR, Laragh JH, Baer L, et al. Essential hypertension: Renin and aldosterone, heart attack and stroke. N Engl J Med 1972;286:441–449.)

nists, as opposed to natriuretic agents (for low-renin patients) such as diuretics or calcium channel blockers (see the following discussion).[32]

Treatment

The goal of treatment of hypertension is to prevent morbidity and mortality associated with high blood pressure. Blood pressure should be controlled by the least intrusive means possible.[5] Modifying other cardiovascular risk factors is as important as controlling blood pressure. One of the difficulties in treating hypertension is that most patients have stage 1 or stage 2 hypertension and are asymptomatic. Compliance is not a trivial problem because patients do not feel sick, and antihypertensive medications may cause unpleasant side effects. This has undoubtedly contributed to the sobering statistic that blood pressure is controlled in only 29% of hypertensive individuals to below 140/90 mmHg.[3]

Lifestyle Modification. Lifestyle modification (Table 15–2) is an important aspect of management of all hypertensive patients and may be sufficient to control blood pressure in individuals with stage 1 hypertension. Although lifestyle modifications have not been studied in large clinical trials to the same extent as drug therapy, they are inexpensive and generally safe. The goals of lifestyle modification are to lower blood pressure and to improve cardiovascular risk factors.

TABLE 15–2. LIFESTYLE MODIFICATIONS FOR HYPERTENSION CONTROL AND/OR OVERALL CARDIOVASCULAR RISK

Lose weight if overweight.

Limit alcohol intake to no more than 0.5 ounce of ethanol per day.

Exercise (aerobic) regularly (30–45 min most days of the week).

Reduce sodium intake to less than 100 mmol per day (<2.4 grams of sodium or <6 grams of sodium chloride).

Maintain adequate dietary potassium, calcium, and magnesium intake.

Stop smoking and reduce dietary saturated fat and cholesterol intake for overall cardiovascular health. Reducing fat intake also helps reduce caloric intake—important for control of weight and Type 2 diabetes.

From The Sixth Report of the Joint National Committee on Prevention, Detection, Evaluation, and Treatment of High Blood Pressure. Arch Intern Med 1997;157:2413–2446.

Obesity and hypertension are closely related, and weight loss reduces blood pressure in a large proportion of overweight hypertensive individuals. Obesity is particularly important in women with hypertension, especially African American women. Weight loss results in lower blood pressure relatively quickly, and loss of as little as 10 pounds may be effective. Weight loss also enhances the efficacy of antihypertensive medication and can favorably modify other cardiovascular risk factors, such as hyperglycemia and hypertriglyceridemia. Analysis of results of the Treatment of Mild Hypertension Study (TOMHS) based on gender suggests that women may be less likely than men to have blood pressure controlled with lifestyle interventions alone, perhaps because they are less successful in losing weight.[33] Although the effects of weight reduction on blood pressure have not been studied extensively in women, small clinical trials clearly demonstrate the expected benefits.[34] Thus, all women with hypertension who are above their ideal weight should be prescribed a weight-reduction program.

Regular aerobic physical activity sufficient to achieve a moderate level of fitness is an important adjunct to diet in achieving weight loss and blood pressure control. Sedentary individuals are at greater risk for development of hypertension, and the effectiveness of physical activity in lowering blood pressure has been well documented, although to a lesser extent in women than in men. Given the beneficial effects of exercise on weight control, prevention of osteoporosis, and insulin and glucose metabolism, increased physical activity is recommended for hypertensive women in the absence of unstable coronary disease. Moderately intense physical activity, such as 30 to 45 minutes of brisk walking most days of the week, is the recommended protocol.

Epidemiologic and clinical trials have demonstrated that blood pressure is positively related to sodium intake, although individual responses to changes in sodium intake may vary. African Americans and older patients are more sensitive to changes in sodium intake.[35] Urinary sodium excretion (24 hours) is a reliable index of sodium intake, and blood pressure decreases on average 6.2 mmHg when urinary sodium excretion is 95 mmol/day, in unselected hypertensive patients. Although the advisability of widespread sodium restriction for all hypertensive patients is a controversial subject, avoidance of high-salt foods is recommended. The most recent guidelines of the Joint National Committee for the Prevention, Detection, Evaluation, and Treatment of High Blood Pressure[3] recommend that hypertensive patients should restrict sodium intake to approximately 100 mmol/day or 2.4 g/day, although this may benefit only salt-sensitive hypertensive patients.

High dietary potassium intake appears to protect against development of hypertension[36] and some of its vascular consequences.[37] Thus, a high-potassium diet, preferably from fresh fruits and vegetables, is advisable.

Low dietary calcium intake has also been associated with an increased risk of hypertension,[27] and some studies have demonstrated a blood pressure–lowering effect of dietary calcium supplementation, especially from food sources.[38] This may be particularly important for women, in whom calcium supplementation is beneficial in the prevention of osteoporosis. Although the magnitude of the blood pressure effect of calcium supplementation may be small, given the risks of osteoporosis, it is reasonable to recommend increased calcium intake to hypertensive women.

Excess alcohol consumption of more than 1 to 2 ounces/day is associated with increased blood pressure. Because women absorb more ethanol than men and generally weigh less, it has been recommended that women limit their consumption to 0.5 ounces of ethanol (one drink) per day.[3]

Other lifestyle modifications that have been investigated for a possible beneficial effect on blood pressure include relaxation and biofeedback. Although harmless, these interventions have not been shown to lower blood pressure on a long-term basis.[39]

Lifestyle modifications that are recommended to hypertensive patients to reduce their overall cardiovascular risk, although they do not lower blood pressure directly, include a low-fat diet and avoidance of tobacco. The latter is especially important in young women, who are at greater risk for sustained tobacco use. Smoking has a pressor effect that is apparent for 15 to 30 minutes after each cigarette, as documented with ambulatory blood pressure monitoring.[40]

Pharmacologic Therapy. The decision to institute antihypertensive medication involves consideration of level of blood pressure as well as the presence of target organ damage, other cardiovascular risk factors, and established cardiovascular disease. Clinical trials have demonstrated that lowering blood pressure with medication reduces the incidence of stroke and congestive heart failure. Coronary heart disease is also prevented, although not as dramatically.

The most recent guidelines for treatment are summarized in Table 15–3. Antihypertensive therapy should be instituted at lower levels of blood pressure when there is established cardiovascular disease or when the patient has significant cardiovascular risk factors. Although hypertensive women may experience fewer adverse cardiovascular events compared with men, there is no evidence to support a higher blood pressure threshold for use of antihypertensive medication in women.

Initial Antihypertensive Therapy. The

TABLE 15–3. GUIDELINES FOR TREATMENT OF HYPERTENSION

BLOOD PRESSURE STAGES (mmHg)	LOW RISK*	MEDIUM RISK†	HIGH RISK‡
High normal (130–139/85–89)	Lifestyle modification	Lifestyle modification	Drug therapy§
Stage 1 (140–159/90–99)	Lifestyle modification (up to 12 months)	Lifestyle modification (up to 6 months)	Drug therapy
Stages 2 and 3 (≥160/≥100)	Drug therapy	Drug therapy	Drug therapy

*No risk factors, no target organ disease, no cardiovascular disease (CVD).
†1 risk factor, no target organ disease, no CVD.
‡Target organ disease, diabetes, other risk factors.
§For those with heart failure, renal insufficiency, or diabetes.
From the Sixth Report of the Joint National Committee on Prevention, Detection, Evaluation, and Treatment of High Blood Pressure. Arch Intern Med 1997;157:2413–2446.

selection of antihypertensive therapy is guided by a number of factors, including evidence based on clinical data, biochemical characteristics, demographics, and coexisting medical conditions. Clinical trials have demonstrated reductions in cardiovascular morbidity and mortality with diuretics and β-blockers as antihypertensive treatment. Thus, the Joint National Committee on Prevention, Detection, Evaluation, and Treatment of High Blood Pressure recommends that these agents be considered first-line therapy unless there are compelling indications for specific agents from other classes.[3] For example, patients with diabetes and proteinuria and patients with congestive heart failure would benefit from an ACE inhibitor. Patients with a history of myocardial infarction should receive a β-blocker.

An alternative to instituting therapy is based on the pretreatment renin profile. The premise of this approach is that essential hypertension is a heterogeneous disorder and that individual patients with comparable degrees of blood pressure elevation may differ in their endocrinologic profiles and in their response to drugs. In this framework, hypertensive patients have been classified as follows[41]:

- Those with primarily a vasoconstrictive component, in whom the plasma renin activity is high
- Those with primarily a sodium-volume component, characterized by a low plasma renin activity
- Those with a medium level of renin, in whom both mechanisms are relevant

In addition, measurement of baseline plasma renin levels identifies two important potentially curable forms of secondary hypertension: (1) primary aldosteronism, characterized by suppressed renin, and (2) renovascular hypertension, characterized by stimulated renin.

Drugs that are effective antirenin agents include ACE inhibitors, β-blockers, and angiotensin II receptor antagonists. Drugs that are effective in low-renin or volume hypertension are diuretics, calcium channel blockers, and α-blockers. Assessment of baseline renin status includes measurement of plasma renin activity in a peripheral venous blood sample along with determination of 24-hour urinary sodium excretion in an untreated patient. This approach requires a reliable laboratory determination of renin level.

Some have suggested that a similar approach can be utilized to guide therapy by predicting the renin status based on demographic characteristics. For example, African Americans tend to have lower plasma renin activity and are thus more likely to respond to diuretics or calcium channel blockers as first-line therapy. Younger patients have higher renin levels compared with older adults and respond more favorably to β-blockers or ACE inhibitors. There do not appear to be any drugs that have particular benefits in women, although there may be gender-specific side effect profiles.[33, 42] For example, women are more likely to develop hyponatremia and hypokalemia in response to diuretic therapy, whereas gout is more likely to occur in men. Also, women are more likely than men to experience cough after taking ACE inhibitors, edema after taking dihydropyridine calcium channel blockers, and intolerable hirsutism after taking minoxidil.

Individual Antihypertensive Agents. The available antihypertensive agents fall into the categories of diuretics, β-blockers, α-blockers, combined α/β-blockers, central α agonists, calcium channel blockers, direct vasodilators, ACE inhibitors, and angiotensin II receptor antagonists.

DIURETICS. All diuretics interfere with sodium reabsorption in different segments of the nephron. The most commonly used diuretic agents in the treatment of hypertension are thiazides, which inhibit sodium and chloride co-transport across the luminal membrane of the distal nephron. Although in the early phase of diuretic use plasma volume is decreased, with chronic use plasma volume returns partially toward normal and peripheral vascular resistance decreases.[43] In patients with renal failure, in whom thiazides are less likely to be effective, loop diuretics are indicated. Diuretics are most likely to be effective in patients with low plasma renin activity, in African Americans, and in older people. Diuretics often potentiate the effect of other antihypertensive agents.[44] Side effects are largely metabolic and include hypokalemia, hyperuricemia, hypercalcemia, hyperglycemia, hyponatremia, and hypomagnesemia.

β-ADRENORECEPTOR BLOCKERS. These agents are competitive agonists of the effects of endogenous catecholamines on β adrenoreceptors. They produce a decrease in cardiac output, renin release, and central sympathetic nervous outflow, and a decrease in peripheral vascular resistance.[45, 46] β-Blockers may be lipid-soluble or insoluble, a feature that determines their pharmacology.[2] Lipid-soluble agents (propranolol, metoprolol) are metabolized by the liver, and are relatively short-acting, in contrast to lipid-insoluble agents, such as atenolol and nadolol, which are excreted mainly by the kidneys and have a longer half-life. Lipid-insoluble β-blockers enter the brain less and cause fewer central nervous system side effects. β-Blockers that are cardioselective (atenolol, acebutolol, metoprolol) antagonize only β_1 receptors and are less likely to cause bronchoconstriction and metabolic disturbances. β-Blockers are more effective for younger and middle-aged hypertensive patients and in those with normal or high plasma renin activity. They are cardioprotective and should be used in patients with known coronary disease.

The most common adverse effects of β-blockers include insomnia, depression, impaired adrenergic responses to hypoglycemia, bronchospasm, and decreased exercise performance. These agents are contraindicated in patients with a history of asthma, although in some cases, cardioselective agents can be administered with caution.

COMBINED β- AND α-ADRENERGIC BLOCKERS. Labetalol is a nonselective β-blocker that also has α-blocking properties. The ratio of α- to β-blocking action is between 1:3 and 1:7. Labetalol results in decreased blood pressure, mainly via a fall in systemic vascular resistance, with a minimal effect on cardiac output.[47] Adverse effects include those mentioned in association with β-blockers (as well as symptomatic orthostatic hypotension) and hepatotoxicity, which may be serious and may lead to liver failure.[48]

α-ADRENERGIC BLOCKERS. Currently marketed drugs in this class are prazosin, terazosin, and doxazosin. Selective α_1-blockers are competitive antagonists of postsynaptic α_1-adrenergic receptors. Their action results in dilation of both resistance and capacitance vessels. Because presynaptic α_2-receptors remain open and capable of binding neurotransmitters, norepinephrine release is inhibited because of direct negative feedback mechanism. Thus there is relatively little tachycardia, and both cardiac output

and plasma renin levels remain stable. α-Blockers have similar efficacy in lowering blood pressure to diuretics, β-blockers, and ACE inhibitors.[49] Adverse effects include hypotension, particularly after the first dose; volume retention; headache; drowsiness; fatigue; and weakness.

CALCIUM CHANNEL BLOCKERS. Calcium channel blockers lower blood pressure by interfering with calcium-dependent contractions of vascular smooth muscle. There are currently four classes of calcium channel blockers available for the treatment of hypertension. Verapamil is related to papaverine. Like diltiazem (a benzothiazepine), it has both negative chronotropic effects and vasodilator actions.

Dihydropyridines (e.g., nifedipine, amlodipine, felodipine) are more powerful in relaxing vascular smooth muscle. One calcium antagonist, mibefradil, was the first calcium channel blocker to block the "T" channel; however, it was withdrawn from the market in 1998. Unlike other vasodilators, calcium channel blockers do not cause sodium retention and, in fact, are mildly natriuretic because of their vasodilator action on the renal afferent arteriole.[50]

Adverse effects include headaches, flushing, ankle edema, and constipation. Verapamil may also contribute to atrioventricular block. It is important to be aware of potential drug interactions: Verapamil and diltiazem increase cyclosporine levels.

ANGIOTENSIN-CONVERTING ENZYME INHIBITORS. Examples of ACE inhibitors include captopril, enalapril, lisinopril, fosinopril, and benazepril. These agents inhibit the activity of ACE, which converts angiotensin I, an inactive peptide, to angiotensin II, a potent vasoconstrictor and stimulus of aldosterone secretion. Thus, these agents interfere with both angiotensin II–mediated vasoconstriction and sodium reabsorption mediated by aldosterone. They are very well tolerated and have additional clinical benefits in treatment of congestive heart failure and prevention of the progression of renal disease. They are very effective in patients with high or normal plasma renin levels and may be less effective in those with primarily volume-mediated hypertension. Adverse effects include elevations in plasma potassium, deterioration in renal function in patients with bilateral renal artery stenosis, and hypotension or prerenal azotemia in the setting of significant volume depletion.

These agents cause a dry cough in as many as 20% of patients, more commonly in women.[51]

ANGIOTENSIN II RECEPTOR ANTAGONISTS. These agents interfere with the actions of angiotensin II by blocking the AT 1 receptor. Unlike ACE inhibitors, they do not increase levels of bradykinin, a property that may be responsible for the absence of cough with these agents. They appear to be as effective as ACE inhibitors and may result in fewer side effects.

VASODILATORS. Hydralazine is a direct-acting vasodilator. It relaxes the smooth muscle in the peripheral arterioles and lowers blood pressure. Its use is associated with an increase in sympathetic discharge, resulting in increases in heart rate and cardiac output, and in sodium retention as a result of lowering blood pressure and stimulation of renin. Thus, hydralazine is rarely used alone; it is usually combined with a diuretic and a β-blocker. Adverse effects include reflex tachycardia, headaches, and flushing as well as a lupus-like reaction.

Minoxidil, a more potent direct-acting vasodilator, also induces vascular smooth muscle cell relaxation by modulating potassium channels. It causes significant fluid retention as well as reflex tachycardia and must be used concomitantly with diuretics and β-blockers. Minoxidil may cause significant hirsutism, an especially bothersome side effect for women. Thus it is a drug of last resort in women.

CENTRAL ADRENERGIC INHIBITORS. Methyldopa is an α_2-adrenoreceptor agonist that acts centrally and results in reduced sympathetic outflow and lower blood pressure, reduced baroreceptor responses leading to a decrease in standing blood pressure, suppression of renin secretion, and a decrease in cardiac output. It is primarily used in pregnancy because of its well-documented safety for the fetus. Adverse effects include sedation, postural hypotension, dry mouth, fever, and liver dysfunction.

Clonidine is another centrally acting agent that effectively lowers blood pressure. It is a relatively long acting drug, but it has some troublesome adverse effects such as dry mouth and drowsiness. Moreover, there may be significant rebound hypertension when it is abruptly discontinued.

COMBINATION THERAPY. To enhance compliance and minimize adverse effects of drugs, the goal of pharmacologic treatment of hypertension is to prescribe the fewest number of drugs in the smallest effective dose and lowest frequency.[52] Monotherapy is desirable because it may minimize adverse effects and cost as well as improve compliance. When monotherapy proves ineffective, combination therapy is indicated. A rational strategy for combination therapy is summarized by Mueller and Laragh.[53] If antirenin therapy (e.g., ACE inhibitor, β-blocker, angiotensin II receptor antagonist) fails to normalize blood pressure, a logical addition would be a volume-reducing agent such as a diuretic. Similarly, if diuretics alone are ineffective, anti–renin system drugs should be added. ACE inhibitors and β-blockers may also be combined successfully with calcium channel blockers.[54] However, caution should be used when combining a β-blocker with a calcium channel blocker that slows atrioventricular conduction such as verapamil or diltiazem. α-Blockers may be successfully combined with calcium channel blockers,[55] ACE inhibitors, or β-blockers.[56]

Secondary Hypertension

Secondary hypertension is due to a known cause. The most common causes of secondary hypertension are renal disease, renovascular hypertension, primary aldosteronism, Cushing's syndrome, and pheochromocytoma. Most studies suggest that between 5% and 10% of hypertensive patients have secondary hypertension. Certain forms of secondary hypertension are more common in women, such as renovascular hypertension caused by fibromuscular dysplasia, and hypertension associated with renal involvement in collagen diseases. The most common forms of secondary hypertension are discussed next.

Renal Disease

Renal disease is the most common cause of secondary hypertension. It may be due to congenital abnormalities, glomerulonephritis, diabetes, systemic lupus erythematosus (SLE), or interstitial nephritis. All women with a new diagnosis of hypertension should be screened for intrinsic renal disease with blood tests for renal function and with urinalysis for detection of proteinuria or hematuria. Hypertensive women with a strong family history of renal disease should be screened with ultrasonography for polycystic kidney disease, which is inherited in an autosomal dominant mode and often presents with hypertension in the third and fourth decades.

Blood pressure control is an integral aspect of management of patients with intrinsic renal disease[57] and, in many cases, is the only therapy employed to prevent progressive deterioration of renal function. In this regard, ACE inhibitors may have additional benefits because they can retard progression of disease in diabetic patients as well as in patients with other forms of renal disease.[58, 59]

Renovascular Hypertension

Renovascular hypertension is caused by anatomic lesions of the renal arteries, leading to diminished blood flow to one or both kidneys, with resulting renal ischemia, stimulation of the renin-angiotensin system, and ensuing hypertension. Not all anatomic lesions of the renal artery result in renovascular hypertension because they may not be severe enough to compromise renal blood flow. Thus, anatomic demonstration of a renal arterial lesion (by angiography) does not establish the presence of renovascular hypertension. Cure of hypertension after revascularization is the most reliable proof of renovascular hypertension.

There are many causes of renovascular hypertension. Atherosclerotic renovascular disease is usually seen in postmenopausal women with a history of tobacco use and diffuse vascular disease, whereas fibromuscular dysplasia is more likely to be present in young women. This lesion is a nonatherosclerotic, noninflammatory vascular occlusive disease, most often caused by medial fibroplasia.[60] Fibromuscular dysplasia is seen three times more often in women and is less common in black or Asian populations. The prevalence of fibromuscular dysplasia in the hypertensive population is approximately 1%.[61] Although the renal arteries are most commonly involved, other vessels (e.g., carotids, coronaries, abdominal aorta, peripheral arteries) may also be affected.

Clinical clues suggestive of renovascular hypertension are severe hypertension, which may be resistant to medical therapy, and which first appears in the second, third, or fourth decades of life. Abdominal bruit and a high peripheral venous plasma renin activity are suggestive findings. Although several noninvasive tests (captopril renography), magnetic resonance angiography (MRA) of the renal arteries,[62] and ultrasonography with Doppler examination of the renal arteries are frequently used to screen patients with suspected renovascular hypertension, renal angiography is usually justified in these individuals because this form of hypertension is potentially curable with either angioplasty or surgery. Furthermore, noninvasive testing may not detect smaller branch lesions, which are not unusual in fibromuscular dysplasia.

The classic angiographic appearance is multiple stenoses with intervening aneurysmal outpouchings, causing a "string of beads" image. Occasionally solitary focal stenoses are present. Renal angioplasty is a highly effective method for treating renal artery lesions due to fibromuscular dysplasia, with a high rate of technical success and a greater than 80% rate of cure or improvement.[63] This form of secondary hypertension should be considered in young hypertensive women who are planning to become pregnant because the prognosis during pregnancy is poor, with a high incidence of early severe preeclampsia and a poor pregnancy outcome.

Aldosteronism

Aldosteronism results from autonomous increased secretion of aldosterone from the adrenal cortex as a result of a solitary adrenal adenoma *(Conn's syndrome)* or bilateral adrenal hyperplasia. Some patients may have a variant of the two *(nodular hyperplasia)* in which both adrenal glands are enlarged or more adenomas secrete most of the aldosterone. A rare form of hereditary aldosteronism is glucocorticoid remediable aldosteronism, a result of a chromosomal crossover that produces a chimeric gene that causes aldosterone to be synthesized by the adrenal fasciculata and regulated by adrenocorticotrophic hormone (ACTH).

Primary aldosteronism is not a rare condition and is frequently missed. The classic clinical features are hypertension, hypokalemia, suppressed plasma renin activity, excessive urinary potassium excretion, hypernatremia, and metabolic alkalosis. These clinical features are not uniformly present, and although hypokalemia is a helpful clue when present, as many as 25% of patients with primary aldosteronism are normokalemic.[64]

The diagnosis is made by demonstration of biochemical and hormonal abnormalities, followed by adrenal gland computed tomography (CT) imaging to determine whether there is an adenoma or hyperplasia. If an adenoma is detected on CT scan, radiologic imaging may be followed by adrenal vein sampling to document unilateral aldosterone secretion prior to surgery.

Surgery is indicated for unilateral disease, with a cure rate of about 65% and an improvement in an additional 33%. Medical therapy with spironolactone or amiloride is usually effective for patients with hyperplasia, although high doses may be necessary. Calcium channel blockers have also been reported to be effective.[65]

Pheochromocytoma

Pheochromocytoma is rare but may have fatal consequences if not recognized. Many pheochromocytomas remain undiagnosed during life, as demonstrated by autopsy studies.[66] Pheochromocytomas are tumors that arise from chromaffin cells, which have differentiated from neural crest stem cells and synthesize and store catecholamines. Although most pheochromocytomas are in the adrenal glands, as many as 10% to 15% are extra-adrenal and may be found in association with sympathetic nerves. Most extra-adrenal pheochromocytomas are in the abdomen or pelvis; they rarely arise in the chest or in the neck.

The clinical manifestations of pheochromocytoma, resulting from excess circulating catecholamines or complications of hypertension, may be dramatic. Common symptoms are headache, sweating, palpitations, and anxiety in association with paroxysmal or sustained hypertension.[67] Additional features include hyperglycemia, orthostatic hypotension, and weight loss.

The most reliable screening procedures are 24-hour urinary metanephrine and plasma catecholamine determinations. If biochemical evidence of pheochromocytoma is present, CT scan or magnetic resonance imaging of the adrenal glands should be performed. Specialized nuclear medicine tests utilizing ^{131}I-metaiodobenzylguanidine may be helpful in identifying extraadrenal pheochromocytomas.

Appropriate treatment includes preoperative α-adrenergic blockade, followed by surgical removal of the tumor.

Cushing's Syndrome

This group of disorders refers to syndromes of excess glucocorticoid production caused by ACTH-independent lesions (e.g., tumors of the adrenal gland or primary nodular hyperplasia) or ACTH-dependent lesions (e.g., pituitary disease or ectopic ACTH). Hypertension is a common feature of Cushing's syndrome and may be due to a variety of mechanisms, including mineralocorticoid effects of cortisol, increased mineralocorticoids, increased angiotensinogen, and increased sensitivity to pressors.[2] Additional clinical features may include bruising, edema, hirsutism, red striae, menstrual irregularity, and truncal obesity. Appropriate workup includes determining the mechanism (dexamethasone suppression, plasma ACTH), followed by radiologic imaging of either adrenal glands or pituitary.

Therapy should include antihypertensive drugs as well as definitive treatment of the syndrome (surgery, chemotherapy, radiation, bromocriptine, cyproheptadine, metyrapone).

Other Endocrine Disturbances Associated With Hypertension

Hypertension is associated with hypothyroidism,[68] hyperthyroidism, and hyperparathyroidism.[69]

Oral Contraceptive Hypertension

The most important—and probably the most common—form of secondary hypertension in women is that caused by oral contraceptive use. A review of data accumulated over the last 24 years suggests that most women taking oral contraceptives experience a small but detectable increase in both systolic and diastolic blood pressures.[70] The magnitude of the increase appears to vary, depending on the population studied as well as on the dose of estrogen and progestin in the preparation. The large Walnut Creek Contraceptive Drug Study, based on data from 11,672 women, demonstrated a pressure elevation of 5 to 6 mmHg systolic and 1 to 2 mmHg diastolic in white women and a lesser rise in black women.[71] A study conducted in developing countries reported similar average changes after 1 year of oral contraceptive use.[72] In some centers, however, marked elevations (10 mmHg systolic, 6.9 mmHg diastolic) were reported.

Hypertension has been reported to be two to three times more common in women taking oral contraceptives than in age-matched women not taking these medications.[73] The risk of contraceptive-induced hypertension increases with age, duration of use, and perhaps with increased body mass. Oral contraceptives currently in use contain lower doses of ethinyl estradiol (30–35 μg) than those available previously. There may be a correlation between both estrogen and progestin dose and blood pressure.[70] Thus, the true incidence of oral contraceptive–induced hypertension may be less than that reported by earlier studies. Nevertheless, data obtained from the Nurses' Health Study suggest that even oral contraceptives with lower doses of estrogen increase the risk of hypertension; the risk increases with duration of use and with increased progestin potency.[74]

The mechanism of the increase in blood pressure attributable to oral contraceptives remains unclear. Increases in body weight, plasma volume, exchangeable sodium, plasma insulin, insulin resistance, and hepatic synthesis of angiotensinogen have been reported. Experimental evidence favors a role for the renin-angiotensin system in the hypertension induced by estrogen.[75] In a rat model of oral contraceptive hypertension, administration of estrogen alone (ethinyl estradiol) caused hypertension and an increase in angiotensinogen and angiotensin II levels.[76] The hypertension induced by estrogen responded to ACE inhibitor treatment. Progestin administration alone also increased blood pressure, although the elevation in blood pressure was of lesser magnitude and of shorter duration and was associated with increased sodium retention.

In view of the aforementioned considerations, a prudent approach to oral contraceptive use is to monitor blood pressure at least every 6 months (dispense only 6 months of pills). If blood pressure rises, a decision to discontinue the pill should be based on the degree of hypertension, the potential hazards of pregnancy, and the overall cardiovascular risk profile. Although it is preferable to avoid oral contraceptives in women with elevated blood pressure, this modality of contraception can be considered in selected individuals when the risks of pregnancy appear greater than the risks of mild hypertension as long as blood pressure and overall cardiovascular status are monitored carefully.

HORMONE REPLACEMENT THERAPY

The effects of hormone replacement therapy (HRT) on blood pressure are not as clear-cut as the effects of oral contraceptive pills. Several reports of an association between estrogen therapy in postmenopausal women and hypertension were published in the 1970s and 1980s.[77–80] Until recently, many physicians considered hypertension to be a contraindication to HRT. Measurements of the components of the renin-angiotensin-aldosterone system implicated increased angiotensinogen generation as well as increased sodium retention in the pathogenesis of HRT-induced hypertension.[81] In fact, estrogen preparations (e.g., Premarin [conjugated estrogens], ethinyl estradiol) that have a greater ability to stimulate hepatic synthesis of angiotensinogen can raise blood pressure to a greater extent than those that have a modest effect on angiotensinogen (natural estradiol, transdermal estrogen).[82, 83] The effects of synthetic progestins on blood pressure have not been extensively studied in postmenopausal women. However, preliminary evidence suggests that they may contribute to increases in blood pressure by increasing sodium retention.[84]

Data obtained largely from prospective clinical trials suggest that the risk of hypertension due to HRT is low, and some studies have even documented a decrease in blood pressure in patients treated with HRT.[85–87] The Postmenopausal Estrogen/Progestin Interventions Trial evaluated cardiovascular risk factors in 875 normotensive postmenopausal women aged 45 to 64 years randomly assigned to treatment with a variety of different regimens of HRT. At 3 years of follow-up, there were no differences in systolic or diastolic blood pressure in any of the treatment groups compared with the placebo group. The patients in this clinical trial were normotensive at the outset, and it is not known whether hypertensive women would be more likely to experience increased blood pressure while taking HRT.

A 1994 prospective study of 75 hypertensive women treated with HRT did not demonstrate an increase in blood pressure after

12 months of follow-up,[88] but data on larger numbers of patients are needed to determine whether HRT is a risk factor for blood pressure elevation in hypertensive postmenopausal women. A limitation of existing data is that reporting mean changes in blood pressure in a population may mask individuals who have a blood pressure increase with HRT. In fact, a 1997 study of ambulatory blood pressure monitoring in normotensive women receiving either transdermal estrogen or oral estrogen showed that although the group as a whole did not have a rise in blood pressure, as many as one third of the individuals showed a 4 mmHg increase in diastolic blood pressure after 6 months of therapy.[83]

In summary, HRT appears to be an uncommon cause of worsening hypertension in postmenopausal women. However, few hypertensive subjects receiving HRT have been followed prospectively. Thus, the incidence of HRT-induced increases in blood pressure in individuals with preexisting hypertension is not known. Subtle increases in blood pressure attributable to HRT might be difficult to detect in women already under treatment for hypertension whose blood pressures may fluctuate with changes in body weight, level of activity, and diet. It is prudent to monitor blood pressure closely in hypertensive women receiving HRT and to consider using preparations with minimal effects on hepatic production of angiotensinogen (transdermal estrogen) if blood pressure control becomes difficult.

References

1. Pickering G. Hypertension: Definitions, natural histories and consequences. Am J Med 1972;52:570–583.
2. Kaplan NM. Hypertension: Prevalence, risks and effect of therapy. Ann Intern Med 1983;98:705–709.
3. The Sixth Report of the Joint National Committee on Prevention, Detection, Evaluation, and Treatment of High Blood Pressure. Arch Intern Med 1997;157:2413–2446.
4. Burt VI, Whelton P, Rocella EJ, et al. Prevalence of hypertension in the U.S. adult population: Results of the Third National Health and Nutrition Examination Survey, 1988–1991. Hypertension 1995;25:305–313.
5. The Fifth Report of the Joint National Committee on Prevention, Detection, Evaluation, and Treatment of High Blood Pressure. Arch Intern Med 1993;153:154–183.
6. Yong LC, Kuller LH, Rutan G, Bunker C. Longitudinal study of blood pressure changes and determinants from adolescence to middle age. The Dormont High School Follow-Up Study, 1957–1963 to 1989–1990. Am J Epidemiol 1993;138:973–983.
7. Stamler J, Stamler R, Riedlinger WF, et al. Hypertension screening of 1 million Americans: Community Hypertension Evaluation Clinic (CHEC) Program, 1973–1975. JAMA 1976;235:2299–2306.
8. Wolf PA, D'Agostino RB, O'Neal MA, et al. Secular trends in stroke incidence and mortality: The Framingham Study. Stroke 1992;23:1551–1555.
9. Kannel WB, Castelli WP, McNamara PM, et al. Role of blood pressure in the development of congestive heart failure: The Framingham Study. N Engl J Med 1972;287:781–787.
10. Collins R, Peto R, MacMahon S, et al. Blood pressure, stroke and coronary heart disease: Part 2. Short term reductions in blood pressure: Overview of randomized drug trials in their epidemiological context. Lancet 1990;335:827–838.
11. Walker WG, Neaton JD, Cutler JA, et al, for the MRFIT Research Group. Renal function change in hypertensive members of the Multiple Risk Factor Intervention Trial: Racial and treatment effects. JAMA 1992;268:3085–3091.
12. SHEP Cooperative Research Group. Prevention of stroke by antihypertensive drug treatment in older persons with isolated systolic hypertension: Final results of the Systolic Hypertension in the Elderly Program (SHEP). JAMA 1991;265:3255–3264.
13. Dahlof B, Lindholm LH, Hansson L, et al. Morbidity and mortality in the Swedish Trial in Old Patients with Hypertension (STOP-Hypertension). Lancet 1991;338:1281–1285.
14. Anastos K, Charney P, Charon RA, et al. Hypertension in women: What is really known? The Women's Caucus Working Group on Women's Health of the Society of General Internal Medicine. Ann Intern Med 1991;115:287–293.
15. Gueyffier F, Boutitie F, Boissel JP, et al. Effect of antihypertensive drug treatment on cardiovascular outcomes in women and men: A meta-analysis of individual patient data from randomized, controlled trials. The INDANA Investigators. Ann Intern Med 1997;126:761–767.
16. Williams GH, Fisher NDL. Genetic approach to diagnostic and therapeutic decisions in human hypertension. Curr Opin Nephrol Hypertens 1997;6:199–204.
17. Jeunemaitre X, Soubrier F, Kotelevstsev YV, et al. Molecular basis of human hypertension: Role of angiotensinogen. Cell 1992;71:169–180.
18. Casari G, Barlassina C, Cusi D, et al. Association of the α-adducin locus with essential hypertension. Hypertension 1995;25:320–326.
19. Sealey JE, Blumenfeld JD, Bell GM, et al. On the renal basis for essential hypertension: Nephron heterogeneity with discordant renin secretion and sodium excretion causing a hypertensive vasoconstriction-volume relationship. J Hypertens 1988;6:763–777.
20. Mackenzie HS, Garcia DL, Anderson S, Brenner BM. The renal abnormality in hypertension: A proposed defect in glomerular filtration surface area. *In* Laragh JL, Brenner BM (eds): Hypertension: Pathophysiology, Diagnosis, and Management, 2nd ed. New York: Raven Press, 1995, pp 1539–1552.
21. Coleman TG, Bower JD, Langford HG, Guyton AC. Regulation of arterial pressure in the anephric state. Circulation 1970;42:509–514.

22. Williams GH, Hollenberg NK. Non-modulating hypertension: A subset of sodium-sensitive hypertension. Hypertension 1991;17(suppl I):I81–I85.

23. Goldstein DS, Kopin IJ. The autonomic nervous system and catecholamines in normal blood pressure control and in hypertension. *In* Laragh JH, Brenner BM (eds): Hypertension: Pathophysiology, Diagnosis and Management. New York: Raven Press, 1990, pp 711–747.

24. Xie P, McDowell TS, Chapleau MW, et al. Rapid baroreceptor resetting in chronic hypertension: Implications for normalization of arterial pressure. Hypertension 1991;17:72–79.

25. DeFronzo RA, Ferrannini E. Insulin resistance: A multifaceted syndrome responsible for NIDDM, obesity, hypertension, dyslipidemia, and atherosclerotic cardiovascular disease. Diabetes Care 1991;14:173–194.

26. Elliott P. Observational studies of salt and blood pressure. Hypertension 1991;17(suppl I):I3–I8.

27. McCarron DA, Morris CD, Henry HJ, Stanton JL. Blood pressure and nutrient intake in the United States. Science 1984;224:1392–1397.

28. Grobee DE, Hofman A. Effect of calcium supplementation on diastolic blood pressure in young people with mild hypertension. Lancet 1986;2:703–707.

29. Appel LJ, Moore TJ, Obarzanek E, et al, for the DASH Collaborative Research Group. A clinical trial of the effects of dietary patterns on blood pressure. N Engl J Med 1997;336:1117–1124.

30. Whelton PK, He J, Cutler JA, et al. Effects of oral potassium on blood pressure: Meta-analysis of randomized controlled clinical trials. JAMA 1997; 277:1624–1632.

31. Working Group on Ambulatory Blood Pressure Monitoring, National High Blood Pressure Education Program Coordinating Committee. National High Blood Pressure Education Program working group report on ambulatory blood pressure monitoring. Arch Intern Med 1990;150:2270–2280.

32. Mueller FB, Laragh JH. Clinical evaluation and differential diagnosis of the individual hypertensive patient. Clin Chem 1991;37:1868–1879.

33. Lewis CI, Grandits GA, Flack J, et al. Efficacy and tolerance of antihypertensive treatment in men and women with stage 1 diastolic hypertension. Arch Intern Med 1996;156:377–385.

34. Kanai H, Tokunaga K, Fujioka S, et al. Decrease in intra-abdominal visceral fat may reduce blood pressure in obese hypertensive women. Hypertension 1996;27:125–129.

35. Elliott P, Stamler J, Nichols R, et al, for the Intersalt Cooperative Research Group. Intersalt revisited: Further analyses of 24 hour sodium excretion and blood pressure within and across populations. BMJ 1996;312:1249–1253.

36. Linas SL. The role of potassium in the pathogenesis and treatment of hypertension. Kidney Int 1991;39:771–786.

37. Khaw K-T, Barett-Connor E. Dietary potassium and stroke associated mortality. A 12-year prospective population study. N Engl J Med 1987;316:235–240.

38. Allender PS, Cutler JA, Follmann D, et al. Dietary calcium and blood pressure: A meta-analysis of randomized clinical trials. Ann Intern Med 1996;124:825–831.

39. van Montfrans GA, Karemaker JM, Wietling W, Dunning AJ. Relaxation therapy and continuous ambulatory blood pressure in mild hypertension: A controlled study. BMJ 1990;300:1368–1372.

40. Mann SJ, James GD, Wang RS, Pickering TG. Elevation of ambulatory systolic blood pressure in hypertensive smokers: A case control study. JAMA 1991;265:2226–2228.

41. Mann SJ, Blumenfeld JD, Laragh JH. Issues, goals, and guidelines for choosing first-line and combination antihypertensive drug therapy. *In* Laragh JH, Brenner BM (eds). Hypertension: Pathophysiology, Diagnosis, and Management, 2nd ed. New York: Raven Press, 1995, pp 2531–2542.

42. Cohen E, Wheat ME, Swiderski DM, Charney P. Hypertension in women. *In* Laragh JH, Brenner BM (eds). Hypertension: Pathophysiology, Diagnosis, and Management, 2nd ed. New York: Raven Press, 1995, pp 159–169.

43. Rose BD. Diuretics. Kidney Int 1991;39:336–352.

44. Burris JF, Weir MR, Oparil S, et al. An assessment of diltiazem and hydrochlorothiazide in hypertension: Application of factorial trial design to a multicenter clinical trial of combination therapy. JAMA 1990;263:1507–1512.

45. Buhler FR, Laragh JH, Baer L, et al. Propranolol inhibition of renin secretion: A specific approach to diagnosis and treatment of renin-dependent hypertensive diseases. N Engl J Med 1972;287:1209–1214.

46. Man in't Veld AJ, Van den Meriacker AH, Schalekamp MA. Do beta blockers really increase peripheral vascular resistance? Review of the literature and new observation under basal conditions. Am J Hypertens 1988;1:91–96.

47. Opie LH. Role of vasodilation in the antihypertensive and antianginal effects of labetalol: Implications for therapy of combined hypertension and angina. Cardiovasc Drugs Ther 1988;2:369–376.

48. Clark JA, Zimmerman HJ, Tanner LA. Labetalol hepatotoxicity. Ann Intern Med 1990;113:210–213.

49. Neaton JD, Grimm RH, Prineas RJ, et al. Treatment of mild hypertension study (TOMHS): Final results. JAMA 1993;270:713–724.

50. Epstein M. Calcium antagonist and the kidney: Implications for renal protection. Am J Hypertens 1991;4:482S–486S.

51. Os I, Bratland B, Dahlof B, et al. Female sex as an important determinant of lisinopril induced cough. Lancet 1992;339–372.

52. Laragh JH. Issues, goals and guidelines in selecting first-line drug therapy for hypertension. Hypertension 1989;13(suppl 1):I103–I112.

53. Mueller FB, Laragh JH. First-line and combination antihypertensive drug therapy. *In* Laragh JH, Brenner BM (eds). Hypertension: Pathophysiology, Diagnosis, and Management. New York: Raven Press, 1990, pp 2107–2115.

54. Mueller FB, Bolli P, Linder L, et al. Calcium antagonists and the second drug for hypertensive therapy. Am J Med 1986;81(suppl 6A):25–29.

55. Elliot HL, Meredith PA, Reid JL. Verapamil and prazosin in essential hypertension: Evidence of a synergistic combination. Abstract presented at the Scientific Meeting of the International Society of Hypertension, 1986.

56. Majid PA, Meeran MK, Benaim ME, et al. Alpha- and beta-adrenoreceptor blockade in the treatment of hypertension. Br Heart J 1974;36:588–596.

57. Lazarus JM, Bourgoignie JJ, Buckaleq VM, et al, for the Modification of Diet in Renal Disease Study

Group. Achievement and safety of a low blood pressure goal in chronic renal disease. Hypertension 1997;29:641–650.

58. Lewis EJ, Hunsicker LG, Bain RP, et al, for the Collaborative Study Group. The effect of angiotensin-converting enzyme inhibition on diabetic nephropathy. N Engl J Med 1993;329:1456–1462.

59. Maschio G, Alberi D, Janin G, et al. Effect of the angiotensin-converting inhibitor benazepril on the progression of chronic renal insufficiency. N Engl J Med 1996;334:939–945.

60. Stanley JC. Arterial fibrodysplasia. *In* Novick AC, Scoble J, Hamilton G (eds): Renal Vascular Disease. London: WB Saunders, 1996, pp 21–35.

61. Wilkinson R. Epidemiology and clinical manifestations. *In* Novick AC, Scoble J, Hamilton G (eds): Renal Vascular Disease. London: WB Saunders, 1996, pp 171–184.

62. Le TT, Haskal ZJ, Holland GA, Townsend R. Endovascular stent placement and magnetic resonance angiography for management of hypertension and renal artery occlusion during pregnancy. Obstet Gynecol 1995;85:822–825.

63. Tegtmeyer CJ, Selby JB, Hartwell GD, et al. Results and complications of angioplasty in fibromuscular disease. Circulation 1991;83:I155–I161.

64. Bravo EL, Tarazi RC, Dustan HP, et al. The changing clinical spectrum of primary aldosteronism. Am J Med 1983;74:641–651.

65. Nadler JL, Hsueh W, Horton R. Therapeutic effect of calcium channel blockade in primary aldosteronism. J Clin Endocrinol Metab 1985;60:896–899.

66. Lie JT, Olney BA, Spittel JA. Perioperative hypertensive crisis and hemorrhagic diathesis: Fatal complication of clinically unsuspected pheochromocytoma. Am Heart J 1980;100:716–722.

67. Manger WM, Gifford RW. Pheochromocytoma: A clinical overview. *In* Laragh JH, Brenner BM (eds). Hypertension: Pathophysiology, Diagnosis, and Management, 2nd ed. New York: Raven Press, 1995, pp 2225–2244.

68. Streeten DHP, Anderson GH, Howland T, et al. Effects of thyroid function on blood pressure: Recognition of hypothyroid hypertension. Hypertension 1988;11:78–83.

69. Lind L, Hvarfner A, Palmer M, et al. Hypertension in primary hyperparathyroidism in relation to histopathology. Eur J Surg 1991;157:457–459.

70. Woods JW. Oral contraceptives and hypertension. Hypertension 1998; II(suppl II):II11–II15.

71. Ramcharan S, Pellegrin FA, Hoag EJ. The occurrence and course of hypertensive disease in users and nonusers of oral contraceptive drugs. *In* Ramcharan S (ed). The Walnut Creek Contraceptive Drug Study: A Prospective Study of the Side Effects of Oral Contraceptives, Vol 2. U.S. Department of Health, Education, and Welfare Pub No. NIH 76–563. Washington, DC: Government Printing Office, 1976, pp 1–16.

72. WHO Task Force on Oral Contraceptives. The WHO Multicentre Trial of the Vasopressor Effects of Combined Oral Contraceptives: 1. Comparisons with IUD. Contraception 1989;40(2):129–145.

73. Royal College of General Practitioners' Oral Contraception Study: Oral Contraceptives and Health. New York: Pitman, NJ, 1974.

74. Chasan-Taber L, Wilett WC, Manson JE, et al. Prospective study of oral contraceptives and hypertension among women in the United States. Circulation 1996;94:483–489.

75. Spellacy WN, Birk SA. The effect of intrauterine devices, oral contraceptives, estrogens, and progestogens on blood pressure. Am J Obstet Gynecol 1972;112:912–919.

76. Byrne KB, Geraghty DP, Stewart BJ, Burcher E. Effect of contraceptive steroid and enalapril treatment on systolic blood pressure and plasma renin-angiotensin in the rat. Clin Exp Hypertens 1994;16(5):627–657.

77. Crane MG, Harris JJ, Winsor W III. Hypertension, oral contraceptive agents, and conjugated estrogens. Ann Intern Med 1971;74:13.

78. Notelovitz M: Effect of natural oestrogens on blood pressure and weight in postmenopausal women. S Afr Med J 49:2251, 1975.

79. Utian WH. Effect of postmenopausal estrogen therapy on diastolic blood pressure and body weight. Maturitas 1978;1:3.

80. Pfeffer RI. Estrogen use, hypertension and stroke in postmenopausal women. J Chron Dis 1977; 31:389–398.

81. Crane MG, Harris JJ. Estrogens and hypertension: Effect of discontinuing estrogens on blood pressure, exchangeable sodium, and the renin-aldosterone system. Am J Med Sci 1978;276:33–55.

82. Wren BG, Routledge DA. Blood pressure changes. Oestrogens in climacteric women. Med J Aust 1981;2:528–531.

83. Akkad AA, Halligan AWF, Abrams K, Al-Azzawi F. Differing responses in blood pressure over 24 hours in normotensive women receiving oral or transdermal estrogen replacement therapy. Obstet Gynecol 1997;89:97–103.

84. Oelkers W, Schoneshofer M, Blumel A. Effects of progesterone and four synthetic progesagens on sodium balance and the renin-aldosterone system in man. J Clin Endocrinol Metab 1974;39:882–890.

85. Lind T, Cameron EC, Hunter WM, et al. A prospective, controlled trial of six forms of hormone replacement therapy given to postmenopausal women. Br J Obstet Gynaecol 1979;86(suppl 3):1–29.

86. Elias AN, Meshkinpour H, Valenta LJ. Attenuation of hypertension by conjugated estrogens. Nephron 1992;30:89–92.

87. PEPI Trial Writing Group. Effects of estrogen or estrogen/progestin regimens on heart disease risk factors in postmenopausal women: The postmenopausal estrogen/progestin interventions (PEPI) trial. JAMA 1995;3:199–208.

88. Lip GYH, Beevers M, Churchill D, Beevers DG. Hormone replacement therapy and blood pressure in hypertensive women. J Hum Hypertens 1994; 8:491–494.

INDEX

• • •

255

ISBN 0-7216-7374-0

90038